A SHOT TO SAVE THE WORLD

ABOUT THE AUTHOR

Gregory Zuckerman is a special writer at the *Wall Street Journal.* He's an investigative reporter who writes about business and investing topics. He's a three-time winner of the Gerald Loeb Award, the highest honour in business journalism. Zuckerman is the author of international bestsellers including *The Man Who Solved the Market: How Jim Simons Launched the Quant Revolution*, *The Frackers: The Outrageous Inside Story of the New Billionaire Wildcatters* and *The Greatest Trade Ever: The Behind-the-Scenes Story of How John Paulson Defied Wall Street and Made Financial History*. He has also written inspirational books for young readers, including *Rising Above: How Eleven Athletes Overcame Challenges in Their Youth to Become Stars*. Zuckerman appears regularly on CNBC, Fox Business and the BBC. He lives with his wife and two sons in West Orange, New Jersey.

A SHOT TO SAVE THE WORLD

The Remarkable Race and Groundbreaking Science Behind the Covid-19 Vaccines

GREGORY ZUCKERMAN

BUSINESS

PENGUIN BUSINESS

UK | USA | Canada | Ireland | Australia
India | New Zealand | South Africa

Penguin Business is part of the Penguin Random House group of companies
whose addresses can be found at global.penguinrandomhouse.com.

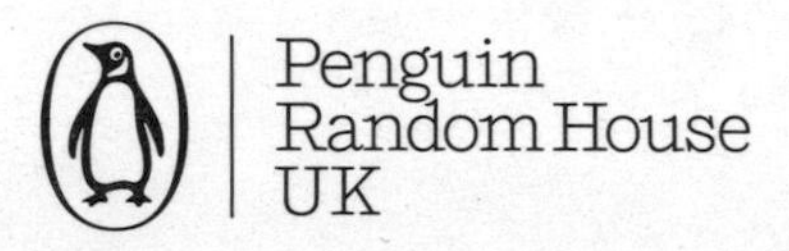

First published in the United States of America by Portfolio / Penguin 2021
First published in Great Britain by Viking 2021
001

Printed and bound in Great Britain by Clays Ltd, Elcograf S.p.A.

The authorized representative in the EEA is Penguin Random House Ireland,
Morrison Chambers, 32 Nassau Street, Dublin D02 YH68

A CIP catalogue record for this book is available from the British Library

HARDBACK ISBN: 978–0–241–53170–9
TRADE PAPERBACK ISBN: 978–0–241–53171–6

Follow us on LinkedIn: https://www.linkedin.com/company/penguin-connect/

www.greenpenguin.co.uk

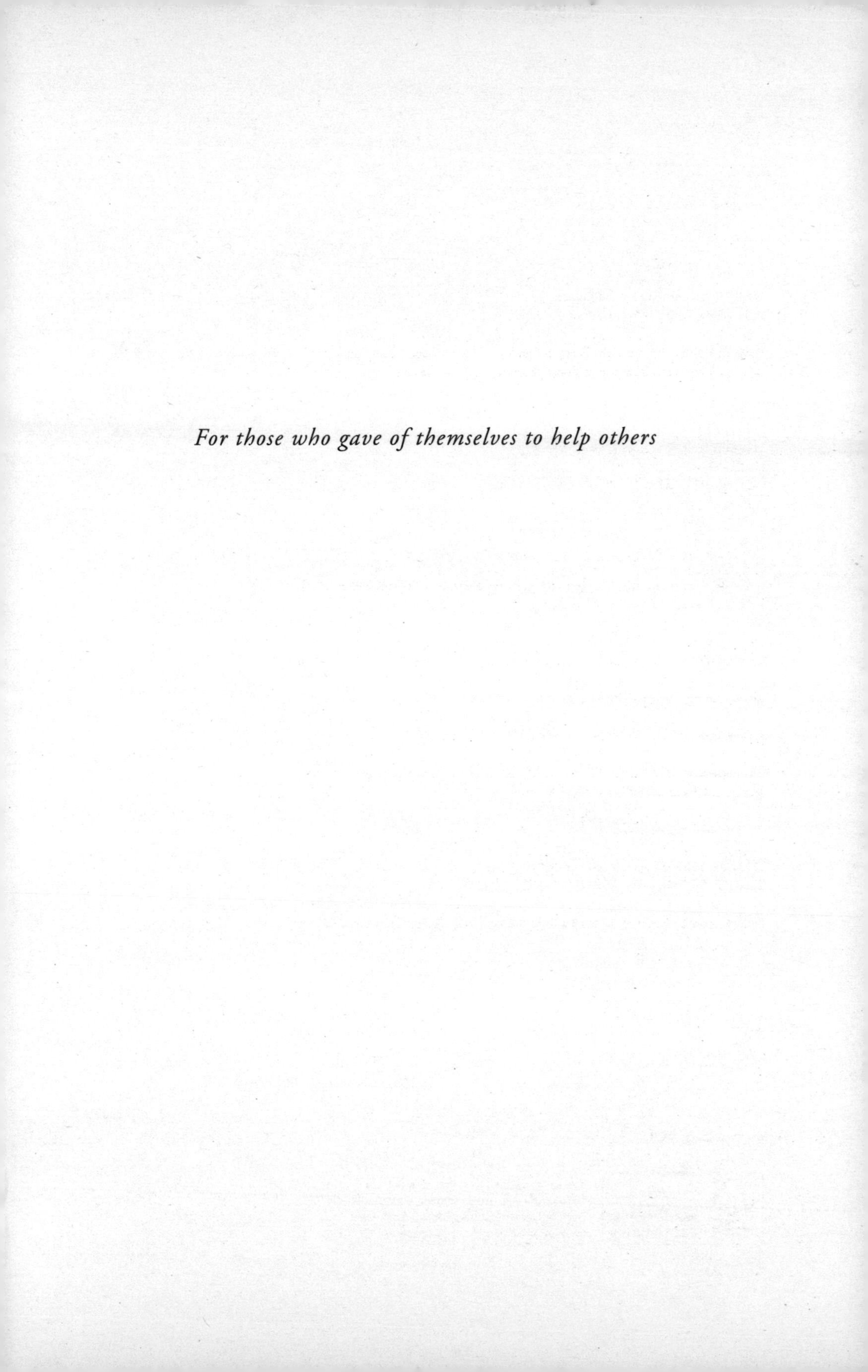

For those who gave of themselves to help others

CONTENTS

CAST OF CHARACTERS

Moderna

STÉPHANE BANCEL—Chief executive and master fundraiser

STEPHEN HOGE—President and ex-McKinsey & Company consultant

ERIC HUANG—Staffer who convinced Moderna to focus on vaccines

KERRY BENENATO—Organic chemist who solved key mRNA challenge

JUAN ANDRES—Head of vaccine manufacturing, stocked up on household supplies in early 2020

ROBERT LANGER—Chemical engineer, helped launch Moderna

NOUBAR AFEYAN—Lebanese-born venture capitalist who hired Bancel

BioNTech

UĞUR ŞAHIN–Cofounder; dreamed of developing cancer immunotherapies

ÖZLEM TÜRECI—Cofounder; cancer researcher

THOMAS STRÜNGMANN—Billionaire backer of Şahin, Türeci, and BioNTech

Pfizer

ALBERT BOURLA—CEO, pushed for fast Covid-19 vaccine

MIKAEL DOLSTEN—Chief scientist, became worried company picked wrong vaccine design

KATHRIN JANSEN—Vaccine-research chief

Beth Israel Deaconess Medical Center

DAN BAROUCH—AIDS researcher, developed vaccine approach employing adenovirus serotype 26, worked with Johnson & Johnson

Oxford University

ADRIAN HILL—Polarizing vaccine researcher who spent his career fighting malaria and being abrasive to his peers

SARAH GILBERT—Chimpanzee-virus specialist who designed Covid-19 vaccine

Novavax

GALE SMITH—Invented vaccine approach using insect viruses, developed AIDS vaccine at MicroGeneSys

STANLEY ERCK—CEO, Vietnam veteran

GREGORY GLENN—President, former physician, hobbyist chicken farmer

Academic Researchers

JON WOLFF—mRNA pioneer at the University of Wisconsin

ELI GILBOA—Achieved early mRNA advances at Duke University

KATALIN KARIKÓ—Hungarian-born researcher and diehard mRNA advocate

DREW WEISSMAN—Worked with Karikó on mRNA breakthrough, feline fan

LUIGI WARREN—Software engineer-turned-biologist

DERRICK ROSSI—mRNA revolutionary, helped found Moderna

JASON MCLELLAN—Structural biologist, discovered way to keep spike protein in ideal form

NIANSHUANG WANG—Native of China, worked on breakthrough coronavirus research

Government Scientists

ANTHONY FAUCI—Top U.S. infectious-disease expert

BARNEY GRAHAM—Deputy director, Vaccine Research Center; chased RSV vaccines, worked with Moderna on Covid-19 vaccine

JOHN MASCOLA—Director of the Vaccine Research Center, part of the National Institutes of Health's National Institute of Allergy and Infectious Diseases (NIAID)

KIZZMEKIA CORBETT—Viral immunologist in Graham's lab

MicroGeneSys

FRANK VOLVOVITZ—Founder, chased AIDS vaccine

INTRODUCTION

In late January 2020, I traveled to Europe and the Middle East with my two sons. We had read reports describing a worrisome virus circulating in central China and likely beyond, but the threat didn't seem immediate or especially worrisome. Walking through Heathrow Airport, my sons insisted on wearing makeshift face masks but I yanked mine off. They were useless, health officials were advising, and might even invite danger. Every few years, it seemed, worries arose about some new virus or other, but the pathogens rarely had broad impact. Besides, I was getting nervous looks from fellow passengers.

Within weeks, the world was held hostage by a virulent virus, and the most calamitous health crisis in decades had begun. Not since the AIDS epidemic of the 1980s, or perhaps the 1918 flu pandemic, did so much of humankind simultaneously fear for its health and wellness. Just as in those earlier periods, fear was accompanied by confusion and uncertainty. No one knew the origins of the novel virus, which eventually was determined to be part of the coronavirus family and was named severe acute respiratory syndrome coronavirus 2, or SARS-CoV-2. It wasn't understood why the virus spread so rapidly and efficiently, or how it could be avoided or stopped. All that was clear was that everyone was a potential victim.

By the late summer of 2021, more than 4.5 million people around the world had died of the resulting disease, which was branded Covid-19, and more than 210 million people had been sickened.[1] The tally included more than 600,000 who perished in the United States, greater than the combined number of Americans who died on the battlefields of World War I, World War II, and the Vietnam War.[2] On many days, more than 3,000 Americans died of the disease, as if the country were experiencing the losses of September 11, 2001, on a regular basis.[3]

Almost every family was affected in some way or fashion, including my own. One of my sons contracted the virus, as did close friends and relatives. An uncle died of Covid-19, as well as a neighbor. So much pain, destruction, and mayhem, and all from an oily bubble of genes with a diameter of about one hundred nanometers, small enough to fit one thousand virus particles across the *width* of a single strand of hair.[4]

Politicians, government officials, business leaders, and public-health professionals were unprepared for the most devastating pandemic in a century. The errors, oversights, and obfuscations witnessed after the mysterious respiratory illness first emerged in Wuhan, China, in January 2020 could fill a book or two. It just won't be this one. This is the story of how science protected humanity from a modern-day plague.

I began tracking the vaccine chase as the world locked down in early spring of 2020 and I retreated deep into my basement office, unable to access *The Wall Street Journal*'s Midtown Manhattan building. Soon I was speaking with extraordinary and often courageous scientists, executives, and government researchers who were going all out to develop shots to stem the pandemic. Their efforts and exploits served as welcome distractions amid the pervading gloom and despair.

The obstacles they confronted were immense. At the start of the pandemic, many health-care experts deemed it unlikely that safe and effective vaccines could be produced, at least in the near term. After all, until 2020, a mumps vaccine was the fastest ever developed, and that took a long four years. The average vaccine was produced in ten years. The stubborn scientists persisted, though, convinced they had a way to save lives. At each turn, they experienced unexpected drama.

I became determined to tell their story. Developing, testing, manufacturing, and then delivering safe and effective vaccines within a single year is a feat unmatched in modern science, and arguably one of humankind's proudest moments. By one count, the Covid-19 vaccines helped prevent 279,000 deaths and averted up to 1.25 million additional hospitalizations, as of summer 2021.[5]

"There's nothing like it in all of history," argues Eric Topol, the director and founder of the Scripps Research Translational Institute in San Diego. "This will go down as one of science and medical research's greatest achievements. Perhaps its most impressive."

If success has many fathers, a historic, lifesaving, improbable triumph like the Covid-19 vaccines has fathers, mothers, grandparents, and all kinds of distant relatives, many of whom have legitimate claims of lineage. The breakthroughs appeared practically overnight, but they all resulted from years of dedication, creativity, and frustration. Pioneering academics laid the groundwork for the shots, often working in the face of deep skepticism, even scorn. Inventive scientists persisted amid years of failure. Imaginative executives jeopardized their careers and reputations to back novel approaches.

Perhaps most intriguing was who *didn't* meet success in the vaccine race. Many of the world's biggest drug and vaccine makers were slow to react to the pandemic or couldn't muster an effective response.

Instead, unlikely and untested individuals stepped up to try to save civilization. A French executive dismissed by some as a fabulist. A Turkish immigrant with little experience working on viruses. A quirky midwesterner obsessed with insect cells. A Boston scientist employing questionable, maybe even dangerous techniques. A British scientist resented by his peers.

Far from the limelight, each had spent years developing innovative vaccine approaches. By 2020, these individuals had little proof of progress. Yet, they and their colleagues wanted to be the ones to stop a virulent virus holding the world hostage. They scrambled to turn their life's work into protective vaccines in a matter of months, each gunning to make the big breakthrough—and to beat one another for the glory that a vaccine guaranteed.

The success of their efforts raises a series of important questions. Why were unheralded scientists the ones who saved civilization? Why were their methods so successful yet overlooked for so long? How can we employ recent advances and approaches to prepare for future pandemics? What distressing diseases might the revolutionary researchers conquer next?

This book, based on interviews with over three hundred scientists, academics, executives, government officials, investors, and others who played important roles in the Covid-19 vaccine achievements or laid the groundwork for their success, attempts to answer those questions and more. I had access to senior officials, researchers, and others at Moderna, BioNTech, Pfizer, Johnson & Johnson, Oxford University, Novavax, and other companies and institutions that made vital, often underappreciated, contributions. The book is based on first-person accounts and recollections of those who personally witnessed or were aware of each of the events I depict. I've done my best to check and confirm every fact, incident, and quote. I owe deep gratitude to each individual who spent time sharing observations, memories, and insights.

This is a story of courage, determination, and death-defying ingenuity. It's also a tale of heated competition, crippling insecurities, and unbridled ambitions. I've tried to tell it in a way that will appeal to general readers as well as to those in the world of science. I will refer to modified nucleosides, structural biology, and lipid nanoparticles, but there will also be vicious rivalries, corporate intrigue, and outsize ambition. Most of all, the Covid-19 vaccine story is one of heroism, dedication, and remarkable persistence.

Ours is an age of outbreaks. Each year, humans encroach on nature, increasing the risks that animal-borne diseases will cross over and threaten humanity. Lessons from the vaccine race will inform scientists, politicians, and others if—or perhaps when—we confront another deadly pathogen.

This is the story of what went right.

PROLOGUE

Uğur Şahin was sweating.

It was early October 2019, and Şahin was standing in a parking lot in Kansas City, Missouri, under a blazing midafternoon sun. By then, Şahin and a few colleagues had spent weeks crisscrossing the United States and Europe, trying to drum up interest among investors for BioNTech, the German biotechnology company Şahin had started.

The trip wasn't going well. Şahin had explained to the investors that BioNTech was developing vaccines and treatments to combat various cancers and infectious diseases. One of its approaches was to use a molecule called messenger RNA, or mRNA, to carry instructions into the body, enabling it to ward off illness. The company needed money from an initial public offering to continue its research.

The investors liked Şahin. He demonstrated an impressive breadth of knowledge, reciting data and citing obscure research papers. They also liked his ambitions for BioNTech and how it planned to develop vaccines for dozens of different diseases. Şahin believed the immune system could be taught to fight disease, and he had spent more than two decades of his life researching how to make it happen.

Soft-spoken and serious, he wore smart business suits to the investor meetings rather than his usual T-shirts. An open-collared dress shirt allowed a glimpse of a Turkish amulet around his neck. Şahin had close-cropped hair, thick eyebrows, and brown eyes that were big, just like his ears. Some investors had done research on Şahin and knew he was a bit different from most other biotech executives. A fifty-three-year-old immigrant from Turkey, Şahin lived in a modest apartment in the German city of Mainz. Each morning, he bicycled to BioNTech, which he ran with his wife, Özlem Türeci, who also was a cancer researcher.

As impressed as they were with Şahin, though, the investors had qualms about his company and its approach. BioNTech had been around for eleven years, but it wasn't close to an approved vaccine. Just one drug was in a medium-stage, phase 2 trial, and only 250 patients had ever been treated with the company's vaccines. Researchers around the world had spent decades trying to work with mRNA without much progress. Some health-care experts thought the idea was pure folly, suggesting BioNTech was wasting its time. And it was an awful time to sell shares—the stock market was under pressure, biotech stocks were wilting, and few investors wanted to pay a lot for a German company with few signs of success.

Standing in the parking lot, his ear to a cell phone, Şahin spoke with yet another investor, trying to gauge his interest in BioNTech. Şahin looked tired and tense. Finishing the conversation, he told his team that the investor would only buy shares if BioNTech reduced the price it was proposing

Şahin and his colleagues had a decision to make. Their choices were ugly—they could scrap the company's IPO or slash its price, hoping enough investors would then be interested. Some of the executives huddled around him, while others sat in their open, black van, hiding from the burning sun. It had been a long trip and they were ready to go home.

"We need to decide," Şahin told his team.

It wasn't a hard decision. His company needed the money and had to sell the shares, no matter the price. A few days later, Şahin rang the bell at the New York Stock Exchange, a wan smile on his face. The company raised $150 million in the IPO, just over half what it had hoped to collect. Even with the discounted price, shares of Şahin's company fell more than 5 percent on their first day of trading.

He didn't mind the reaction from investors. Someday, they and others would fully appreciate what he and his company was trying to do.

Şahin was sure of it.

• • •

Stéphane Bancel faced even more serious doubts in late 2019.

A forty-seven-year-old native of France with full lips, a cleft chin, and a taste for Steve Jobs–inspired turtleneck shirts, Bancel had spent eight years running a Boston-based biotech company called Moderna. By then, Bancel was better known for his powers of persuasion than for any kind of scientific achievement. Bancel had a unique ability to convince investors that Moderna would succeed in its quest to develop safe and effective vaccines and drugs using mRNA. Much of the scientific community snickered at the idea, however. They all knew that mRNA was too unstable to create proteins in the body, at least on a consistent and reliable basis.

If anyone was going to find a way to make mRNA work, it surely wasn't going to be someone like Bancel, the skeptics said. They all knew the stories from the early days at Moderna, when Bancel regularly ripped into his employees, leaving them on edge.

"Fifty percent of you won't be around in a year," Bancel once said matter-of-factly in a meeting to nervous staffers.

By 2019, Bancel was more even keeled. He had built a loyal team and had inspired them with the promise of what mRNA could do. At one point, he told them, their technology would save lives.

"We're going to be the company that can respond to a crisis," he told staffers.

But outside scientists, investors, and some journalists were sure Bancel was exaggerating his company's potential. A few years earlier, a respected scientific publication had even compared Bancel to Elizabeth Holmes, the disgraced chief executive of blood-testing start-up Theranos, who also had an easy way with investors and a predilection for black turtlenecks. There was never any evidence of improper actions by Bancel, yet the suspicions and skepticism persisted.

By the end of 2019, the sniping had taken a toll. Moderna's shares were 15 percent below their own IPO price from a year earlier, making it hard for Bancel to raise new money. Some investors were upset the company had shifted its focus to vaccines, a crowded and challenging field with limited profit potential. Moderna was forced to cut its spending. The criticisms didn't seem fair to Moderna's researchers, who were proud of their progress. They were injecting mRNA molecules packed with genetic instructions, producing proteins in the body capable of teaching the immune system to protect against disease. Moderna was even working with Anthony Fauci, the U.S. government's top infectious-disease authority, and his colleagues, which were becoming intrigued by Moderna's mRNA techniques.

Moderna hadn't tested its vaccines in many people, though. And like Şahin and BioNTech, Bancel's company wasn't close to any approved vaccine. Moderna was planning its very first phase 2 clinical study for a vaccine and was nowhere near a late-stage trial for any of its products. The company *hoped* to have a vaccine in the market by 2023, but even that goal seemed ambitious.

• • •

In late 2019, Bancel flew to Europe with his wife and daughters to spend the holiday season at a home he owned in southern France, after visiting his mother in Paris. It was a chance for him to escape the pressures of running his company and dealing with the doubters.

One morning, just after the New Year, Bancel woke up early and headed to his kitchen, trying not to wake his sleeping daughters. He brewed some Earl Grey tea and grabbed an aging iPad on the kitchen table, checking his emails and scrolling through the latest news. A story stopped him cold: Lung disease was spreading in southern China.

Bancel emailed a senior government scientist.

"Do you know what it is?" Bancel asked.

The researcher had been following the outbreak, too. No one knew its cause.

Bancel couldn't stop thinking about the spreading illness. Maybe his team could do something about it, he thought. Perhaps they could finally prove that mRNA worked. He kept sending messages, each one more urgent than the last.

"What's the latest?"

"Do you know yet?"

"Is it a virus?"

The government scientist promised to let Bancel know as soon as he learned the cause of the sickness. A few days later, as Bancel and his family flew back to Boston, the outbreak remained on his mind. His researchers had spent years preparing to fight viruses, but they hadn't come close to stopping even one of them. He doubted the sickness in China was going to be a huge deal.

But what if it was?

A SHOT TO SAVE THE WORLD

1

1979–1987

Before and after. The epidemic would cleave lives in two, the way a great war or depression presents a commonly understood point of reference around which an entire society defines itself.

—RANDY SHILTS, *AND THE BAND PLAYED ON*[1]

Henry Masur was getting desperate.

The young man before him was short of breath, feverish, and couldn't stop coughing. Masur, a thirty-three-year-old in his first week as an attending physician at New York Hospital on Manhattan's Upper East Side, ran a battery of tests but couldn't make sense of his patient's symptoms. A security guard at a different Manhattan hospital, the man didn't appear to have any underlying diseases. Between gasping breaths, he said he had already visited several New York hospitals and doctors. No one could help him.

The man's heartbeat raced and his oxygen-saturation levels plummeted. Ninety-five percent . . . ninety-four . . . ninety-three. Any lower and death was a risk. Masur couldn't figure out what he was dealing with. A bad strain of tuberculosis? A new fungus? Something more dangerous? He consulted colleagues and scoured medical literature but couldn't find an answer.

Time was running out. Masur still needed more information. He decided to operate, a huge risk given his patient's frail condition.

I have to get a piece of his lung.

Hours later, a hospital pathologist looked up from his microscope and delivered an answer: The young man had pneumocystis carinii pneumonia.

Masur was stunned.

How can that be?

Masur happened to be one of the rare experts on this kind of pneumonia. A few years earlier, when he was starting a fellowship in infectious diseases and tropical medicine, he found himself the most junior recruit in his laboratory, with little choice of which microorganism to study. Malaria and all the other cool, headline-grabbing infections, bugs, and epidemics had already been claimed. Masur got stuck with pneumocystis pneumonia. His colleagues tried to stifle their giggles. At one time, this pneumonia afflicted hundreds of malnourished children each year in Eastern Europe and elsewhere. By the late 1970s, though, it affected only about seventy patients in the entire United States each year, almost always those with compromised immune systems, such as cancer patients. Masur's lab director assured him that there was value in studying the infection, but Masur knew he was unlikely ever to encounter an actual patient dealing with pneumocystis pneumonia.

Now, it was the fall of 1979, and Masur was confronting a case—during his very first week as an attending physician. And his patient was a healthy adult. It didn't seem remotely possible.

Masur decided to administer a drug being tested on childhood-leukemia victims suffering from the same infection. Masur's patient's condition stabilized enough for him to eventually leave the hospital. Before Masur could relax, though, he was confronting additional cases of this rare pneumonia. So were physicians in other New York hospitals, as were doctors in Chicago, Atlanta, Los Angeles, and San Francisco.

Six foot one and rail thin, with a high forehead and jet-black hair, Masur was a ponderer, especially when confronted with important decisions and quandaries. He tended to fixate on problems until he could develop a solution. Walking home after another long day, Masur slowly crossed the street to his one-bedroom hospital-owned apartment, trying to make sense of all the men with the once-rare infection. At night, he and his wife, a nurse at the hospital, debated the cases, searching for an explanation.

Within months, Masur's original patient had died, and more struggling, suffering young men were coming to see Masur and his colleagues around the world. In London, patients battling pneumocystis pneumonia and other puzzling infections and tumors staggered into St. Stephen's Hospital in Chelsea. Doctors at the hundred-year-old institution noticed the patients were likely to be either gay men or intravenous drug users, but those observations didn't explain the nature of the illness or how it could be halted. They knew something was making the men susceptible to these rare illnesses, but they had no idea what it was.

The physicians were reeling. Just a few months earlier, they had been confident and upbeat. In the previous decade or so, enormous progress had been made preventing and treating all kinds of illnesses, including heart disease, diabetes, and some cancers. Powerful antibiotics and accurate diagnostic tests had been introduced, and modern medicine seemed on the verge of wiping out most infectious diseases.

Now the physicians were confronting a malady they couldn't stem, treat, or even understand. Fear and frustration overtook them.

"Apart from compassion and giving some pain relief, we were

completely impotent," recalls Jeremy Farrar, who was a young doctor at St. Stephen's in London. "It leaves a scar the rest of your life."

Infectious-disease experts felt especially helpless. Many had entered the field precisely because they wanted to cure patients, not simply improve a condition or keep illness at bay, which is often the most doctors can hope to do while treating cancer, cardiovascular disease, or certain other sicknesses.

"I like seeing a patient, making a diagnosis, giving treatment, and seeing them get better," says H. Clifford Lane, who worked in a lab at the National Institute of Allergy and Infectious Diseases (NIAID), a part of the National Institutes of Health. "Now, all of a sudden, you're seeing patients your own age and we can't treat them, and we don't even know what it is they're dealing with."

Researchers concluded that most people were contracting the unknown illness through sexual transmission, as a virus crossed mucosal tissues lining the genital tract, rectum, or other body cavities. Others were becoming infected through the bloodstream, sometimes by sharing needles. In 1982, the Centers for Disease Control and Prevention in Atlanta gave the disease a name: acquired immune deficiency syndrome, or AIDS. Investigators at both the Pasteur Institute in Paris and National Cancer Institute in Washington, D.C., determined that a new human retrovirus, eventually named the human immunodeficiency virus, or HIV, was causing AIDS.

The virus spread quickly. At Albert Einstein College of Medicine in New York, five Black infants were admitted showing signs of severe immune deficiency. Anxieties grew, even among professionals accustomed to disease and death. Some pathologists refused to do postmortems, worried they might contract the new disease. Fears raced through the broader society. Later, when an Indiana teenager named Ryan White was infected through contaminated blood products used to treat his hemophilia, anxious parents forced the school to block the boy from attending class.

Government officials tried to understand the disease and how it might be stopped, though some started from positions of remarkable ignorance. In 1983, as staffers and health officials briefed Margaret Heckler, the secretary of health and human services, about the disease, she appeared confused about one way AIDS was transmitted.

"Anal intercourse?" Heckler asked, turning to a close aide who was gay. "You do *that*?"

"I think we better come back and discuss this a little later," another staffer told Heckler.[2]

As scientists gained a better grasp of the disease, some became optimistic they could develop a vaccine, perhaps quickly. Sure, it had taken about five decades to develop shots for typhoid, polio, and measles after their causes had been determined, but medical science was progressing at a rapid clip. At a press conference on April 23, 1984, Heckler voiced confidence a solution was on the horizon.

"We hope to have such a vaccine ready for testing in approximately two years," she told reporters.

Government scientists who followed Heckler to the podium were nearly as sanguine. They had history on their side: Traditionally, vaccines were how most epidemics ended. Indeed, few figures are as revered as those responsible for creating shots capable of wiping out plagues and disease. These scientists often emerged living legends—even when their contributions were a bit exaggerated.

• • •

In the summer of 1774, a farmer in southern England named Benjamin Jesty noticed that one of his dairymaids seemed resistant to smallpox. Earlier that year, the young woman, Anne Notley, had cared for a family afflicted with smallpox, a disease that killed three in ten infected people while causing blindness and other complications in others. Yet, she emerged unscathed. Jesty knew that Notley, like other milkmaids, had previously been infected with a less serious but related pathogen called cowpox, which spread from the udders of infected cows.

Jesty had an idea: He took one of his wife's knitting needles and scraped pus from one of his cows showing signs of cowpox. Then, Jesty intentionally infected his family with the material. Later, when an outbreak of smallpox raged through the region, members of the Jesty family were protected from the disease. Pushing his luck a bit, Jesty deliberately infected his sons with smallpox—still no sign of infection.* Far from impressed, locals were in fear. Some fretted that Jesty's needlework would turn his family into "horned beasts." Eventually the Jesty clan was forced to flee for the Isle of Purbeck on the English Channel.[3]

Word spread about Jesty's inoculations (and how the family remained hornless), and British doctors began attempting similar procedures. In 1796, a physician named Edward Jenner exposed an eight-year-old boy to cowpox; when Jenner later infected the boy with smallpox, the cowpox protected him from the disease without signs of even localized inflammation or infection. Jenner inoculated others as well. Unlike Jesty, Jenner evaluated his subjects, analyzed their results using proper scientific methods, and published his findings. Before long, the country, and later the world, would embrace vaccination as a means to eradicate smallpox. Jesty's ingenuity would be overlooked when Jenner's biographer attributed the genesis of mankind's first vaccine to Jenner's observation that a beautiful local milkmaid was resistant to smallpox. The milkmaid's image proved more memorable than Jesty's dirty needles.

Other vaccine pioneers demonstrated their own originality, even as they generated other kinds of controversy. In the 1940s, for example, a young virologist named Jonas Salk began publishing academic papers that were imaginative in their conclusions, though they

* They did suffer inflammation, but it was probably the result of Mrs. Jesty's dirty needles.

sparked criticism, partly because the stated results were often based on limited data.

"I engaged in extrapolation because I had always felt that it was a legitimate means of provoking scientific thought and discussion," Salk later explained. "I engaged in prediction because I felt it was the *essence* of scientific thought. The fact that neither extrapolation nor prediction was popular in virological circles seemed to me to be a shame."[4]

Salk spent several years searching for a vaccine for polio, an infectious disease that was killing thousands of people a year and paralyzing tens of thousands, many of them children. At the time, most scientists were trying to use live, but weakened, viruses in their vaccines, similar to Jesty's approach with smallpox. Salk tried a different tack: He grew samples of the polio virus in his lab at the University of Pittsburgh and killed, or inactivated, the pathogen by adding formaldehyde, a method that had worked for vaccines for rabies and cholera. Salk tested his shots on thousands of children, and even his own family, showing in 1953 that they worked more than 60 percent of the time. His results sparked singing, dancing, and other celebrations throughout the United States as a grateful nation embraced Salk as a hero, his image appearing on the front pages of newspapers, the covers of glossy magazines, and on television newscasts. Later, Salk's bitter rival, Albert Sabin, introduced an oral polio vaccine based on a weakened, or attenuated, version of the virus, and it too proved effective. Together, the two vaccines effectively ended the scourge of polio for much of the world.

All vaccines work more or less the same way—by teaching and enabling the body's complex immune system to fight off pathogens. The human immune system features two lines of defense. A fast-acting, first-line "innate" immune system is composed of various white blood cells, such as macrophages, dendritic cells, and natural killer cells that stand guard at the body's gateways—the skin, nose, throat, etc.—to detect and fend off viruses and other foreign invaders.

The innate immune system doesn't need prior exposure to a pathogen to be activated against it, but it can have trouble handling especially powerful or clever pathogens. For these difficult battles, the body's "adaptive" immune system joins the fight. Sensing danger, it sends other kinds of white blood cells, including T cells, which can recognize specific pathogens, and B lymphocytes, or B cells, which produce powerful antibodies to battle the pathogens.

These cells do a more efficient job than those of the innate immune system. T cells play important defensive roles, while B cells produce battalions of antibodies specifically trained to take on invaders. The problem is that the adaptive immune system is strong but a bit slow. It takes time deciding whether an invader is dangerous enough for it to send sufficient T cells and B cells to combat the intruder, giving a virus the opportunity to strengthen its hold and infect the body's cells.

That's where vaccines come in. Injected into the body's bloodstream, traditional vaccines contain weakened or killed versions of what would otherwise be powerful pathogens. Once introduced into the body, the invading agents trigger the body's adaptive immune system to pursue and disable them. The pathogen in the vaccine is harmless, but the body fights it off nonetheless, treating the weakling force as if it were a threatening army. The adaptive immune system, unable to shake memories of this simulated battle, continues to send antibodies to patrol for new signs of the pathogen, while training them to return to attack mode if there's an invasion of a genuine foe bearing similarity to the one encountered as part of the vaccine.

Because vaccines usually include weakened viruses, inactivated viruses, or some other facsimile of the real thing, it's rare that they infect the body with the disease they're meant to prevent. Years after Salk's and Sabin's breakthroughs, scientists would introduce vaccines that rely on other approaches, but they would have the same goal: activate and teach the immune system to disable a future intruder.

• • •

Throughout much of the 1980s, scientists were optimistic they could use one of the traditional approaches to develop an effective HIV vaccine, partly because they were making rapid progress understanding the virus. Flossie Wong-Staal, a molecular biologist working in the lab of famed researcher Robert Gallo, helped establish HIV as the cause of AIDS. She then cloned the virus and revealed some of how it worked, showing ways HIV evades the immune system. (Wong-Staal and Gallo even found time to conduct a romantic relationship and have a child together.)[5]

Daunting challenges quickly emerged, however. HIV had an unusually high mutation rate and a devious ability to elude the immune system. Scientists concluded that it was just too dangerous to develop a vaccine using inactivated or watered-down versions of the lethal virus. They feared that if HIV was part of a vaccine, it might replicate uncontrollably or mutate into an even more virulent state. Concerns were heightened because so many of those suffering from the disease already had weakened immune systems. That helps explain why most prominent drug companies, including Merck and Upjohn, had little interest in developing a vaccine—the obstacles seemed too imposing.

Developing drugs to eliminate, or even slow, HIV, proved just as difficult. Among the biggest challenges: Scientists couldn't figure out ways to prevent the virus from replicating in the body. In March 1987, three years after the cause of AIDS was determined, the U.S. Food and Drug Administration approved the first medication to treat it, a drug called azidothymidine, or AZT. The news stirred widespread hope and excitement, but it led to cruel disappointment. A failed cancer drug, AZT stopped helping many patients after several months of treatment, as the virus developed an unusual ability to resist the drug. It was also expensive and could have dangerous side effects, especially in the high doses most doctors prescribed.

• • •

As the AIDS epidemic worsened in the late 1980s, the U.S. armed forces—full of young, sexually active men—were especially hard hit. Military doctors watched helplessly as measures of their patients' CD4+ cells—known as "helper T cells" because they direct the immune system's counterattack—plummeted, a sign their immune systems were deteriorating. So many soldiers were infected with the virus that Walter Reed National Military Medical Center in Washington, D.C., opened an entire ward for AIDS patients.

"They'd get the kind of infection that rarely occurs in a healthy person and it would be over, AZT didn't do squat," says Edmund Tramont, who worked as a senior physician at Walter Reed in the mid-1980s. "Young people would die before our eyes. We couldn't offer them anything but general support."

One day, a three-star general asked to see Tramont in his office at Walter Reed at four a.m., worried about his health. The general was aware that being identified as gay was considered "unbecoming" conduct by the military and potential grounds for dishonorable discharge, so he picked the early-morning hour, hoping no one would be around.

After some awkward pleasantries, Tramont initiated a difficult conversation.

"Sir, if I'm going to help you, I need some information."

The general acknowledged a homosexual experience. He braced himself for Tramont's diagnosis, certain what was coming.

"You have to let your partners know," Tramont said, after telling the general he had AIDS.

"Doc, I've already done that," the general said, sadness in his eyes.

Later, Tramont treated a twenty-year-old woman, the wife of an active-duty soldier. She had acquired the virus from her husband, who had become infected while stationed in Berlin, one of hundreds of soldiers infected with HIV in Europe. Tramont and his colleagues began asking why so many cases were traced to these soldiers, especially those based in Berlin. It turned out the men couldn't afford the prices demanded by local prostitutes, so they frequented women brought from Congo, an early epicenter of HIV. Scientists estimated that as many as 20 percent of the prostitutes favored by U.S. soldiers in Berlin were HIV-positive.

Tramont's patient's condition quickly deteriorated. Unable to provide more than palliative care, he was left shaken by the experience.

"The poor girl gets married and her husband gets stationed in Berlin," Tramont says. "That case really got to me."

Tramont and other hospital staff members were desperate for something, anything, to help those with AIDS. They soon became excited by a promising vaccine being developed by a quirky North Dakota farm boy and a fast-talking East Coast entrepreneur. For a while, it seemed this odd couple had a solution to stem the epidemic.

2

1985–1994

Gale Smith grew up on a ten-thousand-acre alfalfa ranch in Minot, North Dakota, before moving with his family to Williston, a boom-and-bust oil town near the Montana border. As a young boy in the 1950s and '60s, Gale spent hours in his basement working on chemistry sets or building rockets, sometimes with his twin sister, Gayle. He did well in school, even while skipping grades, but he wasn't especially popular with classmates.

"Not everyone likes you when you get good grades," he says.

One day in seventh grade, Gale walked into his school's library and discovered a wall full of science books. For the quiet boy, the library became an oasis, occupying Gale for hours a day while setting him on a career path.

Gale's family was Methodist, but at an early age he began questioning the principles of Christianity. He idolized John F. Kennedy and challenged the more conservative impulses of his neighbors, some of whom were members of the radical John Birch Society.

"I didn't know it was racism, I just thought it was wrong," he says. "The search for truth in an unbiased way motivated me."

Gale saw little purpose remaining in high school, which he found boring, so he dropped out at the beginning of his senior year to take courses at a local college. Nonetheless, top scores and innovative science projects, including one with two local doctors about a gland in the brain, earned Smith a select spot that summer in a prestigious science program for high school students at Brown University in Providence, Rhode Island. The fifteen-year-old, who had never been out of North Dakota, spent two anxious days on a series of connecting trains traveling east. Suspicious of his fellow passengers, Smith kept a watchful eye on his surroundings, barely sleeping the whole trip.

"It was a long two days," he says.

Smith arrived to a campus abuzz over remarkable advances in molecular biology and genetic engineering. He and his classmates listened to lectures by Francis Crick and James Watson, who had been the first to describe the double-helix structure of DNA molecules. They also studied a hand-stapled preprint version of Watson's *Molecular Biology of the Gene* and read from James Crow's *Genetic Notes*, books that would revolutionize the field of genetics.

Smith was hooked.

"I discovered how complex biological systems are, how interrelated everything is," he says.

Smith wanted to attend Brown for college, but he couldn't afford the two-thousand-dollar-a-year tuition, so he enrolled at the University of North Dakota to study biology and chemistry. Smith loved his lab courses but barely showed up for most other classes, preferring to read course materials on his own. Tall, thin, and reserved, Smith spent most of his free time taking photos, listening to classical music in his room, or playing chess with a new group of friends.

By 1981, Smith had started a PhD program in molecular biology at Texas A&M University in College Station. Simultaneously, he was taking graduate courses in the Baylor College of Medicine's virology department in Houston, about a hundred miles away. Some students were preoccupied with partying, football games, and the opposite sex. Smith daydreamed about very different things.

One morning, during an unusually cold Texas winter, Smith was listening to a Baylor professor describe how researchers had cloned the human beta interferon gene, a sticky protein that helps cells defend against foreign invaders. At the time, when most anyone in the academic or pharmaceutical worlds wanted to create interferon or other proteins for a drug or other reasons, they did it in yeast or bacteria. That is, they put DNA instructions for the desired protein in a tube of yeast or bacteria cells, mixed it with a special solution to induce the cells to take up the DNA, and transferred the tube into an enormous vat, where the cells converted the instructions, over time, into multiple copies of a protein, as in a kind of factory.

This way of culturing proteins usually worked, but it wasn't great at making interferon, antibodies, or other complex proteins that can be crucial for drugs. Proteins are folded, meaning they can have three-dimensional structures. They also can be "glycosylated," or decorated with carbohydrates. Yeast and bacteria cells can't produce proteins with many of these structures. In the 1980s, academics were experimenting with using mammalian cells, such as cells from the ovary of a Chinese hamster, to produce such proteins. This approach brought other challenges, though, and there was little evidence it could have commercial value, at least at that time.

Sitting in the Baylor lecture hall, Smith thought he had a better method of producing proteins like interferon: using insect cells. Insects and humans are more alike than most presume, Smith realized. Both require oxygen and have certain anatomical similarities, like brains, hearts, and reproductive organs. Just as important: Their cell structures are similar and both produce similar complex, folded proteins. To Smith, employing a virus that infects insects, called a baculovirus, seemed a perfect way to deliver necessary DNA into those insect cells to create proteins like interferon.

At first blush, it might seem strange, or even dangerous, to use an insect virus to develop medicines for humans. But Smith had been studying insect viruses, and he knew they had been used in pesticides for centuries and were safe for humans. He also realized that baculoviruses were "roomy" enough—meaning they have relatively large DNA chromosomes—for biologists to insert large pieces of genetic information into them.

Smith theorized that insect viruses could be used to infect insect cells to produce specific proteins, according to the DNA instructions. What Smith was contemplating was a brand-new "expression system," or method of producing thousands or even tens of thousands of complex proteins, the kinds that scientists use to develop new drugs and vaccines.

After the lecture, Smith rushed up to John Collins, the professor who had set off his daydream, sharing his idea.

"You're as crazy as I am," Collins told him.

Smith wasn't deterred. He sped back to Texas A&M's campus and headed to an off-campus bar called the Chicken Oil Co., where graduate students met to drink, play pool, and talk science. Smith told pretty much anyone who would listen about his insect-cell notion. Reserved in most social settings, Smith now couldn't stop talking. All it took was a few Lone Star beers and an innovation he thought might revolutionize drug development.

"You think this is pie in the sky?" he asked a labmate named Peter Krell.

Krell told Smith he might be onto something. The HIV epidemic was accelerating, and most biologists and immunologists were focused on the emerging virus, but Smith and Krell had been studying insect viruses, a decidedly unpopular topic. It was time to put their knowledge to work, Krell told his friend.

"Yes, do it," he said to Smith.

Returning to Baylor, Smith hustled to see Joseph Melnick, a

legendary polio researcher who headed the school's department of virology and epidemiology. He had discovered the topic of his PhD thesis, Smith gushed to Melnick.

Melnick looked mystified.

"Why would you want to make proteins in an insect cell?" Melnick asked him.

Smith decided to do his PhD with Texas A&M professor Max Summers, a star in the field, who agreed to let Smith develop the system while working in his laboratory. Smith spent over a year perfecting his method with Summers and a postdoctoral fellow named Malcolm Fraser. Through the grapevine, they became aware that a top scientist in the field, Lois Miller, was working on a similar insect system, adding to their pressure. Most days, Smith, Fraser, and others worked late into the night in the lab, cracking open beers and blasting Beethoven and Mozart to reduce the tension. Smith decided to use the cells of butterflies and moths in his system, reasoning that cells from these insects would be safer than mosquitoes and other biting insects that might have contaminating allergens.

Finally, in 1982, the team met success—they cloned human beta interferon, the protein Smith's professor had been discussing the morning Smith began daydreaming about insects. They produced a surprising amount of the protein, too, which Smith was sure could be injected into the body as a therapeutic. The trio detailed their work in a paper they submitted to a series of journals, none of which had any interest in their work. Using insect cells to develop drugs? Seriously? Finally, in late 1983, the same year Smith, then thirty-four years old, received his PhD, a debut journal called *Molecular and Cellular Biology* published their article.

"They were new and they needed submissions," Smith says of the journal.

Over time, Smith's insect-virus system gained appreciation and companies embraced his approach, first for applications related to agriculture and later for medical research. Much later, popular vaccines and medicines, including those for shingles, flu, and HPV, would rely on Smith's "baculovirus expression-vector system." Because Smith and Summers, together with Texas A&M, had patented their work, they eventually received royalty checks totaling millions of dollars.

That wouldn't happen for years, though. In the immediate aftermath of their breakthrough, Smith was merely eager for the respect of his peers, and he hoped a drug company might see potential in his invention. In August 1982, Smith and Summers traveled to Cornell University in upstate New York to deliver their first talk about their work. The room was packed, and Smith was pumped to meet someone who might want to use his system to make drugs. But only one person lingered around to speak with Smith after the speech: an excitable thirty-two-year-old named Frank Volvovitz.

Volvovitz had heard about Smith and Summers's work and was so intrigued that he drove nearly five hours from his home in West Hartford, Connecticut, for the lecture. In an upbeat mood after discovering a delicious bagel shop in Ithaca before the talk, Volvovitz zeroed in on Smith, hoping to persuade him to join the tiny company he was starting.

Smith immediately liked Volvovitz, who had a boyish face, curly dark hair, oversize wire-framed glasses, and a habit of squinting when he spoke. Volvovitz was a businessman with scientific training who had also worked with interferon. He seemed ambitious and intelligent. Most of all, his face lit up while talking about Smith's insect-virus idea.

"There's a business here!" Volvovitz assured Smith.

By then, Volvovitz had already shuttered one biotech company. He was launching his new company in his parents' basement. His goal was to produce an insecticide for a common pest that attacked Christmas trees. It wasn't exactly cutting-edge stuff.

Smith had no clue about all that, though. Even if he did, it wouldn't have mattered. Volvovitz appreciated Smith's invention. He *got* it. That was all Smith really wanted.

"I was just glad somebody cared," Smith says.

In 1985, Smith moved to Connecticut to help run the scientific effort at Volvovitz's ten-person company, which Volvovitz named MicroGeneSys (pronounced "micro-genesis") and soon relocated to West Haven from the family basement. Before long, Smith and Volvovitz would emerge as unlikely leaders in the quest to discover an AIDS vaccine.

• • •

When Smith approached his new office on his first day of work, he noticed MicroGeneSys was in a building that also housed a furniture warehouse and a helicopter-parts supplier, humdrum surroundings that didn't suggest any kind of medical revolution might be in the offing.[1] Inside, though, Volvovitz brimmed with determination to shake up the scientific world. He already had made a decision that would transform his fledgling start-up into one of America's highest-profile companies.

The AIDS epidemic was worsening. More than one million Americans had been infected with HIV, more than forty thousand had developed the disease, and AIDS had claimed more than sixteen thousand lives. Finally, money was flowing to scientists working to stem the crisis. Sensing opportunity, Volvovitz decided MicroGeneSys would be the one to discover an AIDS vaccine.

At the time, debate raged about the most effective approach to pursue a vaccine. A growing number of AIDS researchers argued for shots using genetically engineered parts of the virus as its antigen—the key substance stimulating the immune system—rather than the old-school approach of using the actual virus. This new kind of vaccine would teach the immune system to recognize the virus's distinctive protein, or even pieces of the protein, so the body would be ready to fight HIV if these viral proteins were ever encountered. This strategy might not work, proponents acknowledged, but it sure seemed safer to rely on shots using synthetic, or recombinant, versions of HIV's protein rather than to inject the deadly virus into the body with traditional shots.

Volvovitz realized this newer approach was perfectly suited for Smith's insect-cell system. Smith, Volvovitz, and their growing team decided to take DNA from HIV, place it in a baculovirus, infect insect cells, and produce proteins that would serve as vaccine antigens. By the late 1980s, scientists had identified the key protein on HIV's surface, known as "envelope," where the virus attached to human cells. Much like the spike protein of coronaviruses—a large family of viruses barely in focus at the time—HIV's envelope protein protruded from its surface and resembled a spike. It enabled the virus to bind to receptors on the surface of human cells so that it could attack the body. Smith and his team at MicroGeneSys focused their vaccine on a form of the envelope protein called gp160.

When government researchers heard what Smith and Volvovitz were up to, they became intrigued, realizing that Smith had gene-splicing talents and that MicroGeneSys's approach was likely safer than using the lethal virus itself. In 1986, Smith was summoned to a meeting at the National Institutes of Health in Bethesda, Maryland. He walked into a cramped office and could hardly believe who sat before him—Anthony Fauci, who ran the government's HIV research effort as director of the NIAID, and three living legends: Jonas Salk, Albert Sabin, and Maurice Hilleman, a prominent vaccinologist.

"What can we do?" a somber Fauci asked Smith and the other scientists. "How can we make an HIV vaccine?"

Three years earlier, Smith had been throwing back Lone Star beers at the Chicken Oil Co. in Texas. Now he was debating approaches with some of history's most accomplished scientists. And they were asking *him* for ideas. It was like being inserted into a starting basketball lineup with Kevin Durant, Kyrie Irving, and James Harden, and being asked to take the team's winning shot.

Smith's inclusion in the meeting was a sign of how few people at the time had experience cloning complex glycosylated proteins, such as those on the outer surface of HIV's coat, which Fauci and others hoped could serve as a vaccine antigen. Smith's presence in the all-star lineup also underscored how desperate the scientific world was for new ideas to fight AIDS.

After receiving the gene for the gp160 protein from an investigator at the NIH named Malcolm Martin, Smith modified it and inserted it into his baculovirus system. Smith and colleagues quickly developed a vaccine, which they called VaxSyn. When animals were given the MicroGeneSys shots, they generated a strong immune response featuring high levels of antibodies, a promising early sign. When Clifford Lane of the NIAID, Ed Tramont at Walter Reed, and other scientists heard about MicroGeneSys's results, they were eager for more testing.

"They moved fast and I was right there with them," Lane says. "My feeling was, 'We're in a pretty bad situation, it's immunogenic, let's see it in volunteers,'" referring to the vaccine's ability to stir the immune system.

In August 1987, MicroGeneSys became the first company to receive permission from the FDA to test an AIDS vaccine on humans. A plan was announced for the NIAID to recruit 81 homosexual men for the trial, news that shocked the pharmaceutical industry, mostly because so few had heard of Volvovitz, Smith, and MicroGeneSys.

"How a company like this one comes out of nowhere—I don't know," a bewildered securities analyst named Gary Hatton said.[2]

Volvovitz embraced the skepticism. Speaking to a gaggle of reporters in Washington, D.C., he oozed confidence, saying the press should keep an eye out for his company's other promising vaccines, too.

"The market potential is enormous," Volvovitz told the reporters. "A company only needs to succeed in one or two of these to be successful. The stakes are very big."[3]

Volvovitz was on his way to solving humanity's most pressing problem. Overcoming challenges and proving skeptics wrong were the two things he relished most. Back in high school, he had read that tropical-fish hobbyists struggled to breed discus fish, which are usually found in the Amazon River. He decided to build a tank in his parents' basement and duplicate conditions found in the Amazon and managed to hatch a school of discus fish.[4] Several years later, after a professor discouraged him from launching a start-up, Volvovitz quit a PhD program in microbiology at New York University to begin his first biotech company.

Now, Volvovitz's vaccine was generating global interest, though it remained years away from regulatory approval. As with any drug or vaccine, there would have to be phase 1 trials to test for safety, phase 2 studies to see if the vaccine had an impact, and a phase 3 trial to test if it actually worked.

Volvovitz was feeling proud. Soon, though, he felt pressure. He needed to raise millions of dollars to build vaccine manufacturing capabilities, pay for laboratory tests connected to the trials, and keep MicroGeneSys going until it had sales. He began scrounging for money, securing funding from private individuals, the state of Connecticut, and a major pharmaceutical company, American Home Products. To get the money, though, he had to give up partial stakes in his company, rights to market the vaccine, and more, sacrifices that deeply pained him.[5]

Volvovitz became preoccupied with his AIDS vaccine. He had few friends or outside interests. After he fathered a child with a MicroGeneSys employee, he built a play area outside his office, so he could spend time near his son as he continued to work.

He began hearing that other biotech companies were making progress on their own AIDS vaccines and drugs and were poised to pass MicroGeneSys. Volvovitz had to come up with still more cash to keep his company afloat. Becoming impatient, Volvovitz began working the phones, hoping for good news.

He called government scientists for updates on early tests they were doing on the vaccine. He asked FDA representatives to allow MicroGeneSys's shots to be approved if they merely showed signs of potentially slowing AIDS. He even asked government scientists for updates on the work other agencies were doing.

"Where are we with the FDA?!" he asked an NIH researcher one day.

Sometimes, Volvovitz hung up and called right back, speaking so quickly it was hard to make out what he was saying.

"What's going on with the studies?!"

Some senior government researchers, like Lane and Tramont, were fine with the hectoring. They appreciated Volvovitz's persistence and his dedication to making his vaccine a success. He wasn't cursing or lying or asking to cut corners. Other companies were badgering them also. Volvovitz just really wanted his vaccine approved, and he wanted it done quickly.

"He was a pain in the ass, but he didn't overstep the boundary," Tramont says. "I didn't mind, I had an idea of what it's like in that world."

Sometimes, Volvovitz turned on the charm, hoping to accelerate the trial or get an update on its progress.

"How's it going?" he asked one day, friendlier than usual. "By the way, did we get any more patients in the study?"

Behind his back, some government researchers made jokes, asking if "the used-car salesman" had called that day.

"There was a buffoonery to him," says Malcolm Martin, the senior scientist at the NIH who produced the clone of the HIV protein at the heart of MicroGeneSys's vaccine. "He was an operator, not a scientist."

Volvovitz's anxieties grew. A phase 2 study of thirty people in early stages of AIDS led by Dr. Robert Redfield at Walter Reed showed MicroGeneSys's vaccine worked, but Redfield came under sharp criticism for overstating the vaccine's therapeutic effects. MicroGeneSys didn't have money to conduct its own studies, which presented a problem. Volvovitz asked for funding from the NIH but was told to get in line—others ahead of him were looking to run studies on malaria, dengue fever, and other pressing diseases.

Volvovitz heard that Genentech, a much larger biotech company, was pushing for government funds for its own HIV vaccine program, a new reason for concern. He needed a definitive trial to prove his own vaccine's efficacy, and he needed it immediately.

His calls became more urgent.

"We've got to get this done! How do we get this done?!" he bellowed to an NIAID staffer.

That's when Volvovitz crossed a boundary. He hired former Louisiana senator Russell Long—the son of Huey Long, the populist and controversial politician of the 1920s and '30s—to lobby for the company. The move initially worked: In 1992, Long helped persuade Congress to give the U.S. Army $20 million to test MicroGeneSys's vaccine. The sum was tiny relative to the army's $253 billion budget that year, and Volvovitz wanted it for a study that might prove the efficacy of his vaccine, which had the potential to help those suffering from AIDS. Some within the NIH sympathized with Volvovitz's plight and were eager to see what a big study might prove.

But the move blew up on Volvovitz. Top AIDS scientists were outraged, and officials at the NIH and the FDA, including Fauci and FDA commissioner David Kessler, criticized MicroGeneSys for subverting the scientific process to get the money. The army and members of Congress would spend over a year quarreling with the FDA and NIH over the decision, as Smith watched from his Connecticut lab, cringing at Volvovitz's maneuvers.

"You couldn't tell Frank anything," Smith says.

With the money still on hold, Volvovitz flew to Los Angeles to try to raise the $20 million he needed for the study. Driving to the hills overlooking Santa Monica Bay, he entered the sprawling home of Michael Roth, a high-profile doctor famous for treating Elizabeth Taylor. There, Volvovitz spoke to a group of well-heeled potential investors, including actor Richard Gere and his then wife Cindy Crawford, discussing the promise of MicroGeneSys's vaccine. He figured that the crowd, which was eager to see an end to the AIDS epidemic and included some who were struggling with the disease, would embrace him.

He was wrong. The meeting turned uncomfortable when guests became outraged that Volvovitz might profit from his AIDS vaccine. He left empty-handed.[6] Later, Volvovitz defended his maneuvers in Washington, D.C., and elsewhere, saying they were simply aimed at proving the efficacy of MicroGeneSys's vaccine. Yes, he would have profited if the company had been able to pull off a lucrative initial public offering at some point, but that was likely well down the road. His primary goal was to stop a worsening epidemic.

"They said we were trying to circumvent the trial process, but lobbying is a way of life in Washington. The money was going to the army for a trial, it wasn't going to our pockets," Volvovitz says.

Volvovitz had clearly crossed an important line, though. If MicroGeneSys had set a precedent for obtaining financing, other drug companies would have followed its lead, coaxing money from various arms of government. If elected officials began telling government scientists which treatments should be tested or deserved backing, the drug development process would likely turn chaotic, and the approval of credible drugs would be delayed.

In 1994, the Pentagon officially canceled the trial Congress had approved, a crushing blow for Volvovitz, Smith, and their company's AIDS shots. Later that year, Volvovitz lost his job at MicroGeneSys. He had become so preoccupied by the vaccine effort that he had lost focus on other activities at the company, staffers said.

Volvovitz, who had built MicroGeneSys and dedicated himself to its vaccine, felt betrayed, he told a friend. On his way out, a board member gave him a painful last dig.

"Make sure you pack your nursery up, too," he told Volvovitz.

Volvovitz would go on to pursue various biotech ventures, including a short-lived effort to develop a drug for schizophrenia and a vaccine for the hookworm, a parasite that spreads illness and death among the world's poor.[7] Years later, studies would show MicroGeneSys's vaccine had limited value, though a Swedish study suggested it held some promise. It was too little, too late, however.

MicroGeneSys changed its name to Protein Sciences Corporation, hoping to erase the blemish left by its AIDS vaccine experience. Decades later, in 2013, the company would introduce a popular flu vaccine based on Smith's insect-cell system. Protein Sciences would be acquired by French drug giant Sanofi for over $650 million.

Smith stayed at Protein Sciences for a few years before leaving to work at a small biotechnology company called Novavax. There, he'd use his insect system to try to develop other vaccines. Eventually, he'd focus on a very different kind of pathogen: a new coronavirus.

3

1996–2008

Mice lie, monkeys mislead, and ferrets are weasels.

—A POPULAR APHORISM AMONG SCIENTISTS

The phone rang in John Shiver's office, startling the young chemist. He picked it up to hear a low growl.

"This is Scolnick—is this Shiver?"

Shiver was sure he was being pranked. Ed Scolnick ran research and development at Merck. He wasn't the company's chief executive, but in some ways he wielded more power. Earlier in his career, Scolnick had discovered a gene that plays a key role in tumorous cells, laying the groundwork for several cancer drugs. He didn't just grab the phone to chat with scientists, let alone one who had received his PhD just a few years earlier and was still new at Merck.

Shiver played along with the joke, enduring a barrage of questions about the progress he and his colleagues were making on HIV. As the grilling continued, Shiver began to take it seriously. Scolnick said he wanted to fight the virus and he sounded determined, even hopeful. In the fall of 1996, he was one of very few sharing much optimism.

The previous year, AIDS had killed a record 42,000 people, and the number of diagnosed patients in the United States had reached half a million. Around the world, over 913,000 had died of the disease. It was painfully clear that researchers were up against one of the most cunning and complex pathogens ever encountered, a key reason most major pharmaceutical companies remained reluctant to work on an AIDS vaccine. Unlike most every other known virus, HIV exists as different genetic sequences in various people, and even within the same individual. The virus displays a devious ability to integrate into the host's DNA, making it that much harder to eliminate. And HIV attacks the immune system itself, invading the very cells that normally fight dangerous pathogens. Once recognized, HIV changes its appearance, adopting a new coat almost hourly to continue its assault. When treated with drugs like AZT, the virus sometimes retreated, but it never fully cleared, remaining hidden in the body.

To those companies focused on a vaccine, including MicroGeneSys, Genentech, and Chiron, HIV's envelope protein had seemed a perfect target for a vaccine. Teach the body to recognize the envelope's spike structure and the next time it is encountered the immune system will know to target and fight it. The problem is, HIV's spike protein is a moving and mutating target, creating enormous challenges for the body's defenses.

There was another important reason few major drug companies were chasing HIV vaccines in the mid-1990s, one that reflected an open secret in the industry: Vaccines usually are losing propositions. Sure, being the first to develop shots for a high-profile disease or virus can deliver prestige and prizes. But the hurdles to gaining regulatory approval are high, government reimbursements can be inadequate, and manufacturing and other costs are imposing. Vaccine makers also contend with significant liability worries if their shots go awry.

Even if a protective vaccine is somehow developed, profits can be scant. Drugs can become a routine; get on a statin and you're likely to be on the medication for life, resulting in a stream of sales for pharmaceutical makers. But vaccines sometimes offer lifetime immunity—great for people, bad for profits. In poorer nations, prices have to be kept low to avoid ugly backlash, another bummer for vaccine companies. As a result, most of those focused on AIDS vaccines were smaller companies with little to lose. For them, success might bring an elevated profile, new investors, and a chance to pursue more lucrative scientific efforts—benefits that outweighed the enormous costs.

By the mid-1990s, some companies and academic institutions had turned their attention to cancer, neurology, and other promising medical fields. Still, a core group of scientists kept working on HIV, scoring under-the-radar advances they hoped might pay off, at least someday. Some of these accomplishments might sound obvious, even mundane, such as achieving a better understanding of the complex workings of the immune system and how it interacts with invading pathogens. In the past, though, this basic knowledge hadn't always been necessary. For all their historic triumphs, vaccine pioneers often employed hit-or-miss approaches. Grab a piece of a pathogen, undertake repeated experiments to weaken or kill it, and try to find the right amount of the virus to use as the basis of a vaccine. Even Jonas Salk, Albert Sabin, and other vaccine heroes usually lacked a mastery of the diseases they were combating or even a full understanding of *why* their vaccines worked. They weren't ashamed to acknowledge the huge role that serendipity, or even dumb luck, played in their discoveries.

Danny Douek, a senior scientist at the Vaccine Research Center, a division of the National Institutes of Health, liked to explain this shared philosophy to his students: "Why is for the rabbis. How is for scientists."

But HIV was different, the investigators realized. They needed to learn much more before they could take on this powerful foe. Researchers began mapping details of how HIV invades cells and replicates, identifying weak spots in the virus that might be targeted by a treatment. Using X-ray crystallography, electron microscopy, and cutting-edge computer modeling, they created detailed three-dimensional images of HIV's viral proteins. With a full view of the virus, scientists had a better chance of creating a vaccine or drug to combat their enemy.

As their grasp of the disease grew, Scolnick turned more optimistic. He assembled a group of nearly two hundred researchers to develop AIDS drugs, racking up a series of successes. Merck and other companies introduced drugs capable of hitting the virus in various stages of its life cycle. Merck's "protease inhibitor," Crixivan, for example, prevented HIV's key protease enzyme from functioning normally, and it worked with other antiviral drugs to inhibit viral replication. Other therapies demonstrated reasonable results with AZT or in combinations with other treatments.

AIDS could now be suppressed, but it wasn't clear for how long. The drugs were expensive and not easily available in many other countries, especially poorer ones. Protease inhibitors could have side effects and there were long-term cardiovascular dangers. And some patients still died from the disease, especially those without access to good health care.

Scolnick's call to Shiver was part of his effort to accelerate work on an AIDS vaccine. Merck's scientists now knew enough about the virus to make it worthwhile to exert a full effort, Scolnick felt, so he was committing resources to make it happen. He was well aware that huge profits likely wouldn't result. But AIDS was a public threat, Scolnick told underlings. Merck had a responsibility to help stem the global epidemic.

Scolnick didn't have to prod Shiver and his colleagues; many of them had been itching to build a vaccine. It was the very reason they had entered the field of medicine. After all, wiping out a disease is a heck of a lot more rewarding than treating it. There was another reason researchers felt compelled to focus on a vaccine: The company's most famous employee was a cantankerous septuagenarian who still roamed the hallways, pushing Merck's scientists to develop shots that might save thousands, even millions of lives, the kinds of breakthroughs that defined his own career.

• • •

Maurice Hilleman grew up during the Great Depression on a huge farm in southeastern Montana, not far from the valley of the Little Bighorn, where Colonel George Custer and over two hundred members of the army's Seventh Cavalry died in one of the most famous battles in U.S. history. Hilleman was born during an outbreak of the Spanish flu, and his mother died two days after birthing him and his stillborn sister. His uncle stepped in, raising the boy and instilling a love of animals and the outdoors.

Early in life, Hilleman demonstrated an independent streak. He was once caught reading Darwin's *On the Origin of Species* during a Sunday sermon, an incident memorably described in Paul Offit's *Vaccinated.* The boy wouldn't let the minister grab his book away, saying it was the property of the local library and couldn't be confiscated.

Hilleman, who was six foot one and lean, with thick, bushy eyebrows and piercing brown eyes, joined Merck in 1957. He was prickly to colleagues, tangled with superiors, and fought government officials. His impatience had its benefits, though. One summer night in 1963, Hilleman's five-year-old daughter, Jeryl Lynn, woke him complaining of a fever, swollen glands, and other obvious symptoms of mumps. Hilleman quickly swabbed the back of her throat and rushed to his lab to freeze the specimen. He cultivated his sample and then attenuated, or weakened it, by passing the virus through chicken eggs and then chicken cells. Four years later, Merck introduced a vaccine for mumps that relied on Jeryl Lynn's sample.

"The right virus was right in my house," he later said.[1]

Salk and Sabin basked in the public's attention, but Hilleman had little use for accolades. By the end of his career, though, he could claim credit for developing more than forty vaccines, including those for measles, chicken pox, rubella, and hepatitis B, achievements that make him among the most important scientists in history.

Approaching his eightieth birthday in 1998, Hilleman remained a powerful presence within Merck's vaccine group in West Point, Pennsylvania, less than thirty miles from Philadelphia, retaining a senior, emeritus role at the company. His behavior amused some colleagues but shocked others. "Goddamnit!" and "Son of a bitch!" were some of his tamer expletives. Once, Hilleman, wearing a white lab coat, lined up for lunch in Merck's cafeteria. He soon became infuriated, grabbing a ladle to bang on a big pot of soup—"What the hell is this goddamn *shit*? It looks like buzzard's *puke*!"

When scientists visited Hilleman's enormous, library-like office, where stacks of research papers were piled high across long, wooden tables, the microbiologist would peer over his reading glasses and make provocative or profane comments, hoping for a reaction.

"What religion do you practice?" he asked Shiver, when he dared a visit one day.

"Presbyterian," Shiver answered warily.

Hilleman nodded in approval, saying Shiver had chosen an intellectual denomination. Hilleman said he preferred Catholics, however.

"The nuns beat you into submission," he said, perfect preparation for working for him at Merck.

Scolnick, Shiver, and others kept dropping by, seeking Hilleman's insights while risking the abuse. They viewed Hilleman's provocations as character tests—he wanted to see which scientists would wilt under his pressure, a likely sign they'd buckle in the lab when times got tough. As Merck made progress on AIDS, Hilleman encouraged Scolnick to keep going, reinforcing his own resolve. Scolnick considered Merck's labs to be the most innovative in the industry, and he yearned for vaccine glory, just like Hilleman had achieved. It was time for Merck to step up.

"We need to be doing something," Scolnick told Shiver.

The Merck team determined they were unlikely to develop shots capable of teaching the body to produce antibodies for HIV's many variants. But they became optimistic they could activate the body's cellular immune response, which involves T cells rather than antibodies, to effectively fight the disease. It made sense to focus on T cells: Patients who seemed to do best dealing with AIDS were those with stronger natural T cell responses, suggesting that a vaccine capable of stimulating a robust T cell reaction stood a good chance at success.

Merck scientists arrived at the idea of cloning genes for three key structural proteins found in HIV and inserting them into the genome of an adenovirus, which would ferry the vaccine into the body. Adenoviruses are common pathogens originally identified in 1953 in human tonsils, or adenoids, though they can be found in other tissues, too, including the gut, or even in animals. These viruses often result in bronchitis, conjunctivitis, or the common cold but generally don't cause serious illness.

Using a virus to get a vaccine into the body was a clever move. Viruses are nature's perfect delivery mechanism. Their whole reason for being is to enter the host's body and replicate by putting their genes into its cells. Merck had long been a fan of adenoviruses. Several years earlier, Hilleman himself had explored employing them to carry a vaccine. Adenoviruses seemed large enough for biologists to insert pieces of DNA into them, much like the insect baculoviruses Gale Smith liked to work with. With an adenovirus carrying a vaccine into the body's cells and then making HIV proteins, the immune system would learn to identify these proteins and be ready to attack if HIV was ever encountered.

Over time, the Merck team tested different types of these viruses, settling on a strain called adenovirus serotype 5, or Ad5, the most ubiquitous and best understood of all the adenoviruses. Merck executives were convinced they could easily purify and manufacture a vaccine relying on an Ad5 vector, or delivery system, producing billions of doses quickly, something necessary to quell the AIDS epidemic.

"It's a good shoveling system," Emilio Emini, the head of Merck's vaccine effort, told a colleague, referring to the adenovirus's ability to deliver a genetic payload into cells.

The Merck team didn't view Ad5 as a perfect delivery mechanism. Because the virus is so common, many people around the world would have been exposed to it and developed an immunity, likely blocking the virus from infecting cells. But most of the Merck researchers figured they'd just screen people for this preexisting immunity or give their vaccine in a high enough dosage for it to be efficacious. Developing an Ad5 vaccine also seemed an easy way to test their concept of relying on adenoviruses.

The executives became intrigued with work being done by a small Dutch company called Crucell based in Leiden, Rembrandt's hometown. A few years earlier, a cancer biologist named Alex van der Eb had figured out that removing a single gene, called E1, from the genome of the Ad5 virus left it unable to replicate in normal cells. The virus could still infect cells, but it couldn't cause too much damage once it got there because it no longer could produce more virus. Now Ad5 was even more attractive to Merck as a vaccine vehicle—the virus was harmless, yet still capable of infecting the body after inoculation, advantages that led the Merck executives to license Crucell's technology.

By 1998, Merck was testing its HIV vaccine in monkeys and a small number of people. The shots weren't great at eliciting an antibody response, but they were quite good at spurring T cell immunity—exactly what the researchers were hoping to achieve. The vaccine didn't block infections, but it seemed to control HIV and prevent death. When Merck executives saw that the virus was undetectable in some monkeys, they got very excited.

"Let's make a real commitment," Scolnick told Shiver. "We have to see if it works in people."

Scolnick demanded regular updates on the vaccine, pushing his team for progress. Staffers struggled to match his intensity. Some whispered about a small, faux-wooden conference-room table that had been worn away over the years as Scolnick, full of nervous energy, dug his fingernails into its surface during meetings, leaving half of it in pieces on the floor. (Scolnick says, "I never damaged my desk with my fingernails.")

By the late 1990s, the AIDS epidemic was ravaging large swaths of Africa. In 1998, HIV infected more than 7 percent of adults in twenty-one African countries, reversing decades of economic progress.[2] But hope was growing as Merck eyed a large-scale trial of thousands of people, a true test of the effectiveness of its vaccine.

By 2003, Scolnick was approaching Merck's mandatory retirement age of sixty-five and preparing to leave the company. But the vaccine program was progressing and optimism was climbing. In 2004, Merck, working with the NIAID, launched a trial of three thousand volunteers in nine countries, mostly in the United States and Latin America. Merck gave the men and women two shots of Ad5: an initial "prime" dose to prompt the body to recognize the virus and stir the immune system to fight it, and a second "booster" shot to stimulate the immune system's memory cells, solidifying and amplifying the immune response.

"I thought this could be the best thing we've ever done," Scolnick says.

Researchers at the NIH's Vaccine Research Center were working on their own AIDS vaccine, which was a twist on Merck's approach, using a gene from both the virus's envelope and its internal proteins.

On September 18, 2007, Shiver was standing in his office when the phone rang. This time, it was a senior colleague sharing breaking news. Shiver struggled to make sense of what he was hearing. He felt energy drain from his body. Needing support, he found a nearby chair, still trying to comprehend the news. Early trial results for Merck's AIDS vaccine had been released, Shiver was told. The shots had no effect. The news got even worse: There were indications that those who had received the vaccine fared *worse* than those in the control group, who had received a placebo.

Word spread within Merck. Scientists grabbed colleagues in the hallway to share the awful news, while others huddled in the company's laboratories.

"It wasn't an easy thing to absorb," Shiver says.

Merck shared details of its depressing data with the public: The company was halting further vaccinations after early data showed its shots didn't prevent infections, didn't decrease the severity of infections, and didn't reduce the amount of HIV in the blood of those infected. Later, a follow-up study confirmed their worst fears: Merck's vaccine somehow made subjects more likely to become infected with HIV—men in the trial who weren't circumcised and had previously caught common colds caused by the Ad5 virus were two to four times as likely as others to become infected if they got the vaccine.[3] Later, the government's own Ad5 trial demonstrated results that were just as disappointing, leaving NIH scientists as despondent as those at Merck. Researchers would never gain a full explanation for the disaster.

Merck shut down its trial and then shuttered its entire HIV vaccine effort, pulling the plug on years of hard work. A few years earlier, the company had received intense criticism after a bestselling painkiller called Vioxx was shown to be connected with serious cardiovascular problems for some people; Merck had to pull the drug. Few Merck executives were eager to fight for their AIDS vaccine program and risk a new round of public opprobrium.

For the gay community, which had cheered Merck's work and was thrilled that a major pharmaceutical company was tackling AIDS, the news came as a body blow.

"We were all just gutted," says Mitchell Warren, executive director of AVAC, an AIDS prevention advocacy group.

Scientists began having second thoughts about the entire idea of using adenoviruses for HIV or anything else. The cure truly seemed worse than the disease.

"The lesson," Anthony Fauci of the NIAID said at the time, "is that you've got to be careful if you use a vector vaccine."[4]

• • •

In early 2008, Fauci convened a meeting at the Bethesda North Marriott Hotel & Conference Center, outside Washington, D.C., for HIV researchers and others involved in the fight against AIDS. The scientists, still reeling from the Merck bombshell, searched for lessons from the fiasco.

Danny Douek dreaded the event. The bearded, bespectacled immunologist had been among the dozens of researchers at the NIAID who had spent years perfecting ways to use adenoviruses and other methods to create an AIDS vaccine. After Merck's news, Douek spent weeks pacing both his office and his Maryland home, struggling to understand what had happened. Douek began hearing "I told you so" from colleagues and others. It never made sense to use the virus as a vehicle for a vaccine, some told him, because so many people have had exposure to Ad5. What were you even thinking?

Heading to the Marriott for the meeting, Douek braced for a new round of reproach, this time in a very public forum. As hundreds of scientists piled into the hotel's largest conference room, Douek grabbed a seat in the very last row, hoping to be as inconspicuous as possible. He felt frustration, embarrassment, and a tinge of anger. Douek didn't see the trials as failures. Science is about developing hypotheses and testing them with experiments. Some confirm the hypotheses, others don't. Douek was convinced important lessons resulted from the trials, but he understood why so many colleagues were eager to place blame.

The self-recrimination began with the day's first speaker—all the things the NIAID should have known, should have done better, and should have realized, just as Douek had feared. He fought the urge to crawl under his chair and hide. The results were so bad, presenters said, that members of the gay community were unlikely to participate in future trials, something the scientists called "vaccine fatigue." It was a concern Douek hadn't even considered. Now he was filled with gloom, even despair. How was an effective treatment going to be developed if no one was willing to participate in new trials?

Then Mitchell Warren, the AIDS activist, took the podium to level a different kind of criticism at the scientists. Enough with the pity party and self-flagellation, he said. Get back in the lab and find a way to stop this plague.

"This is difficult work, we get it," Warren told the group. "But we've got to figure this thing out."

Slowly, Douek could feel the mood in the room shift. He sat a bit taller in his seat. Warren reassured the scientists that the gay community would continue to participate in drug and vaccine trials. Now wasn't the time to give up.

"When you have something good, people will line up," Warren promised the crowd. "Let's get back to work!"

It would take years, but cocktails of antiretroviral pills would prove effective at fighting the virus, allowing AIDS to be transformed into a chronic, manageable disease, at least for those with access to these expensive drugs. For their part, Merck and most other big pharmaceutical companies moved on from HIV, focusing on cancer and other areas that seemed more likely to yield breakthroughs.

Thousands of miles away, though, a few researchers still believed in adenoviruses, those engineered viruses Merck had relied on. These scientists saw flaws in Merck's approach and were convinced they had ways to correct them to create the most effective vaccines yet.

• • •

Stefano Colloca found beauty in chimpanzee feces.

Colleagues in Merck's Pennsylvania offices had focused on human adenoviruses like Ad5, but Colloca and four other scientists at the company's small research office outside Rome were huge fans of animal viruses. They figured most humans would have little exposure to these pathogens, since they mostly affected animals, and therefore would have little preexisting immunity to them, making them ideal vectors to deliver vaccines to human cells.

As Merck executives in 1997 were debating which adenovirus to employ, Colloca had recommended they use a rarer adenovirus that affects only chimpanzees, but his bosses passed on the idea, concluding that it would be hard to produce such a vaccine and that regulators would be wary of approving shots that relied on a chimp virus. The decision had frustrated Colloca, but it hadn't deterred him.

Colloca was among a small group of researchers devoted to animal viruses, particularly those affecting chimpanzees, an affection that can be traced back decades. In the late 1960s, two American virologists, William Hillis and Rosanne Goodman, did something unimaginable to most laypeople: They spent weeks collecting the fecal specimens of chimps. The pair, who were trying to figure out why some hepatitis infections jumped from chimps to humans, swabbed and studied these rancid remains, discovering twenty-two different strains of virus in chimp stool. Who knew chimps were plagued with so many pathogens—or that their poop could prove so popular?

Hillis and Goodman isolated the viruses and shared them with a few researchers. Most peers had little interest in these pathogens, content to rely on weakened or killed human viruses to make vaccines of their own, but over time some came to suspect that chimp viruses might have some value. In 2000, a scientist in Philadelphia named Hildegund Ertl used a chimpanzee adenovirus for potential rabies and AIDS vaccines, a bit before Colloca and his colleagues in Rome began examining chimp and other animal viruses. Their interest was based on sound logic: Chimpanzees are humans' closest living relatives, so a virus that infected these mammals seemed to have a good chance of spreading in humans as well, making it a potential vehicle to chauffeur a vaccine into the human body.

In 2004, Colloca was developing a new strain of the virus from chimp poop when his group was contacted by Adrian Hill, an Irish vaccinologist at the University of Oxford. Hill and a colleague named Sarah Gilbert had spent a decade studying malaria. The redheaded researchers were searching for an ideal vector to shepherd a vaccine containing a piece of the malaria parasite into the body's cells, and were interested in using one of the chimpanzee viruses that Colloca and his colleagues had been working on. They wanted their shots to elicit T cells, in addition to antibodies, based on epidemiological studies suggesting that CD8+ T cells activated by an animal adenovirus would be crucial to developing protection against malaria.[5]

Hill had been fascinated with malaria and other tropical diseases since the early 1980s. As a medical student at the time in Dublin, he liked to spend his vacations visiting an uncle who worked as a priest in a hospital in Rhodesia, which later became the nation of Zimbabwe. Hill was struck by the prevalence of malaria, which hounded the region each spring and affected about 10 percent of Rhodesia's population, and how the disease was compounding troubles facing the country's citizens, who were suffering from a brutal civil war.

"I was really overwhelmed by the scale of the problem," he later said. "Not only was there a huge amount of disease and very little medical care, but also a war."[6]

After training in tropical medicine and completing a doctorate in molecular genetics, Hill joined Oxford, setting out to become the one to find a vaccine to stop malaria, a notoriously challenging disease and one that few big pharmaceutical companies were eager to tackle, partly because it's endemic in developing nations, reducing their potential profits.

Colloca was happy to help, offering Hill and Gilbert a chimp vector that was branded ChAd63. Before long, though, Colloca and his colleagues quit Merck to continue working on animal adenoviruses at their own company, Okairos, a move that scotched a potential partnership with Hill and Gilbert.*

Without a partner to provide a chimp virus, Hill and Gilbert needed someone else to help. In 2010, Hill phoned Göran Wadell, a professor at Sweden's Umeå University, who was a connoisseur when it came to chimp and other adenoviruses, cultivating and using them for his own research. Wadell wanted to help Hill in his quest to discover a malaria vaccine, so he agreed to give Hill an old strain of a chimp virus from his lab.

Hill, who by then had launched the Jenner Institute, a vaccine-research center within Oxford's Nuffield Department of Medicine, worked with Gilbert to use Wadell's strain and develop their own vaccine technology. In a nod to their university sponsor, they called it ChAdOx. For years, Hill and Gilbert would use ChAdOx to try to produce a vaccine technology to defend against malaria, influenza, and many other viruses and diseases. Eventually, they'd even use it to take on a novel coronavirus.

• • •

Dan Barouch was sure he could avoid Merck's mistake.

Barouch was a thirty-one-year-old scientist in 2004, running a small research laboratory at Beth Israel Deaconess Medical Center in

* Okairos eventually was purchased for more than $300 million by the pharmaceutical company GlaxoSmithKline.

Boston. Six feet tall with a full, boyish face and straight jet-black hair, Barouch hungered to discover something big. As a medical student, he had treated desperate AIDS patients, including numerous young children. Now the disease was overwhelming growing parts of Africa. Barouch wanted to be the one to invent an effective vaccine.

Until then, he had sped through life, as if on a mission. The son of an Israeli father and a Chinese mother, he grew up in the town of Potsdam in New York's Adirondack Mountains, finishing high school at sixteen, Harvard University at twenty, a PhD program in immunology at twenty-two, and medical school at twenty-six. Barouch even began playing the violin at the age of four. The achievements hadn't come quickly enough for him, though. He had tried completing his undergraduate education in three years, but Harvard administrators wouldn't approve his plan.

"They require four years of tuition," he says.

Barouch more than held his own at each stop in his education, but he sometimes felt out of place interacting with his older classmates.

"There's something to be said for being the same age as your peers," he says.

A stint as a PhD student in an Oxford University lab with Hill, Gilbert, and other ambitious scientists had cemented Barouch's decision to focus on infectious diseases and vaccines, which he saw as the most powerful way to impact global health. More than anything, Barouch relished an intellectual challenge. He came to see AIDS as modern science's most pressing unsolved mystery.

After starting his lab at Beth Israel Deaconess Medical Center, Barouch traveled to Leiden to spend two months of 2003 working at Crucell, the small Dutch company that had provided Merck with embryonic human cells to grow the protein at the heart of its vaccine. He lived in a room at the Holiday Inn of Leiden, eating hotel food and doing experiments with Crucell's chief scientific officer, Jaap

Goudsmit, a stylish dresser who favored distinctive rounded eye frames. Barouch learned how to grow and purify adenoviruses, becoming convinced they could be effective vaccine vehicles.

By 2004, Barouch was building an AIDS vaccine, just like Merck. He didn't want to work with Ad5 as Merck was doing, though. As the principal investigator of his lab, Barouch felt pressure to raise funding; he knew no one was going to back yet another effort to develop an Ad5 HIV vaccine.

Just as important, Barouch doubted that an Ad5 vaccine would work. While in Crucell's lab, he and Goudsmit had tested blood samples from hundreds of individuals in the United States, Europe, Japan, and Africa. More than 50 percent of these subjects had been exposed to the Ad5 cold virus, the tests showed, suggesting these individuals likely harbored antibodies capable of neutralizing it. Antibodies are great if you want to stop a virus, but they're the last thing you want when building a vaccine dependent on that same virus infecting the body's cells and instructing them to produce a protein. Even more disturbing, Barouch and Goudsmit had determined that close to 90 percent of those tested in the developing world had these antibodies, suggesting that even if an Ad5 vaccine was effective in the United States and Europe, it likely would be of little value in Africa, where an AIDS vaccine was most needed.

Back in Boston, Barouch and his labmates spent a couple years testing a half dozen strains of adenoviruses, settling on serotype 26, or Ad26 for short, a human virus that causes mild colds and is much less prevalent than the Ad5 virus. Years earlier, Merck's scientists had studied Ad26, but they had moved on, just like they did with the chimp adenovirus, something Barouch thought was a blunder. To him, Ad26 seemed adept at invading human cells, suggesting the virus could deliver a payload of genetic material capable of teaching the immune system to block HIV.

Barouch turned to Goudsmit and Crucell for materials and expertise to generate and grow his adenovirus, modified to contain genes for three HIV proteins for use as a vaccine. Goudsmit ran into problems at the office, though. Crucell was a tiny company that couldn't afford big risks. The company's supervisory board didn't want Goudsmit working on an HIV vaccine, especially one relying on an untested adenovirus.

HIV vaccines aren't "commercially viable," a colleague told Goudsmit, echoing the view of most in the industry, while another called his work "preposterous."

Goudsmit didn't want to give up, so he decided to mask his work, hoping to avoid his superiors' notice. He gave his lab notebooks and other materials generic labels, such as "Assay Validations," which he hoped wouldn't tip off nosy colleagues that he was continuing to work on AIDS. He and his colleagues also expanded their work to include another virus, respiratory syncytial virus, or RSV, a more popular vaccine target than HIV.

In 2007, Barouch and Goudsmit had data that was good enough to share with his bosses. With several colleagues, they published a research paper demonstrating that their Ad26-based vaccine generated antibodies in mice. Later, the scientists confirmed that their vaccine provided monkeys with protection from SIV, a monkey virus that's very similar to HIV in humans. The two men grew increasingly optimistic as they prepared for human trials of their AIDS vaccine using the HIV-specific Ad26 courier.

By then, Barouch had become something of a lightning rod in the world of science, stirring both admiration and jealousy in his peers. Among the youngest full professors in the history of Harvard Medical School, Barouch didn't just publish research on a regular basis—his work appeared in top-flight journals. He was a triple threat, teaching, doing research, and treating patients. Some called Barouch a "boy wonder." Nelson Michael, a top researcher at the Walter Reed Army Institute of Research, preferred the nickname "BW," or using military terminology, "Bravo Whiskey."

"Everything he touched was gold," Michael says. "Dan threatened senior scientists, people got jealous."

Then, in 2007, the unthinkable happened. Merck shocked the world with its awful trial results. Instantly, Barouch and Goudsmit's approach, which was seen as similar to Merck's methods, went from attractive to alarming. To Barouch and Goudsmit, Merck's setback was proof of the need to focus on other viral vectors, such as Ad26, not a reason to ditch the entire concept of using adenoviruses.

"The problems are solvable," Goudsmit insisted to a colleague.

No one wanted to hear it. For some rival scientists, it was an opportunity to turn on Barouch. Top scientists emailed and called him, saying he was wasting his time and he should give up the idea of using an adenovirus in a drug or vaccine. Friends pulled Barouch aside at conferences, warning him to drop the work. Rival researchers lobbied the NIH to terminate its financial support of his lab, arguing that the money was being squandered. So much had changed for Barouch, and so quickly.

• • •

Barouch pushed on, preparing for a human trial for his HIV vaccine, scheduled to begin in 2008. Despite Merck's earlier fiasco, he still believed his vaccine approach—using a human virus to ferry viral proteins into the body—could work, if not in AIDS then perhaps against another, less-challenging disease. Adrian Hill at Oxford had just as much faith in his own adenovirus-vaccine strategy.

By then, Gale Smith, the scientist who had worked with Frank Volvovitz and MicroGeneSys, had started his new job with the unheralded Maryland biotech company Novavax. He was still trying to perfect his unorthodox vaccine approach, which relied on an insect virus to carry the genes for viral proteins into cells. Hill, Barouch, and Smith were all unaware of progress being made with a third, even more radical vaccine approach, one that would become the most revolutionary in modern history.

4

1988–1996

Someone's sitting in the shade today because someone planted a tree a long time ago.

—WARREN BUFFETT[1]

Parents, scared and confused, kept making their way to Jon Wolff's office. He was their last resort.

Wolff was completing a clinical fellowship in neuroscience at the University of California, San Diego, in the late 1980s. He had his hands full, but in his spare time, Wolff liked to treat pediatric patients. Bespectacled and bearded, with curly light-blond hair and an infectious grin, Wolff quickly gained a reputation as something of a medical sleuth, identifying rare diseases in young boys and girls that other doctors missed. Word spread and parents were soon lining up to visit the gifted diagnostician. Most were desperate to simply make sense of what was afflicting their children. By then, many had given up hope for an effective treatment.

Humorous and compassionate, Wolff chatted with the parents, examined the children, and frequently identified genetic abnormalities.

Sometimes it was propionic acidemia, an inherited condition that prevents babies from processing proteins and fats; other times, it was phenylketonuria, or PKU, a blood disorder that can lead to delayed development, psychiatric disorders, or early death. Still other children were dealing with muscular dystrophy, a group of genetic diseases that can force patients into wheelchairs by their teens.

These were devastating diagnoses. Coming home to his family in the evening, though, Wolff usually had a smile on his face. Most of his patients had been shunted among specialists, sometimes for years. By identifying their diseases, Wolff provided the families with a measure of relief. He and others in his clinic worked to devise diets capable of making the children's lives bearable, even enjoyable.

Most of Wolff's patients had some kind of metabolic disorder, usually due to a genetic anomaly. A defective gene was unable to make a necessary substance, or otherwise one that didn't operate properly. In his lab at night, Wolff searched for ways to provide help. He received support from the Muscular Dystrophy Association, so he regularly appeared on the organization's televised Labor Day telethons, hosted by Jerry Lewis, explaining to viewers the efforts he and others were making to try to defeat the distressing diseases. Once, Wolff appeared onscreen after a bicycling orangutan. His own young children watched from home, more excited to see the ape than their father.

Over time, he became frustrated by the lack of progress in the area. By the late 1980s, scientists had been studying genes—the physical entities containing deoxyribonucleic acid, or DNA—for nearly a century. They knew DNA molecules helped determine inheritable traits in all living things, from eye and hair color to height and weight. They also understood that DNA is a passive molecule that resides in the cell's nucleus. That knowledge led to a scientific conundrum: How exactly does DNA, stuck in the nucleus, make the proteins that keep us functioning, which are all created in an entirely different compartment of the cell, its cytoplasm?

In 1961, researchers at California Institute of Technology found the answer when they discovered that another molecule, a kind of ribonucleic acid (RNA) called messenger ribonucleic acid, or mRNA, carries a copy of the DNA's genetic instructions to the cytoplasm.[2] There, the instructions are translated into collagen, insulin, antibodies, and millions of other tiny yet crucial proteins.

As Wolff donned his crisp white lab coat to greet his next family in 1988, he itched for a way to heal his young patients' defective genes. Often, he'd see children during the day, come home and talk about his cases with his own young family, and then head back to his lab after dinner, searching for a discovery that could provide some help.

Why can't we cure these kids? Wolff wondered.

The quest occupied Wolff to the point of distraction, which was something of a pattern in his life. A native of the neighborhood of Bayside, in the New York borough of Queens, Wolff spent much of his youth winning science contests and playing schoolyard pickup basketball, intense games that sometimes led to fistfights. Wolff began Cornell University at the age of sixteen as a chemistry major, emerging as one of his class's top students. Dating was a bit of a challenge, though, both due to Wolff's baby face as well as his growing preoccupation with science. Wolff began seeing Katalin Bujdoso, a native of Hungary, but he often turned up late for their dates, apologizing profusely that he had been so absorbed in an experiment that he had lost track of time.

"So sorry, a column ran over!" was a common refrain, referring to tubing he used in the lab.

When Katalin brought Wolff home to meet her parents, he lugged a heavy medical textbook, reading intently on the family couch throughout the visit. Fortunately, Katalin's father was a physician, so he shrugged off Wolff's rudeness. It took Katalin a bit longer to adjust to the impolite idiosyncrasies.

"Eventually, I got used to it," says Katalin, who married Wolff during his first year of medical school at Johns Hopkins University in Baltimore.

In 1988, Wolff and his family moved from San Diego to Madison, Wisconsin, where he assumed a teaching position at the University of Wisconsin–Madison School of Medicine, while also treating pediatric patients and doing research. The family purchased a modest home on the other side of an intramural-sports field from Wolff's new lab. The short walk enabled Wolff to spend even more time on his research. Katalin and the children, who soon numbered two boys and two girls, liked to sit on the front stoop in the early evening and peer across the field to see if a light was on in his lab. If it was off, they knew he'd soon be ambling across the field, his face buried deep in a scientific journal.

As with his scientific pursuits, when Wolff embraced a new hobby, he felt the need to "understand the concept" and discover an improved approach. He threw himself into cross-country skiing: reading books, studying videos, and taking lessons. Eventually, he arrived at a series of steps that helped him cover ground quickly, such as keeping his weight allocated equally between legs, a discovery that led to ribbing from friends.

"Yes, Jon, it's called balance," his friend Patrick Remington teased. "Just ski!"

Wolff's children also rolled their eyes, but it usually was about his fashion sense. Wolff once wore a plaid shirt with plaid pants—each a different pattern of plaid—explaining to his mortified family that his outfit "matched." Katalin came to see her husband's choices as signs of his unusual creativity. Wolff approached life with a beginner's mindset; he was an original thinker who viewed problems from a unique perspective, she concluded.

"Daddy thinks so far out of the box he doesn't see the box," Katalin once said to one of their children.

Wolff began applying his creativity to ways he could help his patients with their distressing and disabling genetic defects. He started from scratch, searching for a fresh approach. He knew that humans are largely composed of proteins, which are complex molecules that do most of the work necessary to live and reproduce. By that time, the way proteins were created was familiar to most anyone with even a passing familiarity with biology, thanks to the earlier advances: Within our cells, DNA is copied, or transcribed, into messenger RNA, which is translated into protein. DNA makes mRNA makes protein makes life; it's a central dogma of science.

Wolff realized that DNA, which contains the basic building blocks of life, is akin to a cell's cookbook. It's full of recipes for making proteins, but it's so thick and bulky that it has to be kept in the library—the cell's nucleus—because it's too heavy to transport. Wolff knew that strings of nucleotides found in the DNA create specific genes, such as those he was struggling to correct. But for any of the protein recipes in the cookbook to get made, the DNA first needs to be transcribed in the cell's nucleus into messenger RNA molecules, which can be seen as temporary copies of a few pages from that heavy cookbook. This mRNA is then easily transported to the cytoplasm, which is akin to the cell's kitchen. There, proteins are made, as instructed, before the mRNA is discarded, its job done.

But if the recipes in someone's DNA are faulty, she could end up missing proteins, with too much or too little of a protein, or with a faulty protein, leading to the types of disease Wolff was trying to treat. He knew that DNA and mRNA are created naturally, but they also can be manufactured, or synthesized, in the lab, much like natural food sweeteners can be engineered.

Wolff wondered: What if we could synthesize and deliver normal DNA or mRNA, without the mistakes, straight into human cells to replace defective genes in his patients? Maybe this way, functional proteins could be created.

When Wolff shared his simple-yet-outlandish idea with peers he didn't exactly blow them away with his originality. *Of course* it had occurred to them that injecting normal DNA or mRNA might be a way to help those suffering from various diseases; the question was how to do it and whether it was even possible. Scientists were beginning to appreciate that if DNA or mRNA could be delivered into the body's cells, they could theoretically read the instructions and make the corresponding protein, potentially curing genetic disease. It was all part of a new potential method of treatment being described as gene therapy.

But hardly anyone was considering injecting straight, or "naked," DNA, an exercise that likely was useless, if not dangerous. There's a reason it's a two-step process—DNA to mRNA to proteins. Within a cell, DNA has to be transcribed into mRNA before it can create useful proteins. It's not easy getting DNA into a cell to begin the protein-creation process. Since DNA is a huge, negatively charged molecule, most researchers expected the cell's membrane to block it from entering the cell. Besides, messing around with DNA, which is the body's permanent instructions, seemed risky.

Wolff's colleagues were even more certain that injecting messenger RNA wouldn't work, largely because it's such an unstable molecule. After moving within the cell to the cytoplasm and providing necessary instructions to create proteins, mRNA is usually degraded, broken down, in a matter of hours. Just as a spare tire can hold up on a short drive but will break down on an arduous cross-country trip, researchers agreed it was folly to expect mRNA to survive a solo trip into the cell, in the hope that it could produce sufficient proteins. Everyone knew that the moment mRNA was injected, it would come into contact with bodily fluids chock-full of enzymes that would immediately chop it up.

Wolff understood the resistance to his idea, but he didn't want to give up. He began looking for ways to get DNA and mRNA into cells to facilitate gene therapy. He became consumed by the intellectual challenge, unable to let it go.

"This was something he never stopped thinking about . . . the scientific puzzle of getting genes into cells," Katalin says.

Recent advances had shown that by mixing DNA or mRNA with certain liquids or fatty lipids prior to adding them to cells, it was possible to induce the cells to absorb the DNA or mRNA. The lipid packaging seemed to protect these two nucleic acids, helping to carry the molecules and their genetic messages through the cell's membrane. But most of the research had been done only on cells growing in a Petri dish. Wolff was an experimentalist, though, so he thought he'd go ahead and inject mice. He didn't have much to lose. It helped that he had ample funding from various sources, including a lawyer for James Watson—the molecular biologist who helped identify the structure of the DNA molecule—who had a son with muscular dystrophy.

Wolff set up a series of experiments to test whether DNA or mRNA injections packaged in crude lipids could create proteins in mice, comparing those shots with a control group of straight DNA and mRNA shots without the lipids.

What Wolff saw was truly astounding. The shots of DNA and mRNA encased by lipids didn't do much to the mice, a disappointing result that was in line with what the naysayers had predicted. But when Wolff directly injected DNA and mRNA into the leg muscles of mice, he found that they were actually successful in creating the desired proteins in the mice cells. The control group had somehow worked better than the experimental group. Excited, Wolff and his colleagues injected a series of additional shots using just DNA and mRNA, showing, once again, that these genetic instructions were absorbed by mice cells and then expressed as proteins that sometimes lasted two months or longer.

Wolff had demonstrated that a functional protein could be created by injecting DNA or mRNA into cells, something that had never before been done. The cell's enzymes were chopping up most of the injected molecule, as expected, but it turned out that enough was slipping by the body's defenses to create a bit of protein. The fact that he could generate protein with notoriously unstable mRNA was especially startling to Wolff and others.

"Wow, messenger RNA is really interesting," Wolff told a colleague, after seeing the results.

Wolff, who was just thirty-three at the time, didn't tell most of his friends about his breakthrough, and he knew he was far from any kind of treatment or cure. It wasn't clear the protein response he had generated was sufficient or capable of fixing any genetic or other problems, nor was it obvious it was beneficial in any other way, such as inhibiting tumor growth or neutralizing a pathogen. Perhaps most important, Wolff's work was in mice, and it was far from clear whether mRNA injections could create proteins in humans.

Still, Wolff's work was eye-opening, especially the results he saw with mRNA, which almost no one expected could remain intact, be absorbed by cells, and be translated into proteins. Wolff had delivered a clear message to fellow researchers: mRNA has more potential than you realize.

In March 1990, Wolff and several colleagues published their work in the prestigious journal *Science*, describing the first successful use of mRNA. His research suggested that mRNA might someday be used as a drug or even a vaccine, since it was now clear the molecule could produce proteins, though Wolff didn't do any work in that area. A bit later, other scientists would show similar results in rats, while still others would directly inject mRNA in mice to generate an immune response, more evidence that the molecule might lead to helpful therapeutics.

There were still many imposing obstacles to overcome for mRNA to consistently produce proteins in humans, Wolff knew. Over the next few years, he focused on developing ways to deliver mRNA into the body's cells and avoid something called RNase, an enzyme that degrades the mRNA molecule, possibly before it's had a full chance to deliver its instructions to cells, something that likely had prevented Wolff from creating ample protein in his earlier experiments. In 1995, Wolff and two other scientists started a company to build sophisticated capsules or other lipid or polymer packaging to make mRNA delivery particles more stable and longer lasting, an improved version of the lipids Wolff first used. A few years later, they sold the start-up for more than $100 million, though the company never managed to produce any mRNA drugs. Wolff took his proceeds and bought a house on a lake in Madison and a new pair of skis, but otherwise maintained his previous lifestyle. He put in long hours in the lab, still searching for a way to insert genes in patients in order to cure muscular dystrophy or other genetic diseases.

Wolff never had the chance to fulfill his goal. In early 2019, he himself became a patient of a difficult disease when he was diagnosed with esophageal cancer. The researcher spent months enduring various treatments, even as he traveled the country to say goodbye to a dozen or so former colleagues, mentors, and close friends. At one point, he began having trouble swallowing, but he rarely complained.

"I can sit around and feel lousy or I can do something and feel lousy," Wolff told a former colleague in California.

In April 2020, as a new kind of coronavirus spread around the globe, Wolff passed away of cancer at the age of sixty-three, his family by his bedside. He couldn't have suspected it at the time, but his earlier work would contribute to a vaccine approach that had a chance to protect against the very virus that was overwhelming much of the world.

• • •

Eli Gilboa just wanted to give the immune system a fighting chance.

Growing up in Israel in the late 1950s and early '60s, Gilboa faced early challenges. His father delivered magazines for a living, hopping on a blue Lambretta scooter to make early morning runs to local cafés, inserting advertisements in the periodicals to pick up some cash. Gilboa's mother was an artisan who made handbags for a well-known fashion house run by Ruth Dayan, the wife of General Moshe Dayan. Eli's parents' careers appeared glamorous, but the couple could barely pay their bills and the Gilboa family was under constant financial pressure. Unable to take sufficient care of Eli, his parents, both recent immigrants from Romania, sent the boy to live in a dormitory on a kibbutz, where he was miserable. Eventually, Ruth Dayan pulled some strings to get Eli a spot in a well-regarded boarding school north of Tel Aviv, where hundreds of disadvantaged children, as well as those from dysfunctional families, studied and worked the fields. At the school, which was called a youth village, Eli proved a mediocre student, but he loved tending to the cows and was thrilled at the chance to help deliver calves.

Gilboa improved in the classroom and eventually trained as a molecular biologist at the Weizmann Institute of Science in Israel, before coming to the United States in 1977 to complete his training in the laboratory of David Baltimore, the Nobel laureate who at the time was at the Massachusetts Institute of Technology. Gilboa spent time working on HIV, but by the time he joined the Duke University Medical Center in 1993, he was focused on aiding the immune system to battle cancer, a challenge that had beset scientists for generations.

The immune system does a better job identifying and eliminating tumor cells than is widely presumed. Autopsy studies have shown that as many as 30 percent of men aged fifty-five or older who die in car accidents show evidence of cancer, and there is similar evidence that a large percentage of women also have cancer cells without realizing it.

"Most of us, probably all of us, have cancer but don't know it and never will," Gilboa says. "There is strong circumstantial evidence that in many instances it is the immune system that keeps it in check."

Too frequently, though, cancer develops elaborate methods to evade the body's defenses and inflict terrible damage. Some tumors, including those related to the lymphatic system, are even centered in the immune system.

Early on at Duke, Gilboa focused on ways to activate immune cells so they might recognize and kill tumors. He staffed his laboratory with scientists from diverse and unorthodox backgrounds, hoping they could help him arrive at an original approach. The team included Smita Nair, an immunology postdoctoral fellow from Mumbai, India, and David Boczkowski, a senior technician who had spent a decade doing blood transfusion and other work in a Pittsburgh hospital.

Gilboa and his team started by placing mouse and human tumor cells in a Petri dish and adding DNA instructions for producing proteins that tend to stimulate the immune system. The goal was to inject the cells back into the mice and eventually into human patients to try to activate dormant parts of the immune system, a so-called cell-based approach.

"Let's try to tickle the immune system," Gilboa told Nair and Boczkowski one day in the lab.

Their early results were mostly mediocre. Over time, Gilboa and Nair tried a different approach: enabling dendritic cells—which play a central role in activating T cells and generating an immune response—to do a better job fighting cancer. Nair took a melanoma tumor grown in a flask and "lysed" it, or blasted it with high-frequency sound waves, creating minuscule pieces of cancerous cells. She added the tumor pieces to a lipid formula in a Petri dish and inserted this blend in dendritic cells, all of it in a tube of liquid. What they had was a mixture—"lysate" in scientific terms or a "gemish" in Gilboa's Yiddish phraseology—of DNA, RNA, proteins, and more from the cancer cells. Nair created various mixtures with slightly different compositions and injected the mostly clear concoctions into mice sick with an aggressive melanoma, hoping to shrink the tumors. Each was an attempt to grab the immune system's attention and teach it to recognize and attack signs of cancer, but Gilboa's team didn't really have a clue which mixture, if any, might work.

"They were a lot of shots in the dark," Gilboa says.

The team didn't get far, but at least Gilboa was a fun guy to be around. He loved to laugh, blared opera music in the lab, and enjoyed jogging so much that he became known for showing up at prestigious medical meetings dripping in perspiration. As a fellow immigrant, Nair felt a special connection to her lab boss. Perhaps most important, Gilboa gave his scientists a lot of leeway, encouraging them to pursue new technologies and novel theories and to conduct independent experiments.

"Can you at least keep me in the loop?" he once asked Nair and Boczkowski, pretending to be upset.

Slowly, the team made some progress. A version of their tumor gemish seemed to shrink mice cancers, though they had no idea why. Gilboa and Nair theorized that a protein component in their mixture was stimulating an immune response, but Boczkowski had a hunch it was something else. Earlier in his career, he had received a master's degree in molecular biology at the University of Pittsburgh in 1993, and he had worked in a lab that studied RNA, including mRNA. Most scientists were wary of using the molecule in experiments because it disappeared so quickly. But Boczkowski and his Pittsburgh colleagues came to see that it was sturdier than most presumed. To him, it was an underrated and overlooked molecule.

"A lot of people didn't want to work with RNA. They thought if you looked at it wrong, it would disintegrate," Boczkowski says. "We had a respect for it but didn't fear it."

Boczkowski wondered if the mice tumors were shriveling because the messenger RNA component of their mixture was stirring the mouse's immune system. That gave him a thought: Maybe mRNA was all that was needed, not all the other elements in their concoction.

On a crisp, fall day in 1995, as Nair prepared another round of experiments, Boczkowski handed her a tube of clear liquid, which he jokingly labeled "the Cure." He asked Nair to test it with all the others.

"Here you go, here's your cure," Boczkowski told her, a mischievous look on his face.

Boczkowski wouldn't tell Nair what was in his mystery tube, but she assumed it was one more mix of tumor proteins and other antigens. A few weeks later, Nair checked on her mice. Those in her control group, which hadn't received any vaccine, had lungs heavy with cancer and had to be euthanized, or "sacrificed," in the language of the scientists. But mice in the experimental group, which had received various vaccine concoctions, were doing better, a positive sign for the researchers. A few were a bit healthier than the rest. When Nair cut the lungs out of the most robust-looking mice and searched for signs of cancer, she didn't see much, surprising her. She weighed their lungs and they seemed entirely tumor-free. Now she was really excited. Checking her charts, Nair realized the healthiest mice had been treated with Boczkowski's secret formula.

Nair rushed to tell her colleagues and Gilboa quickly looked over the results.

"This group looks like it's working!" Gilboa exclaimed.

He and Nair looked at Boczkowski—they were dying to know what he had put in the mysterious vaccine potion.

"It's RNA," Boczkowski told them.

Gilboa gave him a look of astonishment. Boczkowski explained that he had isolated mRNA from the melanoma tumor and included the molecule in the vaccine tube he had given Nair. That was all he had put in there, he said.

Gilboa burst into laughter.

"This is amazing!" he said.

The mRNA-treated mice weren't doing *that* much better than those treated with the tumor gemish, but the results were surprising, nonetheless. At the time, the vast majority of scientists believed mRNA was too unstable to be of much use as a therapeutic or vaccine, no matter what Wolff had discovered a few years earlier. Conventional wisdom held that cell enzymes would chew up the mRNA molecule before it had a chance to stir the immune system.

Could this be right? Gilboa thought.

He needed to repeat the experiment. Once again, the mRNA vaccine shrank the mice tumors. Gilboa and his colleagues concluded that mRNA was instructing the dendritic cells to produce tumor proteins, which in turn were spurring the T cells and B cells in the mouse's immune system to attack the cancer. Yes, much of the mRNA had probably been chopped up by the cells' enzymes, but enough of it was making it into the cytoplasm of the dendritic cells. The mRNA molecule was sturdier than expected, it seemed. Not only was it surviving, but it was helping to shrink the mice's cancer.

Gilboa's face lit up as he sensed enormous possibilities: mRNA could be an effective drug or vaccine.

In August 1996, Gilboa and his colleagues published their results in *The Journal of Experimental Medicine*. It was groundbreaking stuff. Jon Wolff had shown that mRNA can create proteins in mice, while a few others had used mRNA to elicit immune responses. But no one had shrunk a tumor using the much-maligned, short-lived molecule. Sure, Gilboa and his colleagues were working with mice, not humans. And they were removing mice cells, treating them with mRNA in a dish in their laboratory, and then injecting the cells into the body, a complicated course of treatment. Still, their work was a further indication that scientists had underestimated the mRNA molecule.

Big-name scientists were so surprised by the results that some doubted their veracity, a powerful challenge to Gilboa and his colleagues. Injecting mRNA remained a heretical notion; it just shouldn't work, the researchers said. A few months later, Philip Greenberg, among the world's top cancer investigators, stood up in front of dozens of scientists at an academic meeting to address Gilboa's supposed breakthrough. Greenberg said he had tried to reproduce the Duke experiments, but he couldn't get mRNA effectively expressed in the dendritic cells.

"I tried what Eli is doing and couldn't get it to work," Greenberg told the group, as Gilboa felt eyes in the room focus on him.

Later, a junior member of Greenberg's lab spoke with Nair about how she had conducted her experiments and made a few changes, as Nair suggested. Soon Greenberg and his colleagues managed to replicate Gilboa's work, confirming their accuracy and spurring new hope for the idea of using mRNA.

Over the next few years, Gilboa and his colleagues tested mRNA vaccines in clinical trials, eager to find ways to beat brain, prostate, and other cancers. In 2000, Gilboa started a biotech company to produce his own mRNA vaccines. Treating patients proved both exciting and frustrating, however. Sometimes, the Gilboa vaccines worked wonders. A woman with glioblastoma who flew to North Carolina to receive the vaccine at Duke managed to fend off the deadly and aggressive cancer. Nair and Boczkowski were overjoyed to meet someone they had actually helped.

"It was kind of cool," Boczkowski says. "Usually we just see mice."

Most other times, though, their vaccines didn't do enough to help patients, even when an immune response was generated, disappointing Gilboa and his colleagues. They decided they needed more funding to improve their methods.

In September 2005, Gilboa and a newer colleague, Bruce Sullenger, met with Robert Williams, dean of Duke's medical school, to ask for backing for the mRNA effort. By then, Sullenger had become a big believer in the approach and was doing his own work demonstrating how promising mRNA was as a vaccine and drug approach. Sitting across from Williams in a large conference room, Sullenger spent over an hour giving an impassioned presentation about how mRNA could revolutionize patient care. He and Gilboa asked Williams for the money to hire an investigator so they could research using mRNA to fight viruses and other infectious diseases, in addition to cancer.

"This is the *future*," Sullenger told Williams.

Williams wasn't persuaded. A cardiologist with a long list of his own accomplishments, Williams was more excited about genomics, a field that was growing in popularity and involves working with DNA, not mRNA. Duke was hiring dozens of academics with genomic-science expertise, leaving fewer resources for other areas. Gilboa and Sullenger didn't get their money.

For his part, Williams says he had to choose between hundreds of funding requests each year from Duke's academics. Not everyone could get money, he says. Betting on mRNA seemed a dangerous move at the time.

"I was skeptical of RNA," Williams says, referring to the vexing question of how to stabilize it and deliver the molecule to cells. "I thought Eli Gilboa was doing interesting research, but he wasn't leading the gene therapy field."

Walking out of the meeting, Sullenger saw a look of defeat on Gilboa's face.

"I need to leave," Gilboa, discouraged and defeated, told Sullenger.

The next year, Gilboa quit Duke for the University of Miami. Soon he had doubts about his mRNA approach. He suspected that using dendritic cells might not be the way to go. Eventually, he turned his attention to other ways of activating the immune system to attack cancer.

"I gave up on mRNA and left the whole field," he says.

Nair, Boczkowski, and others at Duke kept plugging away, even raising money to purchase a piece of lab equipment called a gene gun so they could do injections of mRNA into skin cells. But they, too, ran into obstacles, especially with funding, and shifted to other areas of research.

"I sometimes regret not sticking with it, but timing is everything in life," Nair says.

Nair and Boczkowski did find other kinds of success: They began a personal relationship that culminated in marriage.

• • •

The work of Gilboa and his colleagues was both eye-opening and trailblazing. To have true practical importance, though, much more was needed. It was too much to ask physicians to draw blood from a patient, isolate cells, treat them in a lab with mRNA, and then reinfuse them back into the same patient. Even Gilboa believed directly injecting mRNA wouldn't work—he was sure the body's enzymes would break up the molecule before it could have a therapeutic impact, no matter what Wolff had done.

It would take an unexpected breakthrough by even more unlikely researchers before mRNA could have a chance of curing illness or stopping disease.

5

1997–2009

Great science is often a group of people.

—MICHAEL HOUGHTON[1]

It took a painfully slow photocopy machine to bring Katalin Karikó and Drew Weissman together.

Karikó and Weissman were researchers at the University of Pennsylvania's medical school in the fall of 1997. Beyond that, they had precious little in common. A gregarious, blue-eyed, floppy-haired immigrant from Hungary working in Penn's neurosurgery department, Karikó couldn't keep her comments and opinions to herself, even when they jeopardized her career. Weissman, a balding, bespectacled professor of medicine from a Boston suburb, was usually so taciturn that his wife once joked that he set a word limit each day, beyond which he didn't dare venture.

For all their differences, Karikó and Weissman shared an affection for an overworked Xerox machine on their floor, trekking over on a regular basis to copy articles from scientific journals, none of which were yet available online. Most days, Karikó and Weissman eyed each other warily, sometimes squabbling over who was next in line.

Eventually, Karikó decided to introduce herself and restart their relationship.

"You're a new guy, right?" she asked. "I'm Kati. I can make any RNA. I can do RNA for you if you want!"

Weissman didn't jump at Karikó's proposal. An immunologist who had come to the Philadelphia school a year earlier to start a research lab, Weissman was working on dendritic cells in culture, much like Gilboa and his colleagues at Duke. But Weissman's goal was to create a vaccine to protect against HIV, not cancer. Like most scientists, Weissman was wary of messenger RNA, no matter the work that Gilboa and a few others were doing. The molecule was hard to make in the lab and couldn't be relied upon in an experiment, since it disappeared so quickly upon entering the cell.

"If you make it I'll try it," Weissman told her halfheartedly.

By then, Karikó had spent nearly a decade trying to excite colleagues about mRNA, pitching over thirty Penn scientists, with little success. Few researchers wanted to work with the molecule. Even fewer wanted to work with Kati Karikó. The indignities didn't bother the forty-three-year-old. She had become accustomed to rejection, disappointment, and humiliation.

Kati was born in Kisújszállás, a small town in central Hungary, where her parents, János and Gőőz, enjoyed a comfortable middle-class life. That changed abruptly in 1957, when Kati was two years old. That year, János publicly criticized the ruling Communist government. Almost immediately, he lost his reliable and well-paid job as a butcher. János spent the rest of his life cobbling work—a stint in a pub, a job building local homes, and farmwork, including shearing sheep. The Karikó family lived in a two-room adobe home that lacked running water, a refrigerator, or a television. For warmth, they stood around a sawdust stove. Despite the privations, János exuded joy and happiness, singing and joking with his family most days, an optimistic attitude that his wife shared and his daughter noted.

In high school, Karikó was assigned to read a book by Austrian-born Hungarian scientist Hans Selye (pronounced "shy-yeh"), who did groundbreaking work on the ways anxiety and tension impact physical health. Resentment and regret were misplaced energy, Selye argued. His lessons, including the importance of living a stress-free life, resonated with the young woman. Karikó vowed to embrace a certain equanimity in life, something Selye called "homeostasis," and to improve her position in life, rather than complain about her lot. Her promise would be tested as Karikó became an adult.

One day, while studying biology at the University of Szeged, Karikó heard a lecture about the underappreciated potential of the mRNA molecule. She became a true believer. At the time, scientists were getting excited about the idea of treating or curing disease by modifying a person's genes, the kind of work Jon Wolff did in Wisconsin. The approach usually meant introducing DNA into the body. Some kind of carrier, or vector, would take the genetic material into cells in the hopes of producing missing or functional proteins. But inserting DNA into the nucleus of the body's cells is tricky and dangerous, Karikó realized, partly because it can create a permanent change. Since DNA needs to be converted into mRNA before a cell reads the instructions and produces a protein, she wondered if it might be easier and more effective skipping a step and injecting mRNA, rather than DNA, to create the necessary proteins.

After earning a PhD in biochemistry at a top Hungarian research university, Karikó landed a prestigious position as a postdoctoral fellow at the Szeged Biological Research Centre, where she began synthetically creating mRNA so it could be used in various experiments. Karikó married an engineer named Béla Francia, and they soon had a daughter.

Karikó lost the job, however, when the institute experienced a cash crunch. She considered searching for a teaching position or another job in the country, where the cost of living was low and she enjoyed child-care help from her parents. But Karikó was dedicated to pursuing her mRNA research and wanted to have some kind of impact on the world. Selye had written about the need to judge one's environment and assess if it was ideally suited for one's personal growth. Hungary didn't seem like that place. It was time for Karikó to leave.

"I wanted to see what more I could do," she says.

In 1985, Karikó decided to move to the United States, though she and Francia barely spoke English. They bought one-way tickets, hoping to force themselves to persevere in their new home, rather than consider returning to Hungary. Boarding a flight in Budapest, Karikó was more nervous than most new immigrants. The Hungarian government prohibited citizens from leaving the country with much cash, so Karikó had sewed the family's savings—about twelve hundred dollars, the proceeds from the sale of their car—into a hole she had carved in the stomach of a teddy bear held by her two-year-old daughter, Susan. The toy escaped notice and the cash was all the family had to rely on when they touched down in New York to restart their life.

Karikó found a position working in the laboratory of Robert Suhadolnik, a professor in the biochemistry department at Temple University School of Medicine working on AIDS treatments. Money was tighter than she had expected. Karikó made seventeen thousand dollars a year, while Francia, who was unable to find an engineering position, made about the same as a facilities manager for a local apartment complex, where he fixed heating and water systems. Their own apartment didn't have a washing machine, so every few days Karikó lugged the family's laundry to the basement of a nearby building.

Karikó didn't mind the challenges, though, because she was expanding her mRNA expertise. With Suhadolnik as her guide, she was perfecting ways to modify mRNA molecules. By altering the building blocks of RNA, which are called nucleosides, new versions of the molecule can be created to produce proteins in the lab. Laboring day and night, she and Suhadolnik published papers in respected scientific journals. Karikó's career appeared not only to be back on track but on a fast track.

That's when she made her first mistake as an academic. Karikó accepted a better-paid position at Johns Hopkins University but didn't think to give Suhadolnik prior warning that she was seeking a new job. When he heard about the offer, he became furious, vowing to do whatever he could to stop his protégée from leaving. In a difficult meeting with Karikó, he made it clear she had two career choices.

"You can work in my lab or go home," he told her.

Suhadolnik followed through on his threat, telling a local immigration office that she was living in the country illegally and should be deported. Karikó and her husband had to hire an expensive lawyer to fight the extradition order. By then, Johns Hopkins had withdrawn its offer, wary of hiring a suspected fugitive. Suhadolnik continued bad-mouthing Karikó, making it impossible for her to get a new position. She tried not to become discouraged, reminding herself of Selye's lessons. Eventually, she met a scientist at a Bethesda Naval Hospital who had his own difficult history with Suhadolnik and was willing to hire her despite her scuffed reputation. A few years later, in the summer of 1989, Karikó landed an even better position as a research-assistant professor in the cardiology department of the University of Pennsylvania's medical school.

She quickly realized she was something of a second-class citizen at the Ivy League school. Her job was to do research and deliver a few lectures for graduate students, but she would never be eligible for tenure, unlike most other faculty members. The cardiology department was composed of physicians who treated patients, did research, and brought in money from grant proposals. PhDs like Karikó were there to help these physician-scientists. The research-assistant professors usually were foreign-born researchers—some faculty members referred to them as "the aliens"—willing to overlook meager salaries for the experience of working in the university's world-class labs and because Penn promised to support their green-card applications.

The second-tier status made life difficult for Karikó. Once she was reprimanded for using deionized water belonging to a senior member of her lab, rather than climb five flights of stairs to get some from a different laboratory. When she applied for grant money, reviewers sometimes questioned her proposals, skeptical of her title. When new colleagues arrived, Karikó proposed working together, suggesting ways her mRNA expertise could be helpful to them. Often, though, her new colleagues would find excuses to cancel meetings, likely after realizing Karikó wasn't a clinician on their level.

"People wondered 'what the hell is wrong with her,' there must be some reason she's not on the faculty," Karikó says.

She didn't dwell on her status. Karikó was thrilled at the chance to pursue her mRNA research. She emerged as a friendly, ebullient presence in the department, lugging Hungarian dishes to the office that she eagerly shared with colleagues. But Karikó also could be sensitive to perceived affronts. Once, while chatting with colleagues at a department Christmas party, a professor mentioned that Karikó was working "for him" on a project. She turned livid.

"You think I'm working *for you*?" she asked him as the scientists around her became uncomfortable. "I'm here to advance science, I'm never, ever, working for you."

More than anything, Karikó cared about pursuing her research, not winning friends, playing politics, or boosting egos. In presentations, she often was the first to point out mistakes in colleagues' work or to critique poorly argued theses. She wasn't intending to be difficult or insulting, she just felt the need to call out mistakes. And she was never going to win tenure, so she didn't worry about the sensitivities of colleagues.

Not that Karikó could have reined herself in, even if she tried. Once, while listening to a public speech by an academic who was a fan of adenovirus vectors, she asked so many challenging questions that Judy Swain, the department head who served as Penn's chief of cardiovascular medicine, ordered her to stop, saying she was being disruptive, Karikó remembers. Another time, when she saw that cells two colleagues had worked on for weeks had degraded and were no longer viable, she discarded them without asking for permission, startling her colleagues.

"This is trash," Karikó told them.

"She was absolutely brilliant, but she challenged people, and that was off-putting to people, especially those who were insecure," says David Langer, a resident in Penn's neurosurgery department in the early 1990s who became a rare supporter of Karikó. "Kati was a pain in the ass. She didn't give a shit about getting a gold star from anyone."

One day, Karikó was told to report to Swain, the department head.

"Everyone's complaining about you," Swain told Karikó, calling her "destructive."

Karikó, who at five foot eleven towered over Swain, stood up to challenge her boss.

"Who's everyone and what's their complaint? Call them now. . . . If I made a mistake, I'd like to hear it."

Swain wouldn't pick up the phone.

At that point, Karikó's salary was about forty thousand dollars a year, compensation that barely budged each year, even as her insurance, commuting, and other expenses climbed. Professors shook their heads about a series of beat-up automobiles that Karikó drove to campus over the years, all of which her husband had salvaged and fixed. After a long day in the lab, she'd return home to write grant applications, proposing to use mRNA to develop treatments for cystic fibrosis, strokes, and other ailments. Because her English wasn't yet fluent, it took her longer than others to compose her proposals. She rarely found success—government bodies and others usually scoffed at the idea of working with mRNA. Without ample data, especially proof that she could produce therapeutic proteins in cells and animals, it was difficult getting grant proposals accepted.

Without funds of her own, Karikó's salary had to come from grants raised by others, usually Elliot Barnathan, a cardiologist who was one of the few faculty members who appreciated Karikó's work and determination. She and Barnathan soon made impressive progress. Inserting mRNA into cells in a cell-culture dish, they managed to instruct the cells to make a protein called the urokinase receptor. For Karikó, the feeling was empowering.

"It was like playing God," she says.

Karikó seemed to be on a roll. More smitten than ever with mRNA, she made plans with Barnathan to use the molecule to improve blood vessels for heart bypass surgery and even extend the life span of human cells.[2]

Her timing wasn't great, though. Around the same time, Karikó's colleagues were becoming enamored with using DNA for their own ambitious experiments. By favoring mRNA, the less celebrated molecule, rather than DNA, she gave her colleagues a fresh reason to dismiss her work.

It was hard to blame the Penn professors for steering clear of RNA. DNA has two strands of nucleotides that wind around each other like a twisted ladder, making it durable. By contrast, mRNA is single-stranded and notoriously labile, or unstable, the reason so many found it hard to work with in the lab. Inside the cell, mRNA usually sticks around only a short while before it is effectively chopped up and eliminated as part of the cell's natural turnover. And since many viruses use RNA as their genetic material, the body has developed elaborate methods to ward off the molecule.

Karikó was hardly the first researcher to become excited about the possibilities of mRNA. Eventually, though, most everyone came to view the molecule as a giant waste of time. Why would you insert mRNA into the body, hoping it created a desired protein, if it was going to disappear within minutes? The same CalTech academics who had discovered mRNA in 1961 included a stark warning about the molecule in the very title of their landmark paper: "An Unstable Intermediate Carrying Information from Genes to Ribosomes to Protein Synthesis." It was as if Columbus sailed to America and wrote a letter home with the title: "New Continent—Not Worth Visiting."

Anyone who dared work with mRNA in the lab knew it was an absolute nightmare. Researchers had to wear gloves just to touch equipment coming in contact with the molecule because enormous amounts of RNases exist on our skin. Just breathing on the instruments made them unusable for mRNA. Glassware used to study the molecule had to be baked in such high heat to destroy the RNases that accidents sometimes resulted. Once a Duke University assistant professor engulfed part of her department in fire—including her department chair's office—while preparing pipettes in a 500 degree oven so they could be used with mRNA. For an academic hoping for tenure, it wasn't the savviest career move.

Karikó had heard all the complaints and criticisms, but she had trained herself to find positives where others saw problems. To her, mRNA was the perfect molecule—it only needed to get into the cell's cytoplasm to create proteins, not all the way into the nucleus, like DNA. She agreed that mRNA was a short-lived molecule, but she thought that might be a *good* thing. Many illnesses and ailments didn't seem to require the introduction of new genes, which can produce permanent changes in the body, as her colleagues were hoping to do with DNA. Sometimes the body just needs a short-term boost or improvement, not a long-term alteration.

For example, to treat patients who are anemic and in need of a temporary blood infusion, Karikó wanted to use mRNA to create a protein called erythropoietin, or EPO, that stimulates red-blood cell production. To test her thesis, she injected laboratory animals with erythropoietin mRNA. They developed so many new red blood cells it was as if the animals had undergone blood transfusions, evidence to Karikó that mRNA could be an effective temporary therapeutic.

She realized that if mRNA molecules were employed to create short-term proteins, they would have to be reapplied on a regular basis, potentially leading to repeated sales of any mRNA-based medication. In other words, the fact that its effects were fleeting could make it more profitable.

"It's *good* it degrades," she told her skeptical colleagues while trying to bring them around to using mRNA.

Karikó became an evangelist for the molecule, offering to create mRNA for colleagues. You're trying to create some kind of helpful protein? Why not use mRNA? They usually gave her a funny look or dissed her behind her back. *There goes that crazy mRNA woman.*

In 1995, Karikó's fortunes took a darker turn. She discovered a lump that doctors suspected was cancer. While she visited doctors and prepared for surgery, her husband became stuck in Hungary for months, dealing with complicated visa issues. That's when Swain called Karikó into her office once again. This time she delivered an ultimatum: Leave Penn or agree to a demotion.

Karikó was taken aback. Yes, her grant proposals weren't finding success and she had to rely on faculty members to pay her salary. And okay, she could be a bit of a pain around the lab. But she was sure she was making progress with her mRNA and that it would yet lead to something big.

At that point, Karikó was forty years old and had few job options. Her daughter, Susan, a top high-school volleyball player, had thoughts of attending Penn. If Karikó left the school, Susan wouldn't be eligible for the tuition discount that Penn offered staff members, and the family wouldn't be able to afford to send her to the school. She swallowed her pride and accepted a new, lower-paid position: senior research investigator. It was a brand-new job title for Penn, but that wasn't something to celebrate: It was new because no one had ever been kicked off the Penn faculty and remained at the school.

Karikó tried to remain upbeat, reminding herself to ignore the affronts. In some ways, the demotion left her feeling liberated.

"It's like *Fight Club*: when you lose everything you are fearless," she says.

She kept improving on her work in the lab, hoping it might lead to success. By then, her previous supporter, Barnathan, had left the school, so she switched to the medical school's neurosurgery department, where she found a new supporter in David Langer, the neurosurgery resident. Karikó appreciated that she still had a "spot on a bench," or a place in a lab to pursue her mRNA work.

If I can still do my experiments, I can still find a way to help people, she thought.

• • •

When Karikó met Drew Weissman at the copy machine in 1997, he was using DNA in his experiments, like so many others at Penn and elsewhere. For months, Weissman had been using DNA to transfect, or load, his dendritic cells with a key HIV protein called "Gag," hoping to teach the immune system to recognize and repel the virus. This meant that Weissman was introducing DNA—in this case, a circular ring of DNA called a plasmid—into the dendritic cells, so they would produce that key HIV protein. That was when Karikó suggested that Weissman use some of her mRNA, instead of relying on DNA, to create the HIV protein.

Weissman had no idea of the drama that surrounded Karikó, nor did he know about her newly diminished status. He likely wouldn't have cared, either. Weissman didn't do office gossip, small talk, or chitchat. He barely had anything to say if it wasn't related to scientific discovery. Once Weissman got going about his experiments or immunology, though, it was hard to get him to stop.

He rarely smiled, or even grinned, even for photos, adopting a serious mien that could be off-putting. The more colleagues got to know him, though, the more his underlying gentleness and kindness became apparent. Weissman was eager to help younger scientists, had a sly sense of humor, and wore blue jeans and white sneakers almost every day, amusing more formally dressed fellow academics.

Others were struck by his remarkable affection for cats. Weissman's daughter adopted sick, unwanted cats from a local shelter, some of whom were so anemic that Weissman felt the need to regularly inject them with the hormone erythropoietin. In time, he became dedicated to the ritual. Once, Weissman barely made a flight to an important conference because he was chasing a cat around his house with a syringe in his hand.

Weissman's empathy and his eagerness to heal his feline friends may have stemmed from his own physical challenges. At the age of six, Weissman was diagnosed with a version of type 1 diabetes; Weissman's blood-glucose levels experienced wild swings, usually without warning. Colleagues sometimes discovered him on the floor of his office after his blood sugar dropped too quickly for him to react. Weissman also lost consciousness and collapsed during meetings outside the office. Sometimes the shift in glucose levels affected his cognitive abilities and he confused colleagues with inexplicable comments. Eventually, his department kept a can of Coca-Cola in an office refrigerator to revive Weissman if his sugar levels suddenly plummeted.

Weissman had learned important lessons early in his career as an AIDS researcher in Anthony Fauci's lab at the NIAID in Washington, D.C. Weissman watched as NIH scientists, frustrated that their grant proposals had been rejected by various government bodies, asked Fauci to use his clout to get them the necessary funding. Each time, Fauci refused. The scientists responded by bad-mouthing Fauci and planting negative stories about him in the press, but he still wouldn't bend the rules.

"He taught me about honesty in science and the importance of not bastardizing data," Weissman says.

In 1998, Weissman and Karikó began working together, but they quickly ran into difficulties. Karikó produced mRNAs that Weissman inserted into human T cells and B cells in a cell-culture dish, but the molecules almost entirely failed to translate, or create proteins. The genetic instructions weren't working, it seemed. When they inserted Karikó's mRNA into Weissman's dendritic cells, though, they saw so much protein creation that it floored them. The mRNA instructed the dendritic cells to produce and display HIV proteins on the outside parts of their cells, immediately triggering an immune response—all of which seemed perfect for a potential vaccine, Weissman thought. The cells, quite literally, lit up: Karikó and Weissman had included mRNA coding for the luciferase enzyme to light up when proteins were produced, and it was generating so much light they could see it with their bare eyes.

The researchers published their work in a scientific journal in 2000, arguing that introducing mRNA into dendritic cells "has the potential to be a potent and effective anti-HIV T cell-activating vaccine." They had demonstrated that mRNA is a more capable molecule than most assumed, confirming the results of Gilboa and his Duke colleagues.

They knew the most realistic way they'd be able to help patients was to deliver direct injections of mRNA, rather than go through the complicated process of inserting mRNA into cells in a cell-culture dish, as the Gilboa team had done. So Karikó and Weissman began injecting mice with their mRNA molecule. They encountered a shocking problem: The mice kept becoming ill, sometimes even dying.

"Nobody knew why," according to Weissman. "All we knew was that the mice got sick. Their fur got ruffled, they hunched up, they stopped eating, they stopped running."[3]

It seemed the mice's innate immune system was identifying the mRNA molecule as a threat and was launching a devastating response to ward off the foreign material. Back when Karikó and Weissman were putting mRNA in cells in tissue culture in the lab, they didn't have to worry about the immune system fighting back. Now that they were injecting it in animals, though, they were setting off inflammatory cytokines, signs that they were inadvertently activating the first line of defense against invading pathogens. It was as if the mice cells were so threatened by the injected molecule and its genetic instructions that they were damaging themselves to avoid having anything to do with it.

Other Penn scientists had little awareness of what was going on in Weissman's lab. That was probably for the best. Had they known about the troubles Karikó and Weissman were encountering they likely would have delivered an "I told you so," or maybe something even less polite. Karikó and Weissman were realizing that mRNA wasn't simply fragile and short-lived. The molecule was setting off a ruinous immune-system reaction, something biologists call "cell death."

They had to find a way to sneak their mRNA past the immune system. Otherwise, it wouldn't have any therapeutic or other value, their work would be deemed a waste of time, and their colleagues would have another reason to snicker. After all, what doctor would want to inject a molecule that could harm, rather than help, a patient?

The scientists' first task was to ascertain the source of their problem. It took over a year, but they eventually identified certain receptors in mammalian cells that act as lookouts, spotting foreign bodies like the mRNA and triggering the harsh immune response that was damaging their mice.

Next, they had to find a way for their mRNA to evade these

receptors. Since the mRNA Karikó had created wasn't working, the scientists thought that maybe they could tweak it to make it efficacious. That wasn't hard to do. Karikó's PhD work had centered on the various modifications of RNA, or changes in its chemical composition, that were possible. Some of these changes, which can occur naturally or be created in a lab, can help a cell survive, though others can lead to cancer or other illness. Karikó knew there were over one hundred ways the four nucleosides that form the molecule's building blocks can be altered. She and Weissman started testing different versions of RNA from both mammalian and bacterial cells, looking for one that elicited little immune response yet still produced proteins.

They noticed an intriguing pattern: The more that the nucleosides of the RNA were modified from their inherent structure, the less they activated the immune system of the cells; the less they were altered, the more they set off the immune system, a surprising, inverse correlation. It dawned on the researchers that when mRNA was modified, either naturally or in the lab, it was able to skirt the dreaded cell receptors, which act as the immune system's sentries, thereby avoiding inflammation.

After doing some experimenting, they realized that whenever one of the building blocks for RNA, a ribonucleoside called uridine, was present in the mRNA, it triggered an immune reaction. But when nature for whatever reason adjusted the uridine, turning it into a slightly different form called pseudouridine, the cell's immune system ignored the mRNA. They wondered: Could the secret to evading the immune system be as simple as swapping uridine for pseudouridine?

To test their theory, Karikó and Weissman created their own slightly modified version of mRNA, one that relied on pseudouridine, which scientists abbreviate with a code Ψ, instead of the usual uridine, or U. They also replaced another nucleoside, cytidine, with 5-methylcytidine. They injected their revamped molecule into mice and were shocked by what they saw: There was no sign of inflammation or other immune response, the exact result they were hoping for. The tweaked mRNA appeared innocuous to the mice's defenses, possibly because the mRNA of viruses and other invaders have few, if any, modifications, so the new, modified mRNA was perceived as self-created and therefore harmless.

The two scientists published their results in a landmark 2005 paper. Later, when they expanded their experiments to include monkeys, they realized the molecule wasn't just sneaking into a cell's cytoplasm—it also was creating huge amounts of EPO, a sign they finally had achieved their goal: creating proteins with mRNA. EPO was the same protein that Karikó had worked with earlier in her career and the protein Weissman was injecting into his sickly cats.

When those results came in, Karikó and Weissman looked at each other. They were the only ones in the lab. For a moment, neither knew what to say. Finally, after all the long hours, years of difficult work, and frustrating experiments, they had produced proteins in animals.

"This is unbelievable!" Weissman said to Karikó.

They finally had their breakthrough: a way to get mRNA past the body's elaborate defenses and into the cells, where the molecule's genetic code was successfully creating ample amounts of protein. Karikó and Weissman were like generals who had spent years watching their warplanes foiled by enemy radar. Now, simply by replacing a small, overlooked piece of equipment on the planes, they were flying undetected into enemy territory.

The researchers congratulated each other, smiling from ear to ear. Later that night, Weissman drove thirty minutes to his home in suburban Wynnewood, Pennsylvania, still in a daze. He hardly slept, thinking of all that he and Karikó would be able to do with their new powers. They had a chance to create almost *any* type of protein—all kinds of drugs, vaccines, and more suddenly were within reach. A new chapter in their careers had begun.

The potential is unlimited, Weissman thought.

• • •

Weissman was certain he and Karikó had fired the starting gun to perhaps the most important race in the history of modern science. Now that they had demonstrated an effective way to produce desired proteins in the body, others would surely rush to develop useful therapeutics, perhaps even those that could save lives. Hoping to stay a step ahead of the competition, they began work on their own biotech company, which they named RNARx. They met with venture-capital investors and won close to a million dollars in small-business grants from the U.S. government for additional animal studies.

But when Weissman looked over his shoulder, he realized hardly anyone was even trying to catch up. Few medical researchers were even bothering to lace up their running shoes. Weissman attended prominent scientific meetings around the country and addressed hundreds of peers who seemed interested in his work. But as he interacted with his peers, he realized their skepticism about mRNA hadn't been shaken. The response was always the same: *Congrats on those papers, really interesting stuff. But man, mRNA is such a pain to work with, I'm still not touching that stuff.*

A reviewer confided that one of the Karikó-Weissman papers had almost been rejected for publication. Too few people had been wowed by the work, the reviewer revealed. Weissman spoke with senior government scientists about working with mRNA, but they "kind of blew me off," he says, questioning how a molecule so unstable could be manufactured in bulk.

Others doubted the Penn researchers had achieved a true breakthrough. Skeptics said that for vaccines, at least, the last thing you wanted to do was avoid or tamp the reactions of the immune system. After all, the goal of a vaccine is to elicit an immune response. Still others asked whether the cell's immune reaction was really such a big problem, and they questioned why Karikó and Weissman hadn't "made something cool" with their technology. A German company called CureVac was testing a vaccine that used the molecule mRNA in its natural, or "naked," form, suggesting that modifications might not be necessary.

Karikó had spent years without the recognition and respect of peers, so the reactions didn't faze her. She and Weissman would just have to build their company and develop world-changing therapeutics, she figured. But Karikó ran into obstacles at Penn once again. The school demanded such a high price to license the technology and work they had developed that it was impossible to raise money from investors.

"They just asked for too much," Weissman says.

At one point, Karikó all but begged an executive of a biotech company to provide her and Weissman with a lipid substance they came to see as likely needed to encase their mRNA so it could deliver enough of a genetic payload to cure disease. The executive refused.

"I was close to getting on my knees," she says. It was "my lowest moment."

Eventually, Penn licensed the work, but not to Karikó and Weissman. It went to a small company in Madison, Wisconsin, called Cellscript, which was working on kits for making mRNA with modified nucleosides. By 2009, Karikó and Weissman had given up on their hopes of starting a biotechnology company. They still believed in mRNA, but few shared their faith. They remained at Penn, but their mRNA research would largely be forgotten.

It would take a British computer engineer with a short fuse and a Canadian globetrotter to demonstrate the value of their work.

6

2007–2010

Science seldom proceeds in the straightforward logical manner imagined by outsiders.

—JAMES D. WATSON

Luigi Warren was having a midlife crisis.

A software engineer living in Los Angeles in the late 1990s, Warren had spent nearly two decades establishing a thriving career in the computer industry. Short, trim, and handsome, he had close-cropped brown hair that he rarely styled yet always seemed rock-star perfect. He made a good living, worked on challenging projects for Sony Pictures, IBM, and other high-profile companies, and he traveled frequently to New York City for work and pleasure. But as Warren approached his fortieth birthday, he felt empty and unfulfilled. Coding was dull and he feared it would become more tedious over time. Desperate for a change, he decided to try to recapture some of the excitement of his youth.

The son of an Italian mother and British father, Warren grew up in Bromley, a London suburb best known as David Bowie's childhood home. Warren's own passions were science fiction and space travel. He devoured the works of Robert Heinlein, Isaac Asimov, and Arthur C. Clarke, and was so captivated by Stanley Kubrick's *2001: A Space Odyssey* that he returned to a local theater nine times to see repeated showings of the movie.*[1] Inspired by NASA's Apollo space program, Warren made plans to become an astronaut, or at the very least, a space engineer.

"I was a bit of a dreamer," he says.

Now, he was bored, middle-aged, and itching for a change. In 2001, the forty-one-year-old Warren moved to New York City, where he rented a four-hundred-square-foot apartment. Shifting careers, he enrolled in Columbia University's School of General Studies, beginning a bachelor's program in biology, a field bursting with activity and possibility. Ambitious biotechnology companies were raising enormous sums of money, and scientists were making dramatic progress mapping the entire human DNA sequence, a feat that promised valuable insights into why people were disposed to certain diseases.

Newly energized, Warren received his degree and moved to Pasadena, California, where he completed a PhD in biology at CalTech in 2007, before beginning postgraduate studies at Stanford University. There, Warren forged a connection with another postdoctoral fellow named Derrick Rossi. A native of Toronto who sported a distinctive soul patch on his chin, Rossi was older than most of his peers, just like Warren. He had traveled the world and appreciated Warren's circuitous journey to their lab. Most of all, he was a huge Bowie fan who was thrilled to learn Warren grew up in Bromley.

Warren's experience as a computer engineer gave him valuable skills in the laboratory. Biological experiments require clear designs, efficient execution, and an efficient debugging process to remove

---

* During his own youth, Bowie also saw *2001: A Space Odyssey* numerous times, writing his classic "Space Oddity" after one showing.

errors and mistakes, much like in computer science. Both fields require repeated experiments until a final product is discovered or developed. Researchers often attempt to program cells by introducing specific stretches of DNA, directing the cells to follow a set of instructions to create various proteins, a bit like computer programmers develop elaborate algorithms to solve problems or reach goals.

Working together in the lab, Rossi could see that Warren was able to design RNA and conduct tricky experiments that frustrated others.

"Luigi was meticulous in his lab work and attentive to details, probably the best I've ever seen," Rossi says.

In 2007, when Rossi was hired by an affiliate of Harvard Medical School's Stem Cell and Regenerative Biology Department as an assistant professor, he asked Warren to be the first hire in a lab Rossi was starting there. Warren accepted the offer and soon moved to Cambridge, Massachusetts, to be a postdoc in Rossi's lab.

Warren had ample reason for optimism. He was still early in his second career, but the forty-seven-year-old was already a key member of a new lab in one of the world's most prestigious universities. Warren was working with a friend who appreciated his unique talents and background. If he did well and helped Rossi's team produce scientific results, he would have a chance for his own academic career. Within months after his arrival, though, Warren got into an explosive fight with an Israeli immunologist, forcing Rossi to officiate the dispute. Later, while speaking with his wife about the incident, Rossi expressed surprise that his lab was gripped by drama so quickly.

Rossi and Warren began an audacious project, with the goal of improving on landmark work by a future Nobel laureate. A year earlier, Shinya Yamanaka, a stem-cell researcher at Japan's Kyoto University, and one of his graduate students had astonished the scientific world by placing genes in retroviruses—viruses that invade host cells and integrate their genomes into the DNA of those cells—to reprogram adult cells. Yamanaka had used this technique to create "pluripotent" forms of the cells, which act much like embryonic stem cells. Yamanaka had, in effect, reverted the cells to their primitive state, turning the clock back on time.

The discovery changed the way scientists viewed cell identity and how fixed it truly was. Just as important, the advance promised to give researchers a new set of extremely useful cells. Embryonic stem cells are prized for their ability to turn into almost any kind of cell, making them valuable for various medical treatments. But because they're usually harvested from embryos discarded during in vitro fertilization treatments, they have long been subject to intense criticism from those who believe embryos should be off-limits to medical experiments. Yamanaka's work, which earned him a Nobel Prize in 2012, raised the tantalizing prospect of sidestepping such controversy by allowing scientists to use these so-called induced pluripotent stem cells, or iPS cells, rather than embryonic cells. Yamanaka's method also promised to produce cells and tissues that could be transplanted without the risk of rejection.

Scientists raced to employ Yamanaka's approach for various medical purposes. Almost immediately, they confronted serious risks. Retroviruses that alter a cell's DNA can be dangerous, because this foreign DNA integrates into a cell's genome, potentially causing dangerous mutations. Years later, researchers took skin cells from a seventy-year-old patient, derived iPS cells from them, and turned them into retinal cells used to treat the patient's macular degeneration. There was some perceived improvement in her eyesight, startling parts of the medical world. But similar work with a second patient was halted abruptly after the scientists checked the genome sequence of their first patient's iPS cells and identified a mutation, which they feared might lead to cancer.[2]

Rossi and Warren hoped to create engineered stem cells or otherwise convert cells into their earlier, pluripotent state, but they too worried about using DNA viruses. Rossi and Warren thought they'd instead try to use messenger RNA molecules, much like Jon Wolff, Eli Gilboa, and Katalin Karikó before them. Since mRNA carries genetic instructions into the cell but can't integrate into the nucleus, Rossi and Warren knew it was likely safer and more efficient to use than DNA.

Because Warren remained something of a newcomer in the world of science, he didn't yet harbor a bias against mRNA and was open to working with the molecule. At the same time, synthesizing mRNA in the lab involves playing with the four single-letter codes that make up the molecule's nucleotides. To Warren, that seemed a lot like computer coding, another reason the approach appealed to him. Best of all, an alternative way of creating stem cells—generating and purifying proteins—takes hours of painstaking work, partly because it can be a challenge getting the proteins into a cell—one more reason Warren was eager to try mRNA in their experiments.

"Proteins are a pain in the ass," Warren says. "And I'm afraid of viruses."

Warren's goal was to insert genetic instructions into adult skin cells via mRNA with the goal of reprogramming them into stem cells. He and Rossi hadn't heard of Karikó and Weissman and didn't know about their mRNA breakthrough. Nonetheless, they weren't deterred by the molecule's notorious instability. They figured they'd just tweak mRNA here or there so it would survive long enough to create their stem cells.

Warren began by attempting to create proteins from mRNA in Rossi's lab, an early test of their approach. He synthesized an mRNA molecule coding for a jellyfish protein called green fluorescent protein, or GFP, and introduced it into human skin cells. The next day, he called Rossi over to look into his microscope. He could see bright green fluorescence emanating from the cells, a sure sign Warren had produced the desired jellyfish protein from mRNA. Who needed DNA when using mRNA worked wonders?

Rossi stood up and smiled at Warren.

"Yeah, this shit really works," Warren said.

Keep going, Rossi told him. Optimistic by nature, Rossi was becoming confident his lab could make stem cells and perhaps other proteins using mRNA. For biochemists, it was the stuff of dreams.

"This is gonna work!" Rossi said one day.

Within weeks, however, Warren was stymied. He produced additional proteins in his Petri dish, but many of the cells died within a day or so, making them of little use. Each repeated dosing of mRNA elicited more troubles for the cells, as if they were self-destructing.

Warren wasn't sure why he was running into so many problems, but he and Rossi deduced that their mRNA might be triggering the cells' immune system to attack his inserted mRNA molecule, putting an end to the proteins. (Their analysis was aided by the Israeli immunologist, who never spoke a word to Warren after their big blowout but continued to communicate with Rossi.) Warren brought their problem to immune-system specialists, including a few at nearby Boston Children's Hospital, who confirmed their hunch—the immune system, believing a virus was attacking the cell, was eliminating the mRNA, suppressing protein expression, and triggering cell death, the same kinds of issues that plagued Karikó and Weissman's research.

Warren had to find a way for his mRNA to avoid an immune reaction so he and Rossi could produce their stem cells. He became consumed by the challenge, dedicating all his waking hours to finding a solution. Warren discovered ways to squeeze even more time in the lab. Each morning, for example, he wore the same outfit: a black blazer, black T-shirt with a V-neck, blue jeans, and black boots. This way, he could avoid wasting precious minutes in his closet deciding what to wear. He went days without changing his clothing, colleagues noticed, and often skipped meals. On Thanksgiving that year, when Rossi invited Warren and his labmates for the holiday meal, Warren shoved so much food into his mouth that his friends were agape.

"He ate enough for four people," says Chad Cowan, a friend of Rossi's who was a Harvard professor. "It was like a snake filling up on a week's calories."

Colleagues were generally amused by Warren's idiosyncrasies, including his habit of staring off into the distance while in conversation, as if he were processing information. Warren almost crackled with energy and intensity, yet he didn't fidget or release his tensions in conventional ways. He concentrated it all on his work, as if his mRNA challenge was the only issue in his life that truly mattered. Warren had a dry, British sense of humor and was a bit of a conspiracy theorist who defended individual rights and had owned a gun in California, but his labmates enjoyed his quirks. As he worked to solve his mRNA problem, though, his friends could see the pressure and anxiety grow. Soon Warren was mired in a months-long funk.

Warren had ample reason to be nervous. Outsiders usually focus on the prestige that comes with a position in an academic or biotech laboratory, and the enormous rewards that can accrue to those who solve important problems or participate in a rousing initial public offering. Scientific work is often intellectually stimulating, colleagues are smart and capable, and medical researchers can improve the world. But anxiety and depression are commonplace in the lab. Investigators pour their hearts into their work, often competing with supersmart rivals around the world, all of whom are focused on finding fault with their latest research.

"We are a skeptical group," Rossi says. "If someone shows data, the first instinct is to find a problem with the experiment—what could they have misinterpreted? And have they found an artifact" rather than a true discovery?

Biology is slow moving and eureka moments are rare, so pressures slowly mount. Take too long to publish your findings and a rival will beat you to the punch, dooming your career.

"You wait to submit your work for publication until you have safely met the burden of proof and are able to say something novel, truthful, and illuminating," says Danny Altmann, who runs a laboratory at Imperial College London, "only to find that some rival in another lab has set their bar lower and pipped you to the post by publishing their version, however less thorough. But they're first to the finish line, so that's the one that counts."

Warren was facing challenges, but at least he wasn't a woman, like Karikó, or a minority. White men have traditionally dominated the world of science, and others can be held to more exacting standards. Part of the problem is there are few objective metrics to judge scientific achievement. Older researchers also can have a tough time, too. Like aging Hollywood movie stars, senior scientists battle insecurities and worry their past successes will be eclipsed and future papers will be rejected.

Some succumb to the pressures. Medicine, especially the field of biology, is littered with fraud.[3] Investigators sometimes fabricate results of experiments to further their careers, while others consciously or unconsciously mold data to fit preconceived conclusions.

"A lot of unwholesome things happen in labs," Warren says.

The deceit, while not commonplace, belies the popular image of scientists as emotionless researchers guided by logic and objectivity. It can involve even well-known researchers and journals.

"You're constantly on your guard in case your career is brutally halted by a bitter competitor or academic employer who spots evidence you've contravened—or one of your students has—one of the many medical regulations governing our work," Altmann says.

The life of a scientist can be grueling, tedious, and unsatisfying. Researchers learn early in their careers that they'll likely make, at most, incremental contributions to their field. Oh, and you can forget about impressing the neighbors at the next barbeque—they're usually not nearly as enamored as you are with infectious diseases and the workings of the immune system.

"There's a limit before people's eyes glaze over," Altmann says.

Once, on a trip to China, Altmann was seated next to a fellow virologist, so he began discussing new T cell research. The colleague pulled a mask over her eyes and grabbed a pair of earphones.

"That was the last I heard from her," says Altmann, who insists he was joking when he suggested chatting about immunity for the duration of their eleven-hour flight.

Much like U.S. politicians, who too frequently spend more time on fundraising than actual policy, medical researchers are on a nonstop hunt for research funding. Anxiety builds as grant proposals are written and rejected. Scientists may have a reputation as bookish nerds, but extroverts, especially those with a bit of swagger and self-confidence, are usually the ones who get ahead. Only by wowing foundations and investors, making dramatic and convincing presentations, and blithely dismissing doubts and critiques can one attract money. Introverts, or even those with a bit of modesty or self-doubt, find raising money a challenge.

A few years ago, the Wellcome Trust, a large U.K. health foundation, conducted a study that suggested it shared the same bias as others in the scientific world toward those with the smoothest sales pitches, forcing a change in the way it handed out money.

"Those with a song and dance left with large suitcases full of money, not the stammering, shy, nervous scientists," says Altmann, who headed Wellcome's infection and immunity strategy at the time of the study.

Scientific work can draw the attention of investors, including venture-capital firms, which can lead to stakes in emerging companies, but the potential for huge paydays magnifies rivalries and jealousies.

"It's a real viper's nest, especially in the Harvard-MIT-Berkeley-Stanford nexus," Warren says. "Their rewards are huge, but they create additional impetus for bad behavior."

As a postdoc, Warren was in an especially difficult position. He lived in Boston, one of the most expensive cities in the country, but he could afford to rent only a tiny studio apartment with his annual salary of about forty thousand dollars. Not that Warren was home very often. Postdocs generally spend more than eighty hours a week in the lab. And his job was a temporary position: Unless a postdoc manages to publish work in a scientific journal, ideally a top-rated one, he or she can have little hope of finding a full-time job or establishing a career.

Not everyone appreciated Warren's skills, which involved constructing RNA, making his challenge even more formidable. Warren still had Rossi in his corner, though. He expressed confidence that Warren would discover a way to deal with the immunity issue.

"You'll figure it out," he told Warren, trying to cheer him up.

It helped that Rossi shared a background that was just as unorthodox as Warren's. Five foot nine with long, unruly hair and colorful tortoiseshell glasses, Rossi resembled the actor Robert Downey Jr. Rossi's parents had both moved to Toronto from the island of Malta, and met as teenagers in the Canadian city's small Maltese community. Neither received much of an education nor did they make much money. Rossi's father, Alfred, managed an auto body shop and came home each evening distant and withdrawn, rarely speaking to Rossi or his four older siblings.

"He was a quiet, simple man, with no life lessons to share," he says. "I don't think I heard him speak more than a thousand words in my life."

Rossi's mother, Agnes, by contrast, was a warm, friendly, and loving presence who attended Catholic mass each day, at least partly for the conversation and companionship she wasn't getting at home. Rossi's older brother, Steve, may have been the biggest influence on his life. Steve had a remarkable passion for exotic animals. Over the years, he kept a great horned owl, some piranha, a squirrel and a raccoon, and a whole lot of snakes in their home. At one point, he even had a four-foot alligator in the bedroom until Steve realized it was a rather impractical pet.

For a while, Rossi was sure he wanted to be a veterinarian. But when a teacher in eleventh grade introduced him to molecular biology, he became utterly fascinated by DNA, genetics, and the inner workings of cells. Rossi had found his calling.

After receiving a bachelor of science degree at the University of Toronto, Rossi felt a need to get on a plane and leave the country. His wanderlust likely resulted from a childhood that featured few vacations or family trips. To escape, the boy had turned to books, including works by Jack Kerouac and Henry Miller, reading about their colorful journeys. Now that Rossi was a young adult, he was eager for his own adventures, preferably in locales as far and different from his own upbringing as possible.

"The world intrigued me, all the different languages and people," he says. "And all the different species of women."

Rossi set out for Central Africa, hitchhiking alone across the continent for five months, an experience that brought several close calls with violence. As Rossi was crossing into Rwanda to see the nation's famed mountain gorillas, Ugandan border guards found evidence that he had exchanged money in the nation's black market during his time in the country. They pointed machine guns at Rossi's face, threatening to throw him into jail for his crime. Rossi immediately realized the real reason for the threats: The Ugandan guards had discovered his secret stash of $125 and were extorting him for the money. But Rossi needed the cash for the rest of the trip.

He launched into a spontaneous lecture, telling the guards how he had spent six weeks in their beautiful country and had planned to urge others to visit Uganda. But their treatment of him would ruin the country's reputation at a time it desperately needed tourists.

"Go ahead, lock me up, but you're fucking it up!" Rossi said.

The guards, feeling a bit ashamed, let Rossi go. Danger averted, Rossi crossed into Rwanda. He almost regretted his resourcefulness a few weeks later. While in the Rwandan jungle, a silverback gorilla, out of nowhere, came charging at Rossi, tearing up the grass to get at him. Yards away, the ape stopped short, his huge face in Rossi's. It all happened so quickly that he didn't even have a chance to be frightened. The incident ended just as quickly. The gorilla, having established his dominance, ambled away.

Still later on his African journey, Rossi was floating down a river in present-day Congo in a canoe, with a fellow traveler from Australia, when he saw an intriguing-looking snake in the water and picked it up with his paddle. He drew the snake closer only to see the distinctive hood of a cobra. The Australian paddled frantically, spinning the canoe in circles as Rossi flung the snake back into the water—but it swam right back into the boat. This time, Rossi lifted the cobra with his paddle and sent it flying, far from the canoe, as he and the Australian paddled for safety.

Rossi returned to the University of Toronto and received a master of science degree before leaving to do a PhD in molecular biology in Paris. He was still restless, though, making it hard for the twenty-eight-year-old to make much progress.

"I got exhausted," he says. "I was having too much fun."

Soon Rossi was off to Dallas to work in a lab at the University of Texas before finally receiving his PhD in 2003 at the University of Helsinki in Finland. By then, he had more life experience than most peers and he was ready to fully focus on his research. Rossi published several impactful academic papers and gained a position in a top stem-cell lab at Stanford University, where he met Warren. Each had come from working-class families and followed unusual paths to the lab, likely why they connected so easily.

"He was this fun guy, a hipster who had traveled across Africa," Warren says. "I thought of him as a friend."

As Warren struggled to overcome the immunity issues related to his mRNA experiments, Rossi provided further encouragement. But Warren soon turned morose. Searching for answers, he sometimes wandered into a nearby lab run by Sun Hur, an assistant professor at Harvard Medical School who was an immune-system specialist. Hur and her colleagues weren't always thrilled by the regular visits, viewing Warren as a bit too intense for their taste, but Hur tried to be collegial and answer his questions about the immune system.

One day in October 2008, Warren asked a young postdoc in Hur's lab named Alys Peisley to meet at a nearby Starbucks. Over coffee, Warren poured out his frustrations, asking why he wasn't getting his mRNA to evade the immune system and create proteins, so the stem cells could be reprogrammed.

"What would you do?" he asked her.

Peisley had thought she was in for a quick coffee, but now the conversation was entering its second hour and she was itching to leave. But Warren was edgy and seemed on the verge of giving up on his project, so Peisley suggested he ask Hur if she had any creative solutions.

A bit later, Hur gave Warren some advice.

"Why don't you try some modifications?" she asked him.

Hur sent Warren a link to the earlier papers written by Karikó and Weissman outlining how they had produced a slightly modified version of the mRNA molecule to generate their own proteins. Most scientists had either forgotten the earlier work or never knew it existed. But immune-system specialists like Hur had been impressed by how Karikó and Weissman had replaced uridine with pseudouridine, injecting the newly tweaked molecule in mice and monkeys to create huge amounts of protein. By tweaking the molecule's building blocks, they had allowed the mRNA to avoid signs of inflammation and other immune responses. Maybe Warren would have luck using a similar approach, Hur suggested.

Warren was elated. He had been considering five other possible solutions to his predicament, but right away he saw that switching the nucleotide was "by far the most promising" of the ideas, Warren wrote in lab notes on October 21. Best of all, it was an easy idea to test. He ordered modified nucleotides from an outside company and worked with others in Rossi's lab to produce an updated version of mRNA. Once again, Warren created a gene sequence to produce the jellyfish GFP protein, but this time he used various combinations of modified nucleosides. He and his colleagues introduced their newly modified molecule into human keratinocytes, which are cells found in the outermost layer of skin, waiting to see what would happen. The next day, their cells were alive, and each was expressing vast amounts of the green fluorescent protein. Even after repeated administrations of the new modified mRNA, the cells thrived and expressed GFP. Their problem had been solved.

A major obstacle now cleared, Warren turned his attention back to deriving the pluripotent stem cells, eventually using five different modified mRNAs encoding five different proteins.

One day in November 2009, Warren hustled into Rossi's office.

"Check it out," Warren said, an impish smile on his face.

Warren led Rossi to a corner of the lab where a microscope was positioned over a Petri dish. Rossi peered in and saw a fluorescent color. It was evidence of nascent colonies of stem like cells. They were tiny and there were just a few of the colonies. But there were robust cells in the dish. Rossi's team had succeeded in converting skin cells into stemlike cells, exactly what they had spent a year and a half trying to produce.

Rossi looked up from the microscope. He was beaming.

"That's it!" he said. "We did it."[4]

Immediately, Rossi realized that his group had accomplished something huge. Not only did they create stemlike cells, but their methods also produced eight kinds of proteins, opening up a world of possibility.

"We were excited as shit," Rossi says.

Karikó and Weissman's papers had been something of a Rosetta stone for Rossi, Warren, and their colleagues, only their work had been in plain sight, not buried in the ground.

Warren felt more relief than joy. He had been consumed by frustration and self-doubt for so long. Career advancement, including a professorship of his own, seemed likely. Finally, Warren was on the verge of enormous success.

• • •

Karikó and Weissman had taken a crucial step, showing that a revolution in molecular biology was possible by tweaking a building block of the mRNA molecule. They had injected synthetic mRNA in mice and monkeys to create EPO proteins. But they hadn't created anything therapeutic or even very useful. They had developed a delicious recipe but never had the chance to cook it up.

By contrast, Warren, Rossi, and their colleagues had used modified mRNA to reprogram adult skin cells into pluripotent cells and produce human proteins. The group had done it in cells in the lab, so they hadn't yet proven that they could create proteins in animals, let alone humans. Still, it was enough for Warren and Rossi to rush to patent their method. Rossi even began making plans to start a company to use some of the techniques he was developing. Warren and his colleagues were sure they now could write an academic paper reporting on their success, one that could shock the world.

The team spent another year doing experiments to validate and expand their idea, and several more months writing a paper describing their breakthrough, and they began considering which scientific journal to submit it to. That's when tensions returned to the lab. Rossi viewed their work as important enough to submit to *Cell*, one of the most respected journals in the field. Warren vehemently disagreed. He had heard rumblings that a German academic group and maybe others were working on similar studies. If another group scooped

Rossi's team, all their remarkable work would be for naught. It wasn't worth taking the risk, Warren told Rossi and others. *Cell* could reject their paper or take many months to publish it. Send it to a lower-quality journal that would quickly publish it, Warren said. It might not make as big a splash, but at least Warren would be assured of having his first published paper.

As the standoff continued, Warren became so infuriated that he threatened to publish the work online, Rossi recalls, shocking the team. One day, he announced he was quitting the lab. Rossi talked him out of the decision, but he couldn't soothe Warren.

"Just submit it!" he told Rossi, showing more anger than his labmates had before seen from him.

Warren was forty-nine years old. He wanted a job as a professor. Publications are currency of the realm in the world of academic science. As a lab leader, Rossi was overseeing dozens of projects, any one of which could be a home-run study, boosting his career. It was a diversified portfolio of promising bets, but all Warren had was the mRNA work. Competitors were getting closer and Warren was growing anxious.

"My career was hanging on this," Warren says. "If someone beats me it doesn't matter how good a job I've done, I get nothing."

To Rossi, Warren's nervousness was unjustified. Their work was complicated and their paper far too sophisticated for someone to easily match. Rossi was proud of what his team had accomplished and wanted to aim high. As the lab leader, he got his way—the paper was submitted to *Cell*. It took just a few days for the journal's editors to reject it, just as Warren had feared. *Cell* suggested that Rossi send the paper to its sister journal, *Cell Stem Cell*, a specialized journal but still the most prestigious in the stem-cell world. Rossi was hopeful even as Warren stewed.

Months later, an editor for *Cell Stem Cell* named Deborah Sweet called Rossi. Reviewers had raised a series of unexpected and thorny questions about the paper. To Rossi and his colleagues, some of the objections seemed excessive, even suspicious. He pushed back on some of the requests but acceded to taking the time to answer others, viewing them as part of the sometimes messy process of getting a paper published. Reviewers are tasked with searching for problems, he told his team.

"It's part of the game," Rossi says. "Reviewers dig deep into their asses and invariably pull out some shit."

Warren was newly infuriated, though. He felt the challenges to the paper proved his original point.

"We should have published," Warren screamed at Rossi. "I told you so!"

Slowly, labmates detected a change in Warren. Before, he was a quirky, dedicated scientist who favored a good conspiracy theory. Now he appeared troubled and agitated.

"You could see a psychological shift," says Cowan, Rossi's friend at Harvard.

One afternoon, Warren walked down the hallway in his building, passing Hur, the professor who had helped him by suggesting he consult the Karikó and Weissman papers. She was eager to hear how his work was coming and if Warren and his colleagues had submitted their paper, so she greeted him with a smile.

"Hi, Luigi!" Hur greeted him.

Warren, his head held low, walked right past Hur, completely ignoring her.

"He looked really down, like he was falling apart," she says. "It was unpleasant."

It all became too much for Warren. One day, while working in the lab, he stormed out and slammed the door, never to return.

"There was tremendous frustration," Warren says.

• • •

Soon it was Rossi's turn to become enraged. One day, Sweet told Rossi her journal would be publishing the team's study. She even suggested it might be chosen for the journal's cover story, thrilling Rossi and members of his lab. A bit later, though, Sweet got in touch with Rossi, once again, to deliver shocking news. An anonymous whistleblower had challenged the veracity of the data in his lab's paper, claiming the results couldn't be repeated.

"Someone has raised questions if they're real or not," Sweet said, referring to the data from Rossi's lab. "You need to find someone to reproduce the results."

Rossi was taken aback. The suggestion that their results weren't real was insulting, even offensive. Others in the lab thought it possible, maybe even likely, that someone was raising challenges to slow their work, perhaps to enable a competitor to publish something similar. Warren's fears might have been justified, after all.

Warren was consulting for a biotech company and no longer in the lab, but Rossi felt he deserved to be updated about the latest obstacle to the publication. Warren turned livid. As he saw it, the doubts about their data were without basis or justification. He was no longer involved in the process, making it hard for him to respond to the challenges, and he worried that, even if the paper were eventually published, his credit would be diluted. Most of all, the accusations were insulting.

"The implication was I was a fraud," Warren says.

Warren realized that his apartment, near Fenway Park, was a short walk from the Technology Square offices of *Cell Stem Cell.* He wondered—why not go and talk to the editor directly? Soon Warren was marching down the street, on his way to the journal's office. Approaching the front door, Warren called Rossi to tell him what he was doing.

"No, no, no, don't do it!" Rossi urged him. "We'll sort it out!"

"I've had enough already, I'm talking to her directly," Warren said, referring to Sweet. Then he hung up on Rossi.

Inside the building, Warren headed to a nearby elevator, taking it five flights up to *Cell Stem Cell*'s offices.

"I need to talk to Debbie Sweet," Warren told a receptionist.

Staffers were rattled. Authors of scientific papers never showed up to dispute reviews. Warren looked upset. The receptionist told him Sweet wasn't in the office. Warren left the building, but the staffers were so shaken up by his visit that they were sent home for the day, according to Rossi, who says he received a phone call from Warren on his way out and became concerned.

"I called the offices of *Cell Stem Cell* to make sure everything was OK," says Rossi. "They told me they were closing for the day to make sure everyone got home safe." (Warren disputes details of the encounter. "I was angry and I did storm over there but nothing much happened," he says.)

Another researcher repeated their experiment and reproduced the original results, reassuring Sweet and her journal. Finally, the paper was published in late September 2010 with Warren as the first author.

Soon Warren had packed up and moved back to California. He was no longer on speaking terms with Rossi and had begun a new leg of his career, consulting in the stem-cell world and then going on to own companies that produced induced pluripotent stem-cell lines for clients.

"I regret that the situation deteriorated," says Warren, who eventually profited from his work.

• • •

The importance of Warren and Rossi's work was instantly understood. They had reprogrammed ordinary cells into pluripotent stem cells simply by injecting them with synthetic mRNA, developing a technology that had "broad applicability for basic research, disease modeling, and regenerative medicine," they argued in their paper. Warren and Rossi were the first to show that something potentially therapeutic could be produced from mRNA, and that they could turn cellular clocks back. The work was named one of 2010's top ten scientific breakthroughs by the journal *Science*, and *Time* magazine included Rossi in its Person of the Year issue, saying his "new method could help move stem cell–based treatments for diseases such as diabetes and Parkinson's more quickly from the lab to the clinic."

Warren was pleased the paper was receiving recognition. He hadn't expected their work to get much publicity or have any kind of broad impact. Science was his second career, yet he already had made a potentially historic contribution. Warren felt new frustration, though. One day that year, he attended a seminar given by Rossi at the Dana-Farber Cancer Institute. A slide at the end of his presentation noted Warren's contributions, but he felt Rossi should have been more generous sharing credit.

"These are my words, my ideas, my problem solving," Warren says. "It was a little distasteful."

For their part, some in Rossi's lab felt Warren had abandoned them by quitting and they resented having to defend the paper to the reviewers without Warren's help, even as they worried he might torpedo them by publishing their data online.

As for Rossi, the period surrounding the paper's publication was tinged with sadness and some disappointment. Just months after it was published, Rossi was giving a talk at the University of California, San Francisco, explaining the science behind his team's breakthrough, when his father, back home in Toronto, collapsed and died, a sudden and unexpected loss.

By then, Rossi was focused on launching a company to employ his lab's new techniques. Several months earlier, Rossi had visited Robert

Tepper, a scientist who cofounded Third Rock Ventures, a three-year-old venture-capital firm in Boston that was gaining a reputation for savvy biotech investments. Rossi gave a lengthy presentation, asking Third Rock to back his start-up proposal.

Tepper wasn't interested. Rossi was an assistant professor who had never pitched a venture-capital firm, so his presentation wasn't very polished. He and his colleagues had shown how mRNA could be used to reprogram cells and create proteins, but they did it in a Petri dish, not in animals or humans. They both knew it might take years to find proof that their techniques could be successful, if they ever could. Tepper said the data Rossi had produced was "interesting," but he passed on an investment.

Rossi arranged to speak with Robert Langer, eager for some advice. Langer was a chemical engineer at the Massachusetts Institute of Technology who had written over one thousand scientific papers and helped launch dozens of companies. Langer hosted Rossi and Timothy Springer, a fellow professor at Harvard Medical School who sometimes invested in biotech companies, in his office.

It was a warm spring afternoon, and the group sat around a conference table in Langer's office, which featured a window looking out to the city of Cambridge. Langer was dressed casually in black jeans and a polo shirt, but his office was intimidating. Every wall was covered, floor to ceiling, with honorary degrees and awards. There didn't seem to be a school in the Western Hemisphere that hadn't honored Langer. Springer, who had made $100 million selling his own biotech company a decade earlier, was a well-known academic and investor in his own right. Rossi knew he'd have to step up his game to grab their interest.

With his long hair pulled up, Rossi took out his laptop and began a presentation mostly focused on his lab's stem-cell work. Rossi shared slides about the stem-cell data his team had collected and outlined three possible business models for his new company: producing research tools for others; converting skin cells to other cell types and providing testing to see what drugs might work; and producing new proteins that could serve as therapeutics. The first two ideas drew little interest. Right away, Rossi was in some trouble. But the possibility of using mRNA to develop proteins intrigued both Langer and Springer.

"You could use this for any protein," Langer said, his interest growing. "This is terrific!"

Later, Springer set up another meeting in Langer's office, this time inviting Noubar Afeyan to join. A bioengineer and Beirut native who had started a venture-capital firm called Flagship Pioneering a decade earlier, Afeyan held a view that big pharmaceutical companies were timid and fearful. Because they spent so much time worrying about wasted time, embarrassing losses, and the resulting blame, most drug companies were too focused on inventing single drugs or making incremental improvements to existing medications, rather than discovering new categories of medicines. That became his firm's goal. In the decade it had been around, though, Flagship had invested in numerous companies, but none had yet produced an approved drug or vaccine, resulting in some skepticism in the venture-capital world. Still, Afeyan remained hopeful.

Listening to Rossi's pitch, Afeyan had trouble mustering much excitement. He didn't see a market for a company that might convert cells or do some of the other things Rossi's group had accomplished.

"I don't know what to do with the Yamanaka factor stuff," he said, referring to the stem-cell work of Rossi's lab.

But Afeyan became intrigued by the idea Rossi had barely touched on: using mRNA to create specific desired proteins within patients. Need a statin, immunosuppressive, or other drug? Just use mRNA to send a message to the body's cells to produce it. In effect, mRNA might be able turn the body into its own laboratory, generating specific medications as needed.

"Can a patient make his own drugs?" Afeyan asked.

"I don't know if anyone has tried," Langer said.

Scientists spent their careers working with living cells in the lab to make proteins. That's how drugs were made. The notion that one might be able to teach the body to make proteins still bordered on heresy, despite the hints of success achieved by Karikó, Weissman, and the earlier researchers. But the more the group discussed the approach, the more it seemed worth trying.

A bit later, a physician-scientist and colleague of Rossi's at Harvard named Kenneth Chien made a key discovery. Chien, who focused on cardiovascular research, had long searched for a way to regenerate heart muscle and vessels as a way to treat victims of heart attacks. Injecting a protein called vascular endothelial growth factor (VEGF) had failed in trials, as it degraded too rapidly to be of much help. But then Chien asked scientists in his Harvard laboratory, working with members of Rossi's lab, to inject modified mRNA into the heart muscle of mice, hoping it might prompt the mice's bodies to create the protein exactly where it was needed.

In one of their very first experiments, conducted at three a.m., bleary-eyed researchers injected mRNA that succeeded in producing luciferase enzymes, a promising sign they might be able to generate different kinds of proteins in the heart. Later, a postdoc working in the lab, Kathy Oi Lan, emailed Chien to deliver truly good news: Their mRNA had served a regenerative role, actually strengthening the hearts of the mice.

"It's exciting because this is the first-time *in vivo* data," she wrote, referring to the process of injecting the mRNA directly in the body. "It means the RNA can be translated *in vivo*" in the heart.

Now there was evidence that injecting mRNA into muscle could generate proteins in the body, not just in a dish in the lab, exciting Rossi and the others about his idea for a start-up. Afeyan agreed to launch the company, with Flagship, Rossi, Langer, and Chien sharing ownership stakes, and Springer becoming an original investor. They didn't spend much time pondering a name. Afeyan simply called it NewcoLS18, signifying the eighteenth life-science company his firm had launched. Afeyan liked to number Flagship's infant companies, rather than name them, partly because it helped prevent him from becoming too attached, in case he had to pull the plug on them.

The company launched in late 2010 with about $2 million in its coffers, just enough money to get the ball rolling. Rossi and his partners were filled with optimism, confident they had a chance to change the course of science. It would prove harder than they expected.

7

2010–2014

Drew Weissman's visitor was getting annoyed.

Months after Derrick Rossi and Noubar Afeyan launched their messenger-RNA start-up in 2010, Weissman was sitting in his office at the University of Pennsylvania with his research partner, Katalin Karikó, when Greg Sieczkiewicz came by for a visit. A young patent attorney at Afeyan's Flagship Pioneering, Sieczkiewicz faced a difficult assignment. His boss's new venture wanted to use mRNA molecules to deliver instructions to the body's cells, directing them to make proteins that might heal ailments or even cure disease.

To have any kind of therapeutic impact, though, Rossi and his partners knew their mRNAs would have to avoid setting off the body's immune system on their way into cells. Several years earlier, Karikó and Weissman had developed techniques enabling mRNA molecules to evade this immune response. But Penn wouldn't license their technology to Flagship, and preliminary patents covering Rossi's research were of limited value. The new partners were in a bind—if their venture couldn't follow the Penn professors' road map, how were they going to make mRNA work as a drug?

Sieczkiewicz traveled down to Philadelphia by Amtrak train to explore other ways Flaghship's start-up might employ Karikó and Weissman's methods, and whether they were devising new approaches or iterations of their existing technology that might provide a solution to the problem. The meeting started out friendly and constructive. They told Sieczkiewicz they were eager for their techniques to be used to develop therapeutics and that they wanted to help Flagship's new effort in whatever way they could.

The conversation quickly spiraled, however. It became clear to Sieczkiewicz that he wasn't going to be able to license their work, there was nothing the professors could do about it, and they didn't have any new technologies or approaches to help the venture.

Sieczkiewicz grew frustrated. Then he got angry, Weissman recalls. Rising to leave, Sieczkiewicz turned to the professors and delivered a vow.

"We're going to do everything we can to get around your patents," Sieczkiewicz said, before storming out of the office.

Weissman and Karikó looked at each other in disbelief, feeling they had been threatened.

(Sieczkiewicz says he didn't mean his comment to sound threatening and that he was pointing out that biotech companies regularly improve on existing technologies.)

Flagship had hit a dead end in Philadelphia, but Afeyan was determined to proceed with the mRNA start-up nonetheless. In 2010, his firm subleased laboratory space in the basement of another Cambridge biotech company to begin scientific work. Rossi, Bob Langer, and the other original founders were eager to help guide their new venture, but they weren't prepared to give up their academic jobs, nor did they have experience operating a business. Instead, Afeyan chose a newly hired scientist on his staff, Jason Schrum, to be the company's first employee, charging Schrum with getting mRNA into cells without relying on Karikó and Weissman's solutions.

The Penn academics had modified mRNA's building blocks so the molecule could escape the notice of the immune system, while Warren and Rossi had demonstrated how the professors' techniques could generate a range of beneficial proteins. It was up to Schrum, laboring in a laboratory in the bowels of an office in Cambridge's Kendall Square neighborhood, to discover other modifications so the new company could have a chance at success.

Schrum seemed well suited for the task. Months earlier, he had received a PhD in biological chemistry at Harvard University, where he had focused on nucleotide chemistry. Schrum even had the look of someone who might do big things. The baby-faced twenty-eight-year-old favored a relaxed, start-up look: khakis, button-downs, and Converse All-Stars.

Schrum felt immediate strain, however. He hadn't told anyone, but he was dealing with intense pain in his hands and joints, a condition that later would be diagnosed as degenerative arthritis. Soon Schrum couldn't bend two fingers on his left hand, making lab work difficult. He volunteered for a drug trial, but the medicine proved useless. Schrum tried corticosteroid injections and anti-inflammatory drugs, but his left hand ached, restricting his experiments.

"It just wasn't useful," Schrum says, referring to his tender hand.

Schrum persisted, nonetheless. Each day in the fall of 2010, he walked through double air-locked doors into a sterile "clean room" before entering a basement lab, where he worked deep into the night designing potential modifications of mRNA nucleosides, hoping to see if they might create proteins. Like all such rooms, there were no windows, so Schrum had to check a clock to know if it was day or night. Sieczkiewicz came to visit once in a while, but most days Schrum was alone.

Some of the company's founders wondered if Schrum could find success, and whether Rossi's results might have been a fluke, suggesting their venture was doomed from the start. Philip Manos, a scientist who had worked on Rossi's breakthrough stem-cell paper, turned down a job with the start-up to join pharmaceutical giant Novartis, dubious of the new company's approach. Perhaps mRNA couldn't produce proteins, after all, at least on a consistent basis.

But as Schrum began testing the modifications in January 2011, he made an immediate discovery. Karikó and Weissman had swapped uridine for pseudouridine to evade the cellular immune response. Schrum found that a variant of pseudouridine called N1-methyl-pseudouridine did an even *better* job reducing innate immune response. Schrum's nucleoside switch enabled even higher protein production than Karikó and Weissman had generated. Schrum's mRNAs lasted longer than either unmodified molecules or the modified mRNA the Penn academics had used, startling the young researcher. Working alone in a dreary basement and through intense pain, he had actually improved on the professors' work. Necessity had truly been the mother of invention.

This was the exact news Afeyan had been hoping to hear. Now there was a potential way for mRNA to produce proteins in large enough quantities to potentially be used as drugs—all without the benefits of Karikó and Weissman's patented methods. Afeyan and his partners were convinced they were onto something special. It was time to name their new company; Rossi branded it Moderna, a mash-up of "modified" and "RNA."*

Afeyan immediately hired additional scientists and leased new office space alongside another Flagship-backed biotech. There was a decidedly unconventional feel to the place and a sense that something revolutionary might be in the offing. Schrum adopted a Shiba Inu puppy named Stella whom he adorned with a matching rose-colored

* A runner-up name: Syndesta, a portmanteau of "synthesize your destiny."

collar and leash and took everywhere, including to the office. Soon he and his colleagues were modifying different mRNAs to produce new proteins. It became so easy, staffers didn't view it as any big deal. By then, Afeyan was searching for a chief executive to lead the enterprise. He seized on a thirty-eight-year-old named Stéphane Bancel and began plotting ways to convince Bancel to join the fledgling company.

• • •

Years earlier, the notion that Bancel might be courted for the top job at a promising biotech company would have seemed improbable, even laughable. Bancel grew up in Marseille, the gritty, colorful city full of immigrants in southern France that serves as a gateway to North Africa and the Mediterranean. Bancel's parents divorced in 1980 when he was eight years old. He had a limited relationship with his father, Lucien, but Bancel's mother, Brigitte, was a constant and loving presence in his life. She set high goals for her son. A physician in a local British Petroleum refinery, Brigitte wanted Stéphane and his younger brother, Christophe, to master the sciences, as she had. But Stéphane brought home awful grades in biology and other subjects, disappointing her. Even more troubling, the boy seemed to forget much of what he had learned, and it wasn't clear why.

"Learning from books was super hard, I mixed things up," he says. "I just couldn't remember stuff."

Later, Bancel would be diagnosed with dyslexia. At the time, though, his difficulties were perplexing. The young man was adept with numbers and did well in math and physics classes, appreciating the logic behind those subjects. It helped that Bancel's grandfather sometimes woke him at six a.m. to quiz him on multiplication tables over baguettes and chocolate milk. But grades of Cs and Ds in biology and other subjects weighed on Brigitte, who feared her son wouldn't gain entrance to a French college, making it hard for him to have a productive career.

Riding a city bus to his downtown school each day, Bancel often dreaded the day ahead. Teachers and school administrators weren't sure how to handle the boy, who demonstrated obvious intelligence yet did so poorly in many of his classes they questioned his future.

"I don't know if Stéphane is stupid or he's pulling my leg," a middle-school administrator told his mother one day.

Brigitte became so frustrated that she sent her son to a farm during spring break one year, to spend two weeks picking asparagus alongside Spanish immigrants, hoping he'd adopt their work ethic.

"It was like a punishment," Bancel says.

The sciences didn't interest Bancel and he hated biology, but technology captivated the boy. He received a computer as a Christmas gift when he was ten years old and threw himself into coding, learning BASIC, C, Pascal, and other languages. Later, after Bancel read a biography of Apple founder Steve Jobs, he decided to become an engineer and maybe even run a company.

"The whole idea that you could use computers to start businesses, literally from a garage with nothing, was actually extremely exciting," he later said.[1]

In high school, though, an administrator made it clear that only the school's top two students would be accepted to a top preparatory school, which Bancel knew was his best chance of becoming an engineer.

Shit, I'm not even in the top ten, he thought.

Bancel had three years to make himself into a top student. His teachers doubted he could do it. A few years later, one teacher told Christophe that she was surprised his brother hadn't dropped out of high school.

"She didn't tell me he was dumb because she was being polite and he's my brother," Christophe recalls. "But she came close."

Bancel developed coping mechanisms to deal with his learning disorder. He became an inveterate note taker, discovering that writing down dates and other facts improved his memory, likely because he was better at processing information visually than in other forms. A conceptual thinker, Bancel began attaching stories and themes to various topics and subjects to compensate for his language challenges. Unusual dedication and perseverance also helped. Bancel found that by setting ambitious long-term goals, he was able to focus and relax his mind. He embraced the goal of running a business one day and spent time researching the steps needed to reach his objective.

"My brain is good at connecting dots, playing out scenarios, how moving one piece affects the rest of the puzzle," he says. "I live in the future."

Bancel succeeded in gaining acceptance to École Centrale Paris, considered France's second-ranked engineering university, barely missing out on the nation's top school. He received a master's degree in 1995, and then enrolled in a master of science program in chemical engineering at the University of Minnesota. Bancel was in a rush to move on to the next stage of his career, so a professor named Wei-Shou Hu allowed him to choose a thesis project that he could complete in just nine months.

In Minnesota, Bancel proved popular with students and faculty, who appreciated his humor and upbeat attitude. He played up his French background, playfully scolding professors for drinking white wine with cheese. Bancel volunteered to build a home page for his program, inserting a photo of himself next to a picture of the Eiffel Tower, adding some personal information: "Single, Available." The language was eventually deleted, but not before eliciting laughs from students and interest from some young women.

After finishing his degree in Minnesota, Bancel decided he needed experience working in Asia if he was going to become a chief executive, so he took a sales and marketing job in Japan for a publicly traded French lab-testing company, bioMérieux SA. Bancel enrolled at Harvard Business School in 1999 but quickly realized he was out of step with most classmates. The internet was raging and students were vying for promising tech jobs. Some dropped out of school to join start-ups, while others were handed generous stock options as inducements to accept job offers, sometimes cashing in millions of dollars even before beginning those positions.

Bancel seemed to exist in a different universe. He wore pressed shirts and sports jackets to class and expressed an eagerness to obtain expertise in manufacturing, which he thought might give him an edge running a drug company someday.

"He was a little more focused, a little more intense, and a little better dressed" than other students, recalls Greg Licholai, a business-school classmate.

After graduating, Bancel joined pharmaceutical giant Eli Lilly & Co. as a senior manufacturing executive, filling that hole in his résumé, and then was hired as bioMérieux's chief executive officer at the age of thirty-three, fulfilling his life's goal at that early age. Bancel engineered sales growth at the six-thousand-person company, learned how to sweet-talk investors and made millions of dollars. But he grew irritated with underlings when they missed key deadlines and ran into resistance from the family-controlled company when he proposed big acquisitions. Soon he was listening to job offers.

Bancel, who had met Afeyan while hunting for acquisitions for bioMérieux, agreed to visit Flagship's offices on a cold February evening in 2011. Sitting across from each other in a large conference room, Afeyan showed Bancel data from Rossi's lab, explaining how Rossi and his colleagues had injected mRNA into ten mice to create erythropoietin, or EPO, the red blood cell–stimulating human protein.

Bancel flashed Afeyan a skeptical look.

"This is not possible," he said, in his French-infused English.

Bancel understood how hard producing proteins could be. He had built proteins in graduate school and at Eli Lilly the old-fashioned way, which involved placing a human gene in bacteria or yeast, a laborious and challenging process. Yes, a "recombinant DNA" revolution had begun in the early 1980s, as upstart companies like San Francisco–area Genentech cut and pasted DNA sequences to create proteins that served as medicines, such as human insulin, and Humira, a new kind of anti-inflammatory that eventually eased Schrum's pain. But not every protein could be produced in the lab. The idea that Rossi had simply injected mRNA into mice and created human protein seemed implausible. Everyone knew mRNA was just too unstable, and that it sets off the immune system. Rossi's data must be some kind of happy accident.

"It's one of those things that happens every day of the week in academia," Bancel said, "a nice paper with data you can't match."

Afeyan grinned. There would be ample time to check Rossi's results, he responded. For now, just presume the data is accurate. What would that mean? Bancel thought for a moment, the wheels in his head turning. He began to list in rapid-fire style all the wonders that would result if mRNA could be injected into the body, make it into the cell, and create proteins. For one thing, making one protein probably means you can make many more, and if it works for one patient, it likely would for most.

"You'd be able to make *hundreds* of medicines," Bancel said, his enthusiasm growing.

Using mRNA for drugs would also mean developing the same fast process each time, relying on a specific sequence of genetic code and cheap enzymes to produce each protein, thereby avoiding the enormous costs that come with building factories and dealing with cells for traditional medicines. DNA wouldn't be directly involved so there wouldn't be a risk of causing mutations that cause cancer, as with gene therapy. And the mRNA approach was so new and unique it likely wouldn't infringe on existing patents, meaning almost every kind of medicine could be produced without legal troubles from drugmakers. Best of all: If patients can make proteins for themselves, it would be like having a medicine factory *in their own bodies.*

Bancel went on and on, growing more animated with each new point. Afeyan just nodded along, hoping Bancel would embrace the concept on his own. When he was done, Afeyan summed up the proposition he was offering Bancel.

"There's a five percent chance of changing medicine forever," Afeyan said, before smiling. "Okay, have a great evening."

Walking home over the Longfellow Bridge toward Beacon Hill that evening, Bancel's head was spinning. He could hardly feel the winter's cold. For the next few days, he barely slept. Later, he met Ken Chien, the Moderna cofounder, and examined his data, becoming even more intrigued.

"It probably won't work," Bancel told his wife over a bottle of wine, as he tried to decide how to respond to Afeyan's offer.

"Stop being so French," she said, encouraging Bancel to take the risk.

If mRNA could work as a drug, he'd kick himself if he turned down the idea of running the new business, Bancel realized. He called Afeyan to accept the job.

• • •

Staffers watched as Bancel walked into Moderna's offices on his first day, a confident, ambitious young man with a distinctive look. Bancel was handsome in an unconventional way, with full lips, a cleft chin, and close-cropped hair that was beginning to thin in the front. His fashion style was a blend of Silicon Valley comfort and Paris chic. Bancel favored Steve Jobs–inspired turtleneck shirts and quarter-zip pullover sweaters, which he matched with form-fitting dark pants and dark shoes, along with an Hermès belt buckle with a distinctive oversize *H.*

Within weeks, Bancel went from cocky to concerned. Using mRNA molecules to produce therapeutic proteins was a rather simple concept, he understood. The academic papers published by Karikó and Rossi were in the public domain, for anyone to see. If mRNA was truly capable of revolutionizing the drug world, pharmaceutical companies, biotech firms, and others were sure to catch on. The German company CureVac already was using mRNA for vaccines, though it wasn't modifying the nucleosides of its mRNA. Another company in that country, BioNTech, was doing its own mRNA experiments.

Moderna needed to prove that its approach worked and raise a ton of money to develop multiple drugs, all before rivals caught up, Bancel decided. Biotech pioneer Genentech had been the first to produce recombinant proteins, introducing human insulin and growth hormone, which became the first biotech drugs. But others quickly joined the game, preventing Genentech from dominating the field. They had squandered an opportunity, Bancel felt. Now Moderna had a chance to own the world of mRNA therapeutics, maybe even do something historic. But it would have to act swiftly.

Bancel convened meetings with the dozen or so scientists Afeyan had hired, handing out ambitious sets of tasks. One group was assigned to run a massive safety study in monkeys to show mRNA wasn't toxic, while others were told to produce one hundred different proteins in mice and rats. It was the first step toward the company's goal of developing therapies that replaced defective proteins, providing patients with missing proteins, and more.

"Let's make all the proteins in the body," Bancel told a staffer.

Moderna began a frenzied effort to file patents, one for each new protein produced, hoping to stake claims before others had a chance. Soon staffers were filing patents even before doing lab experiments proving they could create the proteins, all in a mad rush to accumulate intellectual property so drugs could be rolled out, at least down the road.

Bancel began meeting with executives of larger pharmaceutical companies, hoping to work out partnerships that could bring Moderna needed cash. He raced back to the office, ordering his team to produce proteins that his potential partners were most interested in, to convince them that mRNA was for real. But Bancel had never been involved in drug discovery before, so he had unrealistic expectations. After meeting with Eli Lilly executives, Bancel gave his team two weeks to use mRNA to produce insulin, work that usually took over a month. When the Eli Lilly deadline was missed, he turned furious.

"You're not doing your job!" he told staffers, who were left shaken by the unexpected criticism.

Soon Bancel was complaining about employees, cursing in both English and French, and sending nasty emails to underlings, often in all caps.

"He just swore at everyone," a staffer recalls. "'How did you fucking mess that up,' 'Why is this fucking late.'"

Bancel could be demeaning.

"This is a stupid idea," he told one staffer who had disappointed him.

"You're incompetent, you don't know what you're doing," he told another.

Employees grew fearful of disappointing Bancel and eager to avoid his criticism. It didn't help that he publicly spoke of the need to upgrade Moderna's staff, to improve its scientific capabilities and accelerate the pace of drug development, all of which suggested he going to be replacing employees.

Complaints about the difficult work environment began appearing on Glassdoor, a website where current and former employees anonymously review companies, helping to shape a view of Bancel as a difficult boss. Eventually, the criticisms reached the board of directors and Moderna's founders, some of whom worried about morale at the company.[2] Someone created a Wiki page about Bancel that included bogus biographical facts, such as that he had studied ballet in Paris, which were removed.

By 2012, employees were trying to match Bancel's pace and meet his expectations. They, too, sensed the new company had a unique opportunity to change medicine and felt pressure to make progress before others caught up. Sometimes they pushed themselves harder than was reasonable. One young scientist, Summar Siddiqui, fell to the floor in the office kitchen while working a twelve-hour day and was rushed to an emergency room for treatment.

"I guess I had the flu but didn't want to admit I wasn't feeling well," she says. "It was work, work, work, we were motivated by where the company was going and I had just started at Moderna and didn't want to lose my job."

Another stressed-out scientist collapsed at home, hitting his head on a table, knocking himself unconscious. He woke in a pool of blood and was taken to an emergency room. Still another passed out in the shower. One researcher fainted in a parking lot near Moderna's office. After being revived by a colleague, she insisted on heading into the office but was persuaded to check into nearby Mount Auburn Hospital.

Sometimes Moderna staffers made embarrassing flubs, exasperating Bancel. One day, two young scientists misunderstood a passing comment from Justin Quinn, a twenty-eight-year-old responsible for improving the mRNA manufacturing process, and they stopped using an enzyme that allows mRNA to be used in experiments, free of DNA. The mistake jeopardized weeks of work, compelling Bancel to fire Quinn.

"You're gone," he told Quinn.

Colleagues watched Quinn, in tears, vacate the office.

"I was so sad, I felt I let him down," Quinn says. "Stéphane is all business, a stone-cold killer, but I really liked him."

In Bancel's view, the ire and impatience were necessary. Moderna had a chance to revolutionize health care and he was sure competition was around the bend, so he had to push his team to move as fast as possible. As for the criticisms, they weren't aimed at being cruel, he says, so he didn't feel much responsibility.

"It's not mean if the intent isn't to hurt," Bancel says.

Bancel had risked a lot to join Moderna, turning down well-paid job offers from big, established companies, and he had invested a chunk of his life savings into the new company. Moderna would need huge amounts of money to stay ahead of the field and develop drugs in a proper way, and Bancel didn't know how long Flagship would fund the business, adding to his worries. He came from the world of Big Pharma, and now he found himself in a tiny office, surrounded by secondhand microscopes and aging equipment.

Soon he and Schrum were butting heads. Once, after Schrum worked past three a.m. in the lab, he went home to grab some sleep. He returned to the office just before nine a.m., passing Bancel on his way back to the lab.

"Where have you been?" Bancel demanded. "Why isn't anyone here already?"

Schrum tried to explain that he and others had worked through the night, but Bancel didn't seem to care.

"It was very discouraging," Schrum says.

A year later, Schrum quit to take a different job.

Bancel's mood swings put the team on edge. When they received an important patent or achieved another goal, Bancel was upbeat, complimentary, and fun to be around. Those days, he came home and told his wife that he felt on top of the world.

"When we met patent, filing, or other deadlines, he would thank the team and take people out or pay for a team lunch," says Kenechi Ejebe, a scientist who joined Moderna early on. "When he was happy, he was very nice."

But when his scientists met frustration or produced disappointing data, Bancel's mood soured, often abruptly, as his mind found a dark place.

Shit, this won't work, he thought.

At one point, Bancel told his wife he might have made a mistake taking the job.

"I wonder if I did the right thing," he told her.

Staffers developed strategies to deal with Bancel's emotions.

"He had a hard time managing his anger. His moods were all over the place," says Ejebe. "You would basically avoid him. That was my strategy. I'd close my office door."

Other employees shrugged off the harsh language and scoldings. They appreciated that Bancel was honest about their work and thrived in the pressure-packed atmosphere. Science is a combative field; harsh criticisms are commonplace; even physical confrontations occur. Some fights, such as the time a furious Rosalind Franklin came from behind a lab bench at Cambridge University to charge at a cowering James D. Watson, just before they unveiled DNA's double-helix structure, are legendary.[3]

Bancel expected a lot from himself. Staffers could see that he genuinely believed Moderna had a unique chance to improve the way patients received medicines and that he worried about squandering an enormous opportunity, a concern many of them shared. He impressed these staffers with his focus on the future. He began speaking of the need to build manufacturing capabilities, rather than rely on others, since mRNA would likely require sophisticated production methods. Above all, Bancel was almost evangelical about the possibilities of mRNA and the role Moderna could play in public health, and his enthusiasm inspired some of the scientists.

"This is the software of life," he told a researcher, referring to mRNA.

One day, Bancel spoke to his team about future pandemics, and how the technology the company was developing could save lives, partly because mRNA is so much faster than other drug and vaccine approaches.

"We just have to be ready," he told them.

Moderna moved into new office space on First Street in Cambridge, sharing the building with the Cambridge School of Culinary Arts. It was an incongruous pairing. On their way in, bookish scientists sometimes passed tattooed would-be chefs smoking cigarettes and discussing veal cordon bleu. Even if they wanted to stop and chat, the Moderna team had been trained to avoid conversations. The company was still in stealth mode. It didn't have a website, wouldn't talk to the press, and forced employees to sign confidentiality agreements preventing them from sharing information, even with spouses.[4] The researchers were accumulating valuable data, but Afeyan and Bancel didn't want it published in scientific journals, as most other biotechs did. Bancel didn't want to tip potential rivals off to what his team was up to, nor did he want to alert big drug companies, which might then shift dozens of their scientists to focus on mRNA work.

"All we need is for Genentech to find out" what the company was doing, Bancel told a colleague.

For a while, Moderna's founders shared suggestions to improve the company's operations. Some had more time and inclination to help than others. Langer, the MIT chemical engineer, was in a perpetual rush between meetings with MIT students, biotech companies, and others. Once he drove to Moderna's offices for a board meeting, parked his red C-class Mercedes-Benz sports car in front—with the car's engine still on and its lights flashing—and bolted inside, unable to find parking. "Can you park it?" he asked a Moderna assistant. Langer was happy to guide Moderna staffers when they sought help or had a question, but he preferred a hands-off role.

By contrast, Rossi emailed, called, or came by on a regular basis, asking researchers like Schrum and Tony de Fougerolles, Moderna's new chief scientific officer, about their progress. Upbeat and enthusiastic, Rossi had so many recommendations they sometimes overwhelmed members of the team.

Over time, he and Bancel locked horns. Rossi wanted to have input into the company's direction and didn't like what he was hearing about how Bancel was treating staffers. Rossi says that Bancel asked him to disclose his new research at Boston Children's Hospital so that Moderna could file patents on that work.

"The work is their property, he was asking me to steal from a hospital that treats children," Rossi says. "Stéphane is someone without a moral compass."

For his part, Bancel says he asked Rossi not to do mRNA work at Boston Children's that could compete with Moderna's research, viewing such work as a potential conflict of interest for Rossi, since he owned Moderna shares. Bancel told others that Rossi had no experience running a company or getting medicines made and that his suggestions were distracting the team. At one point, Rossi called a meeting of Moderna's founders to try to reclaim power from Bancel but found little support.

"He was under the mistaken impression that when you start a company, you run it," says Chien, the Moderna cofounder.

Bancel reasserted his authority and Rossi eventually sold some of his Moderna shares to refocus on his own research and other scientific ventures, though he stayed in touch with Moderna staffers and the other founders.

Now that Bancel had a free hand running the company, his strategy began to flounder. He had hoped to find a Big Pharma partner willing to pump money into Moderna in exchange for rights to one of the drugs it was developing, but he kept striking out. Eli Lilly and Roche Holding AG both turned down opportunities to work with Moderna, expressing varying degrees of skepticism about mRNA's capabilities and concern that Moderna was years away from even testing its science in humans. In 2012, Bancel managed to raise $25 million from some wealthy families, but Moderna needed a lot more money to have any shot at fulfilling its hope of producing a series of drugs.

One day, Rossi told Chien there was chatter at Moderna that he wasn't doing enough to help the company and that his vested shares were at risk. Based on his earlier work using mRNA to create the VegF protein, Chien had become an adviser to British drug giant AstraZeneca, which had suffered a series of clinical failures that resulted in layoffs of over one thousand scientists. The company's new chief executive, Pascal Soriot, was under pressure to discover new drugs to fill an empty pipeline. Chien connected Bancel with AstraZeneca's head of research and development, Martin Mackay. Soon Bancel was on a plane to Wilmington, Delaware, near AstraZeneca's U.S. offices, for a breakfast meeting with Soriot and Mackay. To save his company money, Bancel stayed at a nearby Motel 6 on I-95, but he was composed and confident the next morning for the big meeting.

Right away, Soriot loved the idea of using mRNA to develop drugs and was impressed by Chien's earlier data showing that the VEGF protein could be produced with mRNA. Most of all, Soriot was taken with Bancel, a fellow Frenchman bursting with ambition. When Soriot asked Bancel why Moderna needed cash, Bancel told him: "We want to dominate the space."

Bancel had the nerve to ask for *a lot* of money. AstraZeneca eventually agreed to pay Moderna $240 million for an option on the rights to dozens of mRNA drugs, if they were ever produced, including a cardiovascular therapy. They promised another $180 million if Moderna achieved certain technical milestones. Suddenly, Moderna's coffer was full and Afeyan's and Bancel's dream was alive once again.

The deal left mouths agape in the biotech and venture-capital worlds. AstraZeneca had paid all that money and didn't get a drug, intellectual property of any kind, or even Moderna shares. Bancel was soon signing deals with other companies, raising hundreds of millions of dollars in the process. He also upgraded Moderna's talent, hiring experienced scientists to a team that now included Stephen Hoge, a partner at McKinsey & Company and former physician.

After the AstraZeneca deal was completed, Bancel met Afeyan for a beer at an outside café in Cambridge. Bancel was almost giddy, feeling Moderna was finally on its way to leading a revolution. Afeyan stopped him short, saying Bancel had overlooked something important.

"Now everyone in town will hate you."

Bancel looked stunned, even a bit hurt.

"Every board of directors of every biotech is going to ask their CEO why they can't get a deal like Moderna," Afeyan said.

Bancel thought about it for a while.

"Shit, you're right."

Moderna had oodles of money. But Bancel had inadvertently placed a target on the company's back.

• • •

Bancel made enemies in other ways, too. In late October 2013, he flew to the historic German city of Tübingen for his first encounter with others in the small but now growing world of mRNA. Tübingen is a town of less than one hundred thousand residents best known for its cobblestone streets, Renaissance architecture, and rich tradition of noteworthy science. Back in 1869, Friedrich Miescher, a Swiss biochemistry student at the University of Tübingen, had first identified nucleic acids, the group of molecules that includes DNA and RNA. The school's reputation had been sullied when it lent scientific backing to Nazi policies. In more recent years, academics at the University of Tübingen had been working with mRNA to try to develop various drugs.

Over one hundred attendees piled into a majestic hall in a fourteenth-century castle to hear leaders in the field. A headline speaker was Ingmar Hoerr, a founder of CureVac, which was based a few miles away and by then had been working on mRNA approaches for over thirteen years. Katalin Karikó was there, too, as was Michael Heartlein, who ran Shire Pharmaceuticals's mRNA efforts. Uğur Şahin, founder of BioNTech, came to give a talk, as did Bancel.

Bancel quickly infuriated the crowd. Unlike the other speakers, he refused to give details about Moderna's work. He spoke about how much money he had raised, made vague promises about how Moderna was going to introduce a new generation of medicines, and told the mRNA devotees they had "a responsibility" not to screw things up. Bancel pointed to a slide showing the cover page of a paper written by James W. Wilson, a U.S. researcher who ran a laboratory at the University of Pennsylvania in 1999, when his team injected a young man with an experimental treatment to treat a rare metabolic liver disease. The virus used in the vaccine, which was shuttling a working copy of the teenager's broken gene, threw his immune system into overdrive, killing him within days, a tragedy that ended work on gene therapy for years.[5]

Similar mistakes would set mRNA back "by five years," Bancel warned.

Scientists in the audience rolled their eyes. There even was a groan. *We know all about the Wilson fiasco*, the researchers were thinking. *We don't need you lecturing us about it.* During a conference break, Heartlein approached Bancel with a colleague, hoping to compare notes about their companies' progress. Bancel stuck a hand in his face, spun around, and walked away.

"He gave us the Heisman," Heartlein says, referring to the stiff-arm gesture delivered by the miniature bronze running back on the trophy given annually to the best player in U.S. college football. Bancel and Moderna "wanted to collaborate with everyone, but it was a one-way street." (Bancel says "it is pure fiction" that he put his hand in Heartlein's face.)

Bancel and Moderna had become the bad boys of biotech. But an even bigger problem was emerging back in the lab: They couldn't get their mRNA to work.

• • •

When Moderna's scientists first began doing experiments, they used "naked" mRNA, meaning they created a version of the molecule in the lab that encoded for a particular protein and injected it into the body with nothing more than a crude chemical encasement, hoping for the best. Naked mRNA was used on a repeated basis to produce the VEGF in mice, demonstrating enough of that protein to get AstraZeneca excited that a cardiovascular medicine could be manufactured using Moderna's mRNA technique.

By early 2013, though, it was clear that the VEGF protein was a rare exception. As the Moderna team tried developing mRNA molecules for several other rare diseases, they found they couldn't produce nearly enough protein to be of much help to anyone. Almost all their mRNA was getting cut up and eliminated by an enzyme called a nuclease, well before the molecule could get into the cell. To address this problem, the Moderna researchers began inserting their mRNA in lipid nanoparticles, or LNPs, which are tiny balls of cholesterol and fat that act to protect genetic material on its way into the cells. Back in the 1970s, Langer and others had begun experimenting with lipids and other substances, eventually finding that they helped protect big, complex molecules like DNA and RNA, and made them easier to deliver into the body. Wrapping mRNA in LNPs helped Moderna create a more potent molecule. When injected into the muscle, the LNP delivered the mRNA directly to the lymph nodes in the underarm, hitching a ride into the heart of the immune system.

But the scientists ran into a huge new problem. When they first administrated their mRNA encased in LNP to mice and monkey test subjects, it generated impressive amounts of protein, exciting the team. Within a week or so, though, subsequent administrations saw the protein production plummet. It was as if the body's defenses had learned to fend off the injected molecule and its genetic payload.

Karikó, Rossi, and other mRNA pioneers had never done repeated dosings, nor were they trying to produce enough protein for potential drugs, so they didn't need to surround their mRNA in complex LNPs and they never experienced this "transient protein expression" issue. The Moderna scientists were shocked by what they were seeing: They checked the mice and monkeys two weeks or so after the dosings and barely any of the desired protein was detected in the animals. On their own, modifications of the mRNA's building blocks weren't enough to evade the immune system, it turned out.

The researchers couldn't figure out what was going wrong—was it the mRNAs or had the LNP gone awry? Were proteins not being made or were they being eliminated so quickly they weren't useful? There were no solutions, and the team was growing frustrated, some so glum that they moped around the office. How were they going to create useful drugs to replace missing or defective proteins if their therapeutic proteins disappeared in a few short days? Using naked mRNA appeared to be Moderna's only reliable way of making drugs, and only one or two injections seemed possible. It seemed there would be very few diseases the company could ever hope to address.

The news made Bancel visibly irritated, and some staffers worried they were going to lose their jobs.

"Why can't we repeat the dosing?" Bancel asked one day. "Why isn't this moving forward?!"

Stephen Hoge, who ran the scientific effort and usually was a calm and upbeat presence in the office, began to fret he had made a big mistake leaving a well-paid job at McKinsey for Moderna. Hoge paced his office, nervously tossing a football in the air to himself, trying to come up with a solution. He asked a senior scientific staffer named Eric Huang to take a fresh look at their dilemma, to see if there was something they were missing.

Huang took on the assignment, even as he dealt with Bancel's growing impatience. Early on, he consulted a mentor who reminded him that scientific discovery takes time.

"Science moves at the speed of science," she told Huang, who was reassured by the words but knew enough not to share the maxim with Bancel.

Huang was a glass-half-full kind of guy who tried to emphasize the positive aspects of life. When he was fourteen and living in Taiwan, he left the country to go to school in the United States. Huang didn't speak any English and was homesick for months, but his parents wanted him to stay, eager for him to get a good education. Alone and depressed, Huang decided to see his new circumstances as an opportunity.

It's not like my parents will let me come home, he thought.

Eventually, he received a PhD in parasitology at New York University, and then a master's in business administration. Now, as he confronted Moderna's existential dosing problem, he decided to come at it from a different direction. Everyone at Moderna was looking at what their mRNA *couldn't* do, namely create potent and plentiful proteins after repeated dosings. Huang focused on what it *could* do: get into cells and create ample, if short-lived, proteins, before the mRNA was eliminated. Somehow their mRNA/LNP combinations, when injected in the muscle, were delivering a payload to the lymph nodes that was eliciting a strong immune response, even at very low doses. Yes, the proteins weren't being created on a sustained basis, but maybe that wasn't an awful thing, Huang thought.

Earlier in his career, Huang worked with malaria vaccines. What was happening to Moderna's mRNAs reminded Huang of what effective vaccines all do: teach the immune system to recognize the virus and then disappear. The duration of protein production doesn't matter as much with vaccines—just the immune response. Moderna's scientists were disappointed that their mRNAs had trouble creating long-lasting medicines, but maybe they had it all wrong. Limited protein production wasn't a bug of their technology, and neither was the strong immune response being generated. They were features.

This is the perfect vaccine, Huang thought.

In the late spring of 2013, Huang brought his idea to Hoge: Moderna should be making vaccines, not drugs. If proteins made by mRNAs are inherently immunogenic, let's take advantage of that feature in the molecule, Huang said.

Hoge found Huang's argument persuasive, but he had serious qualms about focusing on vaccines. Moderna had sold itself to investors and partners as a company that could produce proteins to help those suffering from diseases. Its goal was developing a pipeline of medicines, not vaccines. Heck, the name of the company was Moderna *Therapeutics*, not vaccines. CureVac had already spent years working on vaccines, with little apparent luck. Moderna executives had already considered vaccine work but had decided against it—everyone knew vaccines were a low-margin, boring business.

Nevertheless, Hoge asked Huang to build an influenza vaccine using mRNA and test it in mice. They wouldn't tell anyone until they were certain their new approach worked. Only if their mRNA vaccine produced more impressive results than alternatives would they advocate for a radical shift of the company's focus.

A few days before the Thanksgiving holiday that year, Huang was sitting in his office when a researcher at a testing company called to say he was sending a computer file with Huang's influenza-test results from an experiment he'd been running with mice. Huang stared at the data, unable to utter a word for what seemed like an eternity.

"Is this right?!" he eventually asked.

Huang was assured that the data was entirely accurate. His mRNA, which stimulated an immune response by producing a key influenza protein in the mice, had achieved startling antibody levels, or titers, in blood. The mice's protection was one hundred times higher than existing flu vaccines, including CureVac's, as well as other flu-vaccine approaches, such as using naked mRNA.

Someone must have screwed something up, Huang thought.

He repeated the experiments but found they were indeed correct. When the mice were infected with influenza, the vaccine seemed to fully protect them. Later, Huang and Hoge saw the same impressive results after testing the vaccine in monkeys.

A bit later, Hoge approached Bancel in an office hallway.

"I have something I need to tell you," Hoge said.

Bancel was thrilled to hear about the vaccine data and the potential solution to their problem. So was Afeyan, Moderna's board of directors, and the company's early backers. Vaccines weren't their first choice for a product. But they were striking out with drug research. And the data from Huang and Hoge was pretty remarkable. If a flu vaccine could work, then others might, too. Finally, they had a shot at something special.

8

2015–2017

Jason McLellan was just a few years out of graduate school, but he already claimed a crucial role in breakthrough medical research. A productive stint at the National Institutes of Health had provided him with enviable connections in his field. In 2015, the thirty-two-year-old secured a prestigious position as an assistant professor at Dartmouth College's Geisel School of Medicine in Hanover, New Hampshire, where he ran his own laboratory.

He couldn't find any funding, however. He spent months applying for research grants from the federal government and other bodies, meeting rejection after rejection. By the fall of 2015, McLellan was truly worried—without backing, his lab and career were in jeopardy.

McLellan was a different kind of scientist than Katalin Karikó, Derrick Rossi, and most of the Moderna team. A structural biologist, McLellan studied the atomic shapes of proteins, nucleic acids, and carbohydrates, determining how altering them could change their function and behavior. For years, researchers held out hope that a detailed understanding of the structures of disease-related molecules would help them design effective drugs and vaccines to target these pathogens. They had few signs of definitive success, but McLellan and others were still trying.[1]

McLellan had been building and dismantling structures for years. Growing up, he owned multiple Lego sets, spending hours at a time manipulating the multicolored plastic bricks to create impressive edifices with surprising speed. An athletic boy with talent on the soccer field, McLellan was even more gifted at Tetris, the tile-matching video game, and others that require spatial visualization and reasoning. It wasn't apparent at the time, but he was honing skills that he'd later apply in the lab, where he and others in his field would rotate long strands of small molecules called amino acids to adjust the structure of proteins.

The son of a grocery-store manager and a part-time office administrator, McLellan grew up in St. Clair Shores, a lower-middle-class neighborhood thirteen miles from Detroit. McLellan was the valedictorian of his high school class, but his parents didn't have resources to pay for a private college or the University of Michigan. Instead, McLellan enrolled at Wayne State University, a public school in Detroit, which offered him a full scholarship. McLellan completed a bachelor of science degree in chemistry in 2003, becoming the first in his family to graduate college, before starting a PhD program at the Johns Hopkins School of Medicine.

Broad-shouldered with a youthful face and an easy smile, McLellan in 2008 joined a lab run by Peter Kwong, a well-known scientist at the NIH's Vaccine Research Center, who was tweaking the configurations of HIV proteins to develop a vaccine. Kwong didn't have room for another postdoc in his fourth-floor lab, though, so McLellan was shunted to an annex on the building's second floor, near a lab run by Barney Graham, an infectious-disease specialist.

Graham was a true presence at the VRC. Six foot five with a thick, graying goatee and neatly parted hair, Graham looked like a cleaned-up version of the actor Jeff Bridges. A few years earlier, on a visit to the VRC, President George W. Bush saw Graham, sized him up, and called out to the scientist in a slow Texas drawl: "Big Baaahney," a nickname that stuck. Graham dressed more formally than his colleagues, usually in khaki pants and a button-down plaid shirt, and he sometimes even wore a tie and sports jacket. Colleagues, who too often were stressed out and overworked, liked listening to Graham speak about science, his family, his trips to Africa, or most anything else. His soothing tone reminded them of a kind grandfather telling a story around a family fireplace.

Graham might have had a calm veneer, but he was a bit of a glutton for punishment. By the time McLellan pulled up a lab stool to chat in 2008, Graham had spent two frustrating decades trying to develop vaccines for two of the most intractable and deadly viruses mankind has encountered: HIV and respiratory syncytial virus. This common yet terrifying respiratory virus hospitalizes millions of infants each year and is responsible for nearly 7 percent of the deaths of babies one month to one year of age, and also is lethal to some older people.[2]

Efforts to discover an RSV vaccine had long been linked to tragedy. In 1966, a decade after the virus was discovered, NIH researchers were testing a vaccine made from a killed version of the pathogen. Hope turned to horror when two infants died after contracting RSV, months after vaccination, while others landed in the hospital, tragedies that suggested the shots weren't protective and might even have enhanced the disease. The disaster would dissuade drug companies and most others from chasing the virus for years to come.

Graham kept at it, though, trying to understand why the earlier vaccine had failed. Difficult problems captivated Graham, who grew up on a farm in Kansas with quarter horses, cattle, and thousands of hogs.

"On a farm, you spend half the day fixing equipment in order to get the work done on the back end of the day," Graham says.[3]

Graham was introduced to RSV in the mid-1980s when he trained at Vanderbilt University. Tasked with growing RSV in the lab so mice could be infected with the disease, Graham spent seven months on the project in his little cubicle, becoming attached to the subject.

"You make progress on something and you feel ownership," he says. "I became an RSV guy."

One day in 2008, McLellan wandered into Graham's office and got to chatting about RSV. Graham asked McLellan if he might like to work on a vaccine with Graham's team, which didn't include any structural-biology specialists. The idea appealed to McLellan, though Kwong warned him that studying a low-profile virus with a checkered history could be a career killer.

The challenge facing Graham and McLellan was clear: The earlier, failed vaccine had successfully introduced RSV's key protein—which is named the F protein because it fuses the virus with human cells to infect them—to the immune system. The earlier RSV vaccine also managed to produce ample antibodies capable of binding to the protein, which exists on the surface of an RSV particle. The problem was these weren't neutralizing antibodies, the kinds that fend off infection.

Here was the issue: The F protein rearranges itself while invading a cell, McLellan and Graham determined, hiding vulnerable spots on the virus targeted by antibodies. By attacking the postfusion, rearranged form of the protein, not the prefusion protein, the RSV vaccine had flooded lungs with nonneutralizing antibodies, which were causing inflammation and a deadlier version of the disease upon natural RSV infection. In other words, the earlier vaccine had the right protein but in the wrong shape, or conformation.

To build a protective vaccine, Graham and McLellan realized they'd have to somehow lock the F protein in its prefusion form so that neutralizing antibodies could be activated. That was easier said than done: The F protein is notoriously unstable, meaning it frequently changes shape and is therefore hard to pin down.

McLellan spent over a year employing various X-ray crystallography techniques, some developed to study HIV's envelope protein, becoming the first person to produce a reliable image of the F protein's prefusion shape, which he decided looked a bit like a Nerf football.[4] In early 2013, McLellan, Graham, Kwong, and others at the VRC used that image to design a new F protein. They tweaked the genetic sequence of the protein, swapping four amino acids with others that could fill open space in the protein's structure and keep the molecule together, preventing it from changing shape.[5]

McLellan infected mammalian cells with his modified DNA to produce the prefusion protein, which became the antigen of a new vaccine that produced levels of neutralizing antibodies in animals that were as much as forty times higher than those previously generated by an RSV vaccine. The group's study showing how to stabilize the protein would be published in *Science* in November 2013, becoming a runner-up choice for breakthrough of the year. By the summer of 2021, several companies would be closing in on potential RSV vaccines using the work of McLellan, Graham, and their colleagues.

Back in 2013, however, as McLellan began his first faculty position at Dartmouth, he couldn't get any funding. Three times over the next year or so, he sent proposals for NIH grants related to his RSV research, but he was turned down each time. McLellan became discouraged about his future and fretted about whether he'd be able to pay the salaries of the PhD students and postdocs in his lab.

"It was my lowest point," says McLellan.

McLellan called Graham for advice. In his soothing tone, Graham suggested that McLellan focus on a different type of pathogen: coronaviruses. These viruses didn't usually grab the attention of the public, nor did most scientists care too much about them, but they are ancestrally related to RSV, so Graham thought McLellan's recent work might prove useful. Both RSV and coronaviruses have genomes made of RNA, rely on proteins to fuse with cells, and spread through particle droplets. A dangerous coronavirus seemed to emerge every decade or so, Graham noted. In fact, there were concerning reports of a new kind of coronavirus spreading just then in the Middle East.

McLellan heeded Graham's advice. Before long he was diving into a true scientific backwater.

• • •

For decades, coronaviruses were viewed as obscure and largely inconsequential. These pathogens could cause severe sickness in pigs, chickens, dogs, cats, and mice. For humans, though, they were responsible for little more than cause the common cold.

Specialists in the field didn't mind that no one cared about the area. To them, coronaviruses were unusual and interesting pathogens that expressed their genes and proteins in unique ways, satisfying the researchers' intellectual curiosity. For some, the relative obscurity of these pathogens made them *more* intriguing. Dedicated experts had the field to themselves, boosting their chances of making discoveries. Much like treasure hunters, scientists are happiest when they can uncover something new. The possibility of a new find keeps many seventy- and even eighty-year-old researchers from hanging up their lab coats for good.

The coronavirus field attracted microbiologists who preferred to remain out of the limelight rather than make headlines or launch billion-dollar start-ups. Their papers rarely were accepted for publication by top journals, so the specialists usually focused on journals read by those with interest in these pathogens. Sometimes it gave them a better chance to be published.

"I liked that no one cared about it," says Susan Weiss, who began focusing on coronaviruses in the late 1970s and later became a professor at the University of Pennsylvania.

Coronavirus chasers, scattered around the world, were collegial and collaborative, even as fierce rivalries developed in other scientific areas. In 1980, the world's experts, a grand total of about sixty people, gathered for a conference in an ancient castle in Würzburg, Germany. The meeting was as memorable for the socializing and delicious food and wine served as for the captivating presentations delivered.

By then, a view had emerged that the human coronavirus, called OC43, likely arose in the nineteenth century, perhaps jumping from cows to humans before melting into civilization's background as one of the causes of the common cold. The surfaces of these spherical viruses are marked by a halo of crown-like protein projections that bear a resemblance to spikes. That explains why British virologists David Tyrrell and June Almeida in 1968 dubbed them coronaviruses—"corona" means crown in Latin.[6]

Tyrrell was determined to find a cure for the common cold. In 1957, he became the head of the Common Cold Unit in the city of Wiltshire, where a team collected nasal secretions from children and other volunteers inoculated with an original cold specimen. To demonstrate how easily the virus spread, the researchers trickled a solution of fluorescent dye into the nose of a laboratory staffer before the group played a game of cards. Later, they turned off the lights and turned on a fluorescent lamp. To their shock, the dye was on cards, fingers, tables, and pretty much every other spot in the room.[7]

Tyrrell grew frustrated that so few cared about stopping the coronavirus that caused the cold. He liked to quote a poem by English humorist A. P. Herbert chiding doctors for ignoring the most common of pathogens and for saying that colds need to run their course.

> But I reply with frank chagrin
> "Why must the blasted thing BEGIN?"[8]

Eventually, coronavirus vaccines were introduced for some livestock, protecting their vulnerable respiratory and gastrointestinal systems from the virus, but most scoffed at the notion of focusing precious resources to prevent runny noses, sore throats, and other minor annoyances in humans. Over time, scientists did gain a better understanding of these viruses, though. In the 1970s, researchers including Kathryn Holmes, working with a coronavirus that affects mice, identified the spike protein on the surface of the virus particle that allowed it to attach to host cells. The tip of the spike binds to receptors on the host cell's surface, Holmes found, and the base of each spike protein contains the fusion machinery that allows the virus membrane to fuse with the host's cell membrane and start infection. The genome of a coronavirus was determined to be longer than that of other RNA viruses, about three times that of HIV's and twice as long as the influenza virus's genome.

In 2002, a very different kind of coronavirus emerged in Guangdong Province in southern China, likely from bat poop that reached humans via catlike mammals called civets. The virus infected food workers and then spread to hospital staffers, one of whom unwittingly brought the virus to a Hong Kong hotel. Soon it was in many Asian countries and around the world. The pathogen was named SARS-associated coronavirus, or SARS-CoV, and the disease it caused was called SARS, short for severe acute respiratory syndrome. Soon it was killing people, reaching a mortality rate of 10 percent.

Coronavirus-obsessives were absolutely stunned. They had no idea that a version of the pathogen they were so passionate about could kill humans. Suddenly, their field was the talk of the scientific world and beyond.

"*Can you believe it's a coronavirus?*" Weiss emailed a colleague at the time.

SARS-CoV disappeared in about eight months, though, killing fewer than one thousand people. Early adoption of mask wearing, handwashing, and temperature-taking ended the epidemic. And the virus was primarily spread by those who were ill, not asymptomatic people, so isolation and contact tracing were effective public-health measures. Several companies tried developing SARS vaccines, including GlaxoSmithKline and the small Maryland biotech that Gale Smith of MicroGeneSys had joined, Novavax, but the epidemic's rapid end made their efforts unnecessary.

SARS-CoV hung around long enough for scientists to further their understanding of coronaviruses, though. It turned out that the tip of the virus's spike protein attached to cells in the body by binding to a cellular membrane enzyme called ACE2, which the virus appropriated as a receptor. This knowledge suggested that the spike protein could be an important target for future coronavirus vaccines. It also was now clear that coronaviruses mutated and could jump from animals to humans, and from one human to another.

After SARS ebbed, funding to the field slowed, restoring order in the scientific world. Then, in 2012, a few people in Saudi Arabia began complaining of fever, cough, and shortness of breath. A viral respiratory disease was identified as Middle East respiratory syndrome, or MERS, stemming from another new coronavirus transmitted from bats, this time via camels. MERS was even more lethal than SARS, with a 36 percent mortality rate, though it wasn't as transmissible among humans.

Soon a global health crisis was under way, as the virus causing the disease, MERS-CoV, spread to dozens of countries, sparking renewed interest in coronaviruses that eventually helped McLellan receive the funding he needed for his growing Dartmouth lab.

McLellan and Graham began focusing on a vaccine for MERS, helped in part by a young researcher from China who would play a crucial role in their effort.

• • •

Nianshuang Wang grew up in the 1990s in a tiny village in Shandong Province on China's east coast, the son of peasant farmers who grew wheat, corn, and other crops while also laboring in local factories.

The family had enough food to survive, but they avoided extravagances, such as meat or milk. Wang often dreaded going to school. Winters could be brutal and his classrooms were never heated, so Wang and his schoolmates bundled up and shivered. Some days, his hands and feet were in such deep pain that he couldn't grab a pencil. When he got an answer wrong, he'd brace for a smack from a teacher, a disciplinary method that made him a better student, Wang concedes.

"It worked but it also hurt," he says.

The education Wang most enjoyed came from exploring nature, both in his village and in surrounding areas. He would wander the neighborhood, capturing scorpions, locusts, and other insects, and examining fish and plants. He'd ask endless questions about the scientific rules and principles governing animal and plant life.

"I wanted to know the stories behind the animals," he says. "I didn't care too much about academics, but I was curious about science."

Wang's high school entrance test scores were so high that he received a scholarship that provided free tuition and some spending cash. Later, after winning a spot at Ocean University of China, Wang chose biology as a major, hoping to answer some of the questions of his youth. Moving to Qingdao, a port city of 9 million, was rough. Visiting a supermarket for the first time, Wang resisted putting food in a basket, worried he'd be arrested for stealing. On a bus, he couldn't figure out how to pay his fare, and Wang's roommates teased him for struggling with a video-game console.

"They thought I was stupid," he says.

Wang's top grades boosted his confidence, though, and in 2009 he moved to Tsinghua University in Beijing to begin a PhD program in structural biology at the school some consider the nation's most prestigious. By 2013, Wang had decided to focus on coronaviruses. A decade earlier, China had been at the center of the SARS-CoV outbreak, which infected more than 5,000 people in the country, killing 349 individuals and causing broad socioeconomic unrest. China had been caught unprepared for the epidemic, which had occurred less than five decades after Mao Zedong bade "Farewell to the God of Plagues."[9]

As signs emerged that MERS-CoV was spreading in the Middle East, Wang became part of a group at Tsinghua that raced to determine the configuration of the receptor-binding area of the new virus's spike protein, the spot through which the pathogen infected the body's cells. Wang's group beat competing academic groups to the finish line, his first huge scientific achievement.

Wang, who had a full face and spikey dark hair, was convinced coronaviruses would continue to threaten global health, and he was disturbed by how little was known about them. After reading about McLellan's RSV breakthrough, he applied for an appointment in McLellan's Dartmouth lab, hoping to further develop his expertise in the area and maybe devise a coronavirus vaccine.

Moving to Dartmouth, Wang immediately felt comfortable. He appreciated McLellan's easy sense of humor and the fact that he wore T-shirts and jeans most days. If McLellan disagreed with someone, he usually did little more than raise his eyebrows just a bit. And Wang loved that McLellan was even-keeled, no matter the crisis in the lab, despite the unusual, military-produced caffeine gum he chewed all day for an energy boost.*

Most of all, Wang fell in love with Dartmouth's serene campus, nestled in the woods of Hanover, New Hampshire, where bears, bats, and moose roamed, reminding Wang of the wildlife he remembered from his home village.

By early 2015, Wang and McLellan were working on ways to develop a vaccine for MERS-CoV, focusing on how to teach the immune system

* "Coffee is too slow, the caffeine has to be absorbed by the gut/intestines," McLellan explains about this gum predilection. "Gum causes the caffeine to enter via the gums and circulates within five minutes. Plus no calories."

to recognize the pathogen's spike protein. Their strategy made sense. The body's adaptive immune system sometimes needs help recognizing both friends and foes. Once educated, though, it tends to remember its lessons well, remaining primed to fight its enemies for months or even years after the initial tutorial. The challenge is finding a way to teach the body how to detect a pathogen. Ideally, there's some part of the virus so distinctive that the immune system will recognize the virus just by getting a look at it, or even a piece of the pathogen. Just as many of us can identify Tom Brady simply by seeing his cleft chin, Angelina Jolie by her full lips, or Kim Kardashian by, well, the outline of her derrière, the immune system needs to see only a small, unique portion of a virus to recognize it.[10] But scientists first have to identify what piece or pieces of a virus are its most distinctive feature, the equivalents of Brady's chin, Jolie's lips, and Kardashian's tush.

That's what the spike protein is—the coronavirus's most distinctive trait. McLellan and Wang knew if they could build a version of MERS-CoV's spike protein and expose it to the body's immune system, protective antibodies would be generated and they wouldn't have to inject a piece or version of the actual virus as part of a vaccine.

For months, they met frustration, though. Much like RSV's F protein, the spike protein on the surface of MERS-CoV wouldn't sit still, changing shape before and after infecting cells, a bit like how the spring-loaded coil in a jack-in-the-box jumps to life. Wang and McLellan, along with members of Graham's lab, inserted genetic code to produce the spike protein in cells originally derived from a human fetus or the ovary of a Chinese hamster, but copies of the spike protein weren't potent enough to act as an antigen for a vaccine.

They kept tweaking their code, each change taking weeks to create and test, but they didn't get very far. The immune system needed to see the protein in its prefusion stage to produce protective antibodies, but protein modifications that had worked for RSV weren't locking MERS-CoV's spike protein in place, nor were other, more traditional techniques McLellan and Wang tried.

Graham shared some new advice: Why not take a break and study a more benign coronavirus called HKU1, which causes the flu? A young researcher in Graham's lab had become infected with HKU1, so they had easy access to antibodies. McLellan and Wang began working with Andrew Ward, a young professor at the Scripps Research in La Jolla, California, who used cryo-electron microscopy to get the first detailed picture of the molecular details of the spike protein, including the key helix-shaped area in its stem, which seemed similar to the stem area of MERS-CoV's spike protein.

Now that they had a fuller picture of the structure of these proteins, McLellan and Wang felt confident shifting back to MERS. They were eager to test an idea they had developed to keep the virus's spike protein in the ideal prefusion shape. Sitting in front of his computer, Wang designed a genetic sequence that added two rigid amino acids, called prolines, to the stem of MERS-CoV's spike protein. Like contractors redesigning a building, Wang and McLellan were adding scaffolding to keep their structure from collapsing.

In February 2016, Wang took their digital genetic code, inserted it into a culture of human cells, and found that it produced a stable version of the spike protein—and in large quantities, too.

"We got it," he emailed McLellan.

Kizzmekia Corbett, a newly hired viral immunologist in Graham's lab, began testing their new vaccine in mice, demonstrating that the shots produced five times as many titers as the unstabilized spike protein. They had yet to show it provided other animals with protection, let alone humans, but McLellan and Graham were convinced they had determined an effective vaccine antigen for MERS-CoV, a huge accomplishment.

They entire team was elated. Well, everyone but Wang.

• • •

In his short time in the country, Wang had helped achieve a better understanding of HKU1 and determine ways to attack that virus. Now he had helped design the genetic sequence to produce MERS-CoV's spike protein in a perfect shape, one that could teach the immune system to ward off the virus. Perhaps most important, Wang and his colleagues were sure their techniques could be applied to the next, inevitable outbreak of a coronavirus, or any other similar pathogen that relies on a spike protein.

Then, in March 2016, a month after his breakthrough, Wang and his wife, who used the English name Joy, welcomed their first child, a daughter named Grace—still more good news.

Instead of elation, though, Wang was despondent.

Working with McLellan, Corbett, and others in Graham and Ward's labs, Wang had submitted a paper detailing their MERS research, demonstrating a potentially universal method of stabilizing the coronavirus's spike protein to enable an effective vaccine, but the paper had been rejected by all five of the leading scientific journals. One reviewer called their data an "artifact," while another decided they "did not provide a broad conceptual advance."

Ouch.

Wang wanted a senior academic position of his own and to lead his own lab someday, but he knew there was no way he was going to get ahead without published work. Joy tried to cheer him up, as did McLellan. Sometimes it takes time for peers to appreciate new research, McLellan told him. But Wang continued to spiral. He felt pressure outside the lab, too. He had spent so much time on the MERS vaccine and writing the paper that he had neglected Joy and his newborn.

"You need to contribute more to this family," Joy told him one evening.

Wang promised to do more to help at home, but said he needed to wait until his paper was published.

"This can change the field," he told her unconvincingly. "It can help us prepare for another pandemic."

To Wang, each rejection felt like a fresh blow. He wasn't the first author on the HKU1 paper, so he needed one that belonged to him. Wang became resigned to finding an entirely new project. He'd have to devote many more years to research and then write a new paper in order to get a new job. When McLellan accepted a senior faculty position at the University of Texas at Austin, Wang reluctantly joined his lab there, quickly finding that he missed Dartmouth's easygoing environment.

The worries piled up. As a postdoc, Wang didn't make much money, and now he faced additional expenses related to his child. He and Joy didn't have green cards allowing them to permanently stay in the country, and he feared being sent back to China after his visa expired, with too little to show for all his hard work in the United States.

The group's paper eventually was accepted for publication by a respected, though second-tier, journal, but most scientists ignored the research, many still uninterested in coronaviruses, a reaction that left Wang further dejected.

"People will find it," McLellan told him, trying to cheer him up.

At night, Wang found it hard to sleep. In the morning, he couldn't get out of bed, overcome with sadness and exhaustion. Sensing her husband was battling depression, Joy urged him to see a therapist, an idea McLellan backed.

Wang visited a local therapist who put Wang on antidepressants. His mood improved, but Wang had trouble stringing his thoughts together, so he stopped taking the medicine, which left him on edge and led to frequent squabbles with his wife and McLellan.

"I became really sensitive," Wang says. "I had conflicts with the two people trying to help me."

Slowly, Wang emerged from his darkness. He decided that devoting himself to his family would be his goal and that he'd worry a little less about what peers thought of his work. Publications don't define talent and achievement, he realized.

"I accepted myself and struggled to climb from the bottom," he says.

Around the same time in late 2017, his research with McLellan began to receive more recognition, at least among coronavirus specialists. Wang, McLellan, Graham, and their colleagues had achieved an understanding of the structure of coronaviruses and how to tame their unstable spike protein. They also had a blueprint for a potentially effective MERS vaccine.

The researchers didn't have proof their approach worked, though. And they'd need a lot of help to make it into an effective vaccine. Just as architects draw up plans that look great on paper but still need to be translated into an actual product, they and their colleagues needed a company to produce their MERS shots and find an effective way to consistently get it into the body's cells.

Graham was becoming enthused about Stéphane Bancel and Moderna, convinced that using messenger RNA was an ideal vaccine approach and that the company was onto something special.

He had no idea of the trouble Moderna was dealing with.

9

2014–2017

Kerry Benenato was struggling to solve Moderna's biggest problem.

Three years earlier, in 2014, Eric Huang and Stephen Hoge had convinced Stéphane Bancel and the rest of Moderna's leadership to shift the company's focus to vaccines from drugs, a pivot that seemed to save Moderna from failure. By 2017, Moderna and Barney Graham's group at the National Institutes of Health were discussing working together to develop messenger RNA–based vaccines, a partnership that Moderna's executives hoped would prove valuable.

There remained a huge obstacle in Moderna's way, however. It was up to Benenato, a forty-year-old organic chemist, to find a way out of their difficulty. Benenato got an early hint of the hurdle three years earlier, when she was first hired. When a colleague gave her a company tour, she was introduced to Moderna's chief scientific officer, Joseph Bolen, who seemed unusually excited to meet her.

"Oh, great!" Bolen said with a smile. "She's the one who's gonna solve delivery."

Bolen gave a hearty laugh and walked away, but Benenato detected seriousness in his quip.

Solve delivery?

It was a lot to expect from a young scientist already dealing with insecurities and self-doubt. Benenato was an accomplished researcher who most recently had worked at AstraZeneca after completing postdoctoral studies at Harvard University. Despite her impressive credentials, Benenato battled a lack of confidence that sometimes got in her way. Performance reviews from past employers had been positive, but they usually produced similar critiques: Be more vocal. Do a better job advocating for your ideas. Give us more, Kerry.

Benenato was petite and soft-spoken. She sometimes stuttered or relied on "ums" and "ahs" when she became nervous, especially in front of groups, part of why she sometimes didn't feel comfortable speaking up.

"I'm an introvert," she says. "Self-confidence is something that's always been an issue."

Soon after assuming a spot in Moderna's lab in late 2014, Benenato got a sense of why the company needed so much help. Its vaccine approach seemed promising—the team was packaging mRNAs in microscopic fatty-acid compounds called lipid nanoparticles, or LNPs, that protected the molecules on their way into cells. Moderna's shots should have been producing ample and long-lasting proteins. But the company's scientists were alarmed—they were injecting shots deep into the muscle of mice, but their immune systems were mounting spirited responses to the foreign components of the LNPs. The body wasn't tolerating the microscopic encasements, especially upon repeated dosing.

Moderna's mRNAs were stirring the immune system—exactly what got Huang so excited a few years earlier. But the molecules were also producing drastic side-effects, as the body reacted to the LNPs. This toxicity was a huge issue for the Moderna team: A vaccine or drug that caused sharp pain and awful fevers wasn't going to prove very popular.

Delivering mRNA into cells had long bedeviled scientists, of course.

Katalin Karikó and Drew Weissman had introduced modifications to mRNA's chemical building blocks so the molecule wouldn't set off the immune system as it passed through the cell membrane into the cytoplasm. Jason Schrum and others at Moderna had introduced important improvements to Karikó and Weissman's methods. But the complications hadn't been fully resolved—mRNA still had to be wrapped in the fatty nanoparticles to have a chance at producing plentiful proteins. It was this mRNA encasement that was now causing all the hand-wringing within Moderna.

Scientists had long struggled to find the perfect packaging for mRNA molecules. During the 1970s, Bob Langer, the Moderna cofounder, was among those who had helped pioneer early approaches to delivering large molecules, like DNA and RNA, overcoming deep skepticism from academics and others who were sure they were too big and fragile to make the journey from outside the body to the inside of a human cell. Langer and the others developed ways to wrap nucleic acids in tiny particles, including tiny polymer or lipid particles, which protected them from destruction by the body's enzymes.

Over the next three decades, various academics and companies improved on these methods. Their work helped lay the foundation for a company called Alnylam Pharmaceuticals, which in the 2000s managed to get RNA molecules into cells in LNPs. Alnylam succeeded in shutting off unhealthy gene expression, something called RNA interference, an important early sign of the benefits of LNPs. Later, a Canadian company invented a different kind of lipid encasement that did a good job shielding mRNA, a technology that Moderna had licensed.

But all LNP packaging, including the one from the Canadians, can generate problematic reactions as lipids accumulate in injection sites, something the Moderna team was now realizing. The company's scientists had done everything they could to try to make the molecule's swathing material disappear soon after entering the cells, in order to avoid the unfortunate side effects, such as chills and headaches, but they weren't making much headway and frustration was mounting. Somehow, the researchers needed to find a way to get the encasements—made of little balls of fat, cholesterol, and other substances—to deliver their payload mRNA and then quickly vanish, like a parent dropping a teenager off at a party, to avoid setting off the immune system in unpleasant ways, even as the RNA and the proteins the molecule created stuck around.

Benenato needed to find a solution.

She wasn't entirely shocked by the challenges Moderna was facing. One of the reasons she had joined the upstart company was to help develop its delivery technology. She just didn't realize how pressing the issue was, or how stymied the researchers had become. Benenato also didn't know that Moderna board members were among those most discouraged by the delivery issue. In board meetings, some of them pointed out that pharmaceutical giants like Roche Holding and Novartis had worked on similar issues and hadn't managed to develop lipid nanoparticles that were both effective and well tolerated by the body. Why would Moderna have any more luck?

Stephen Hoge insisted the company could yet find a solution.

"There's no way the only innovations in LNP are going to come from some academics and a small Canadian company," insisted Hoge, who convinced the executives that hiring Benenato might help deliver an answer.

Benenato got to work, quickly realizing that while Moderna might have been a hot Boston-area start-up, it wasn't set up to do the chemistry necessary to solve their LNP problem. Much of its equipment was old or secondhand, and it was the kind used to tinker with mRNAs, not lipids.

"It was scary," she says.

When Benenato saw the company had a nuclear magnetic resonance spectrometer, which allows chemists to see the molecular structure of material, she let out a sigh of relief. Then Benenato inspected the machine and realized it was a jalopy. The hulking, aging instrument had been decommissioned and left behind by a previous tenant, too old and banged up to bring with them. Benenato began experimenting with different chemical changes for Moderna's LNPs, but without a working spectrometer she and her colleagues had to have samples ready by noon each day, so they could be picked up by an outside company that would perform the necessary analysis. After a few weeks, her superiors received an enormous bill for the outsourced work and decided to pay to get the old spectrometer running again.

After a few months of futility, Benenato became impatient. An overachiever who could be hard on herself, she was eager to impress her new bosses.

Benenato felt pressure outside the office, as well. She was married with a preschool-age daughter and an eighteen-month-old son. In her last job, Benenato's commute had been a twenty-minute trip to AstraZeneca's office in Waltham, outside Boston; now she was traveling an hour to Moderna's Cambridge offices. She became anxious—how was she going to devote the long hours she realized were necessary to solve their LNP quandary while providing her children proper care? Joining Moderna was beginning to feel like a possible mistake.

She turned to her husband and father for help. They reminded her of the hard work she had devoted to establishing her career and said it would be a shame if she couldn't take on the new challenge. Benenato's husband said he was happy to stay home with the kids, alleviating some of her concerns.

Back in the office, she got to work. She wanted to make lipids that were easier for the body to chop into smaller pieces, so they could be eliminated by the body's enzymes. Until then, Moderna, like most others, relied on all kinds of complicated chemicals to hold its LNP packaging together. They weren't natural, though, so the body was having a hard time breaking them down, causing the toxicity.

Benenato began experimenting with simpler chemicals. She inserted "ester bonds"—compounds referred to in chemical circles as "handles" because the body easily grabs them and breaks them apart. Ester bonds had two things going for them: They were strong enough to help ensure the LNP remained stable, acting much like a drop of oil in water, but they also gave the body's enzymes something to target and break down as soon as the LNP entered the cell, a way to quickly rid the body of the potentially toxic LNP components. Benenato thought the inclusion of these chemicals might speed the elimination of the LNP delivery material.

This idea, Benenato realized, was nothing more than traditional, medicinal chemistry. Most people didn't use ester bonds because they were pretty unsophisticated. But, hey, the tricky stuff wasn't working, so Benenato thought she'd see if the simple stuff worked.

Benenato also wanted to try to replace a group of unnatural chemicals in the LNP that was contributing to the spirited and unwelcome response from the immune system. Benenato set out to build a new and improved chemical combination. She began with ethanolamine, a colorless, natural chemical, an obvious start for any chemist hoping to build a more complex chemical combination. No one relied on ethanolamine on its own. Benenato was curious, though. What would happen if she used just these two simple modifications to the LNP: ethanolamine with the ester bonds?

Right away, Benenato noticed her new, supersimple compound helped mRNA create some protein in animals. It wasn't much, but it was a surprising and positive sign. Benenato spent over a year refining her solution, testing more than one hundred variations, all using ethanolamine and ester bonds, showing improvements with each new version of LNP. After finishing her 102nd version of the lipid molecule, which she named SM102, Benenato was confident enough in her work to show it to Hoge and others.

They immediately got excited. The team kept tweaking the composition of the lipid encasement. In 2017, they wrapped it around mRNA molecules and injected the new combination in mice and then monkeys. They saw plentiful, potent proteins were being produced *and* the lipids were quickly being eliminated, just as Benenato and her colleagues had hoped. They had their special sauce.

That year, Benenato was asked to deliver a presentation to Bancel, Noubar Afeyan, and Moderna's executive committee to explain why it made sense to use the new, simpler LNP formulation for all its mRNA vaccines. She still needed approval from the executives to make the change. Ahead of the meeting, she was apprehensive, as some of her earlier anxieties returned. But an unusual calm came over her as she began speaking to the group. Benenato explained how experimenting with basic, overlooked chemicals had led to her discovery. She said she had merely stumbled onto the company's solution, though her bosses understood the efforts that had been necessary for the breakthrough. The board complimented her work and agreed with the idea of switching to the new LNP. Benenato beamed with pride.

"As a scientist, serendipity has been my best friend," she told the executives.

• • •

Barney Graham watched Moderna's progress in 2017 with keen interest. Graham was a vaccine guy who'd long been intrigued by the idea of developing mRNA shots. He wanted shots that could be rolled out quickly to combat a new epidemic or even pandemic, and he viewed the older approaches as too slow and costly. Killing or weakening an actual virus and then growing cells and building manufacturing plants to produce proteins for old-school vaccines can take months, if not years.

Yes, elsewhere in the country, Dan Barouch was hard at work perfecting vaccines using the Ad26 adenovirus for HIV, while over in Oxford, England, Adrian Hill was plugging away on his chimpanzee-adenovirus shots. Graham agreed that those vaccines had potential. But he also remembered how Merck's Ad5 HIV shots back in the early 2000s failed in an awful way, in some cases worsening test subjects' conditions. He understood that Barouch and Hill were developing shots with very different adenoviruses, but he still worried about antivector cellular immunity, or the concern that a segment of the population has already developed antibodies against adenoviruses. That was the issue that had caused Merck's AIDS shot to go so wrong, resulting in tragedy.

By contrast, the idea that an mRNA molecule could ferry genetic messages into cells, allowing the body to make proteins, effectively turning it into a vaccine factory, held tremendous appeal.

"I'm thinking that using this technology may be a quicker way to screen our antigen design for flu, RSV, HIV, MERS, etc.," Graham wrote a colleague after first being introduced to Moderna back in September 2015. "It is more potent than DNA and probably faster than vectors."

With mRNA vaccines, Graham and his colleagues only needed to provide cells with a set of genetic instructions to spur them to make proteins that could serve as vaccine antigens.

"RNA is the most elemental way to make a protein," Graham says.

By 2017, Moderna had produced an early version of an mRNA flu vaccine that looked promising. But the company struggled in its attempts to produce an effective Zika vaccine, suggesting it might need some help. That year, Moderna and Graham's team agreed to join forces to develop vaccines. The government scientists would design the genetic code at the heart of the shots, while Moderna would produce the mRNA molecules, wrapping them with Benenato's new lipids.

The two partners immediately produced a vaccine for MERS-CoV, the coronavirus that was causing MERS. Their shots generated impressive levels of antibodies in tests on mice and monkeys, but before testing on humans could proceed, the MERS epidemic died out. Nevertheless, the two teams were pretty sure their shots would have proven effective, and maybe would have been enough to halt that coronavirus.

They vowed to team up, once again, if a similar virus ever emerged.

• • •

Bancel was convinced his company was making progress. Outsiders were dubious.

Bancel and Moderna had long attracted skeptics, initially because the company was betting on its ability to shepherd mRNA molecules into the body to create proteins for drugs, something that had never before been done. A few years earlier, when Orn Almarsson, a senior Moderna scientist, traveled to the West Coast to try to hire drug veteran James Cunningham, he was blunt about why he wouldn't work at Moderna.

"I don't believe it, you've got nothing," Cunningham told him, Almarsson recalls. "How are you going to make mRNA? I don't see how you're going to be able to do that."

Over time, the skepticism became outright suspicion. There was something about Bancel that most everyone in the biotech and research communities didn't like. He wasn't a scientist, for one thing. Bancel and Moderna were still super secretive, avoiding conferences and refraining from publishing in scientific journals. Promising to develop breakthrough drugs, but then shifting to vaccines, made others wary. Bancel was a foreign-born CEO with a thick French accent, which probably didn't help matters.

Some snickered that Moderna was a "VC creation," suggesting it was merely an effort by its founding backers, including Noubar Afeyan and Flagship Pioneering, to create some hype, raise money, and then bring the company public before they exited with big profits. Some resented that Bancel spent so much time highlighting all the money he had raised—one year, he even brought it up at Moderna's

Christmas party—an emphasis that seemed unbecoming for someone running a company that was trying to save lives.

There was something else going on, too. In October 2015, *The Wall Street Journal*'s John Carreyrou had begun a series of investigative stories raising serious questions about a high-flying blood-testing start-up, Theranos Inc., and its chief executive, Elizabeth Holmes. Eventually, Theranos would be exposed as a fraud.

Now some journalists, investors, and others in the scientific world were on the lookout for the next Theranos. Holmes and Bancel were both smooth and telegenic salespeople who had raised a shocking amount of cash, sometimes from investors with limited scientific backgrounds. They ran secretive companies. And weirdly, Holmes and Bancel both favored turtlenecks, à la Apple founder Steve Jobs. Moderna vowed to change the world but wouldn't share a shred of proof to back its claims; it wasn't a good look.

Sometimes the detractors made it harder for Moderna to hire top researchers, a huge problem in an industry that viciously competes for talent. In 2015, when Melissa Moore was courted to join the company in a senior position, she loved the idea of pursuing mRNA medicines but was nervous about the Theranos chatter. Moore's wife, who had heard the accusations about Bancel and Moderna, urged her not to accept the job. The couple had only made it through the 2008 financial crisis thanks to Moore's tenured academic position at the University of Massachusetts Medical School. Now she was going to give it up for a company that might be a fraud?

"It took me a year to convince her," Moore says.

The whisper campaign took an emotional toll on Moderna's senior scientists and executives, including Hoge. He saw the scientific advances his colleagues were making and couldn't understand the nonstop accusations.

Why do people hate us so much?

By 2016, the doubt was spilling out into the open. In February of that year, top-tier life-science journal *Nature Biotechnology* published a devastating piece criticizing Moderna's lack of openness about its work, noting that the company hadn't published a single research paper about its therapeutics work. A few years earlier, Ken Chien, the Moderna cofounder, had published a paper in that very journal, work that became the basis for the AstraZeneca deal. But that was a rare exception for a company that was trying its best to avoid providing hints of the details of its progress to its competitors.

The *Nature Biotechnology* article, entitled "Research Not Fit to Print," not only compared Bancel and Moderna to Holmes and Theranos, but it went on to argue that Moderna even bore a resemblance to Kadmon Holdings, the drug company founded by Sam Waksal, a notorious executive who had served five years in federal prison in the mid-2000s for insider trading and other crimes.[1]

"Moderna, Theranos, Kadmon and companies like them may think they are better off if no one knows what they do or how they do it," the journal said. "But there will come a time when they have to decide whether to trust the community with their data. If they don't, the community may start to ask whether these companies themselves can be trusted."

As always, Bancel and Moderna dismissed the criticism. They didn't want rivals hearing about their activities, but at some point, when they were more comfortable their competitors couldn't catch up, they were committed to sharing details about their research.

The most biting criticism came from the well-read health-care website STAT in September 2016, when it published a punishing piece with the headline: "Ego, Ambition, and Turmoil: Inside One of Biotech's Most Secretive Startups."[2] In the nearly three-thousand-word article, author Damian Garde described a "caustic work environment" at Moderna that was chasing talent away. He said there were signs Moderna was running into problems with various vaccine projects, citing interviews with more than twenty current and former employees, and others.

"Bancel has hampered progress at Moderna because of his ego, his need to assert control and his impatience," Garde wrote, adding that Moderna had a "culture of recrimination" and that Bancel "prized the company's ever-increasing valuation, now approaching $5 billion, over its science."

There was barely an aspect of the company's operations, or of Bancel's leadership, the article didn't disparage, cementing a view of Bancel and Moderna as money-hungry renegades likely to fail.

• • •

In January 2017, Bancel flew to San Francisco to speak at a mega conference hosted by JPMorgan Chase, an annual gathering that serves as the health-care industry's Woodstock, though money, not music, is on everyone's mind. That week, thousands of executives and investors piled into the elegant Westin St. Francis on Union Square, with others in nearby downtown hotels, many paying more than a thousand dollars a night to hear a week of pitches from top executives of the world's drug companies about their products and plans.

It had been four months since STAT published its critical article, and Bancel hoped to convince attendees that Moderna was making headway. He had helped raise billions of dollars in private sales of the company's shares and Moderna was worth billions, but expenses were piling up. Bancel knew the company would have to sell shares in an initial public offering to have a chance of producing any vaccines or drugs, so drumming up investor interest was crucial.

He gave an upbeat address, describing Moderna's first potential products, including its vaccines, as well as the VEGF therapy for heart failure being developed with AstraZeneca in the first phase of clinical trials. Some in the audience were enthused about Moderna's prospects, and Bancel was hopeful he and Moderna were moving past the bad publicity.

A day later, though, Garde and STAT published a new article, this one describing "troubling safety problems" associated with a treatment Moderna was developing with biotech giant Alexion Pharmaceuticals for a rare and debilitating disease known as Crigler-Najjar syndrome. The drug had been indefinitely delayed, Garde reported, forcing Moderna to focus on its "less lucrative" vaccines.

Later that day, in a room Moderna rented in a nearby hotel so the company could host private meetings with investors, a downcast Bancel met with biotech investor Brad Loncar. It was a business conversation, but Loncar brought a beer and a bottle opener, hoping to lift Bancel's spirits. He accepted the drink and they shared it together.

"I felt so bad for him," Loncar says.

The drumbeat of criticism got so loud Noubar Afeyan felt compelled to publicly back Bancel.

"Stéphane is often cited for the amount of capital he's raised," Afeyan said in a Moderna press release. "But I think what's often overshadowed by that big number is the pioneering mRNA-therapeutics technology that is at the root of Moderna."

Afeyan didn't share any details about the company's research efforts, so most scientists ignored his defense.

• • •

Bancel heard carping and criticism, and he knew some in the industry suspected he was pulling off an enormous fraud. The accusations bothered some Moderna executives and scientists, including Hoge, and Bancel's family and friends also expressed concern. Not so much, Bancel. He had a remarkable amount of self-assuredness and was able to shrug off the criticism quickler than his colleagues.

Bancel had more pressing worries on his mind. By late 2017, he was starting to feel competition closing in. Moderna was making progress in its various mRNA vaccines and there was reason to hope it could yet figure out a way to develop effective drugs. But Bancel feared Moderna wasn't moving fast enough, though few of his colleagues shared his concerns.

Executives at the company sometimes half joked that one day, a big pharmaceutical company would seize on the possibilities of mRNA, and then Moderna would be in true trouble.

"Someday, Pfizer will wake up and pour money into this," a Moderna executive told a colleague one day. He didn't actually *expect* that to happen, though. Working with mRNA was still über-unpopular and it didn't seem likely a major drugmaker would risk investor backlash by attempting to develop the molecule for vaccines or drugs.

Over time, though, Bancel became increasingly convinced that someone was going to catch up to Moderna. Starting a successful company was never his goal—Bancel was already wealthy and accomplished. He wanted to *dominate* a new industry in a way Genentech never could. That was the point of all that cash he worked so hard to raise; Moderna needed it to establish a stranglehold on the mRNA industry.

"Time is your enemy," Bancel told staffers at the company, over and over again. "If we're not ahead we're behind."

Bancel read a book about the growth of Uber Technologies. Others who knew the book usually focused on how ruthless and rough-edged the ride-sharing service's original chief executive, Travis Kalanick, had been, but that wasn't Bancel's concern. Instead, he was struck by how swiftly the company had acted to grab market share before inevitable fierce competition emerged. In meeting after meeting at the office, Bancel kept coming back to the company.

"Uber didn't invent taxis, they didn't invent ride-sharing," Bancel said to senior executives. "What did they do?"

Bancel scanned the room, as if quizzing his team, before providing his own answer.

"They scaled quicker than anyone else!"

Every minute counts, every second counts, Bancel kept emphasizing. We're in a race, he said.

Some of the executives thought the exhortations were a bit much, even hackneyed. *We get it, Stéphane, we need to move fast. But there's no one bearing down on us. Relax a bit.*

"It was jarring to a lot of people, there didn't seem like a lot of people in the race," says Greg Licholai, Bancel's former business school classmate who headed Moderna's efforts to find medicines and vaccines for rare diseases. "He was talking like we were Coke, but there wasn't a Pepsi."

Underlings may have rolled their eyes, but Bancel was onto something. There indeed was another company, nearly four thousand miles and a huge ocean away, making its own progress working with mRNA. Before long, that company would emerge as a genuine rival, exactly what Bancel most feared.

10

2001–2017

Uğur Şahin had no idea what was coming for him.

It was the summer of 1968 and the three-year-old was kicking a soccer ball down a narrow street in İskenderun, a mountainous Turkish port city on the Mediterranean coast, not far from the Syrian border. Decades earlier, Uğur's family, like others in the neighborhood, had moved from the island of Crete, settling in a town of seventy-five thousand marked by clustered neighborhoods and unusually close relations between its Muslim, Christian, and Jewish residents.

It was late afternoon, and the sun was setting as Uğur ambled along, passing a group of older women on wooden chairs relaxing and chatting after another hard day. Out of nowhere, a car turned a nearby corner at high speed, bearing down on the young boy, who was oblivious to the danger. Just then, one of the women leapt from her chair and grabbed the boy by his arm, yanking him to safety. Uğur Şahin's life had been spared. He would dedicate himself to saving others.

Not long after that eventful afternoon, Uğur and his mother,

Kadriye, moved to the Turkish city of Niğde before joining Uğur's father, Ihsan, in West Germany. That nation, which was enjoying an economic boom, had invited Turkish citizens to be guest workers, or Gastarbeiter. The immigrants provided a new source of cheap labor as their own economic opportunities. The Şahin family settled near Cologne, where Uğur's father worked on the floor of a local Ford Motor Company factory and his mother found a job in the factory's cafeteria.

Growing up, Uğur had two main interests: soccer and science. He and friends played hours-long games that frequently started as six-on-six friendly matches and ended as hard-fought, fifteen-on-fifteen battles. Uğur was a top midfielder in a Cologne youth league, but his success on the pitch was sometimes tinged with pain.[1] The local boys could be insulting and physically intimidating, Uğur later told a friend, often leaving the boy with bruises. Uğur vowed to escape the rough area and leave his own mark.

On the field, Uğur demonstrated a competitive streak that startled teammates. "If he lost he would get sad and cry," recalls Recep Aydin, a friend at the time. "Then he'd get even more ambitious."

At home, Uğur was sensitive and unusually observant. He was troubled when members of his extended family became seriously ill with the disease and noticed how fearful adults were about developing cancer.

Why don't people do something about cancer? he wondered.

Uğur became interested in how the body's defenses sometimes successfully fight cancer, and he was captivated by an animated German television show detailing the immune system. Soon Uğur was heading to a local library, where he devoured books about how the body is constructed, as well as the basics behind rockets, trains, and planets.

"I was curious, I wanted to understand things," he says. "The principles, the basics, how things worked. I loved soccer and I loved books."

As he grew older, Uğur told friends he wanted to be a physician. His parents provided encouragement, instilling their son with a rare self-confidence. Uğur's grades were mediocre, however, so he wasn't selected to attend an advanced, college-preparatory high school, called a gymnasium, setting the young man on an almost-certain path toward a blue-collar career. But a neighbor who saw potential in Uğur stepped in to advocate for him, helping hm gain a spot at Cologne's Erich Kästner-Gymnasium, becoming the first child of a guest worker to attend the school. There, Uğur blossomed, winning regional competitions and graduating atop his class in 1984.

After studying at the University of Cologne and receiving a PhD in cancer immunotherapy, Şahin was accepted as a trainee-doctor in a hospital in the German state of Saarland, becoming a resident on a cancer ward in the early 1990s. There, a patient once asked Şahin to explain the potential benefit of joining a trial for a new drug that promised to lengthen the patient's life a bit but couldn't cure his cancer. Şahin struggled with an answer, becoming determined to discover better methods of helping those with the disease, and specifically to find ways to activate the body's immune system to destroy cancer cells.

"We have to have better medicine," he told a colleague.

Early on, Şahin supervised Özlem Türeci, a young physician also of Turkish heritage, though her family was from the metropolis of Istanbul. They quickly bonded over a shared love of science and an eagerness to find ways to aid their patients. Türeci had enjoyed an early exposure to the world of medicine. Her father had been recruited to be a surgeon in a small hospital in the city of Lastrup while also running a local medical practice, and her mother was a biologist. The family lived across the street from the local hospital, and Türeci often accompanied her father to work, viewing an appendectomy at the age of six.[2]

As a girl, Türeci declared her intention of becoming a nun, which came as a surprise to her family, since she wasn't especially religious. They eventually understood her motivation: Türeci's father's hospital was in a repurposed monastery, and local nuns assumed various roles in the institution, including caring for patients. To Türeci, serving as a nun and healing patients seemed the ideal career.

"It was my early dream," she says. "But it was a big misunderstanding."

A few years later, Türeci realized that she was better suited to be a physician or a scientist. Studying for a medical degree at Saarland University Faculty of Medicine in Hamburg, she became attracted to the idea of exploring new medical technologies, something else that connected her with Şahin, who became her serious boyfriend.

Türeci, who completed a PhD dissertation on molecular biology, saw that physicians were developing a better understanding of the mechanisms of cancer, yet the pace of drug development was molasses slow. While treating patients in cancer wards, she, too, vowed to find ways to translate the expanding knowledge in the field into new drugs.

We should be able to offer so much more, Türeci thought.

They were a distinctive-looking couple. Şahin had close-cropped hair and thick, dark eyebrows. Around his neck, he wore a traditional Turkish amulet, known as a Nazar in Arabic, that's meant to protect against evil. Türeci had green eyes, wore glasses, and kept her wavy, dark hair short. Both about five foot five and soft-spoken, the young scientists shared an easy banter and were unusually respectful and supportive of each other's work and aspirations.

Şahin and Türeci were chosen by Michael Pfreundschuh, a lymphoma expert who was Şahin's thesis adviser, to be part of a small team in Pfreundschuh's Hamburg laboratory, where they worked on new methods to identify tumor-specific antigens, which are proteins or molecules found on cancer cells. Others focused on writing academic papers that might be accepted in scientific journals, but Şahin and Türeci were intent on translating their knowledge into concrete ways to help those suffering from cancer.

The couple's closeness became a problem, however, as did their competitiveness. Pfreundschuh bred intense rivalries among young scientists in his lab, believing that conflict and pressure lead to breakthroughs. He hosted weekly meetings in which he encouraged researchers to criticize one another's work, stoking various clashes. Şahin and Türeci embraced the intense environment and were viewed by others as overly ambitious. Labmates enjoyed discussing progress they were making on various projects and comparing techniques, but Şahin and Türeci rarely shared details of their own work, sparking resentment from peers.

"They kept to themselves and took the competition more seriously than others," says Bjöern Cochlovius, a colleague at the time.

Şahin exhibited similar impulses outside the lab. Each year, the scientists left for a day of exercise and fun in a nearby park, an outing highlighted by a relay race, four legs of four hundred meters each. Most viewed the day as a rare opportunity for bonding and relaxation. Not Şahin. He hungered to win each year's competition, and he usually succeeded. One time, though, his team lost by a nose, with Şahin running the anchor leg. He was stunned by the result, so upset after the race that he told a teammate he needed time to calm himself, taking a half-hour walk so his anger could dissipate.

Back in the lab, someone asked Şahin how he was doing.

"I'm *fine*," he said, demonstrating an irritation that told a very different story.

"The race mattered to him in some important way," says Thomas Brunk, a labmate.

Others found Şahin's reaction distasteful, but Brunk saw it as a sign he'd likely go far in science.

"The research world is one big competition," Brunk says.

As Şahin and Türeci assumed senior roles in Pfreundschuh's lab in the 1990s, they made progress in their research. They developed a technology called SEREX, which demonstrated that a variety of cancerous tumors spark specific responses from the immune system. The technology suggested there may be ways to introduce vaccines enabling the immune system to fight cancer. They searched for ways to inject antigens into the skin, an approach that didn't work but showed a creativity that impressed some in the field.

Over time, Şahin and Türeci became friendlier presences in the lab, helping younger scientists with their research and even their personal lives. After Brunk went through a difficult breakup with his girlfriend, they were supportive, reducing some of the pressures he faced at work, providing encouragement as Brunk finished his PhD thesis, and lending an ear as he detailed his relationship drama.

"I wasn't in good shape, but they treated me like a family member," Brunk says.

A bit later, Şahin and Türeci moved to Mainz, a German city on the Rhine River that's best known as the home of Johannes Gutenberg, the father of modern typography. The couple had been wooed by a rival of Pfreundschuh named Christopher Huber, who ran a lab and was chairman of the department of hematology and oncology at the Johannes Gutenberg University Mainz. A native of Vienna, Huber had come to Mainz to establish a hub of immunotherapy research in the university town. He offered Şahin and Türeci the chance to build their own research group, promising support from the government and other bodies. Charismatic and well connected, Huber became a mentor to the scientists, teaching Şahin and Türeci how close connections to politicians and financial support from investors and others could enable breakthroughs.

Şahin, Türeci, and Huber spent several years creating genetically modified lymphocytes, which are important immune cells, identifying markers on tumors that could stir the immune system, and doing other work to try to teach the immune system to fight off cancer. In 2000, Şahin spent time at the University of Zurich, where he worked in the lab of Rolf Zinkernagel, a 1996 Nobel Prize winner, and Hans Hengartner, an upbeat immunologist who detected something different in Şahin. Some postdocs are well versed in the scientific literature, while others are skilled at developing innovative ideas in the lab. But Şahin showed a unique ability to analyze existing data, extract the most important ideas from scientific literature, and apply them to his own work.

As Hengartner got to know Türeci, he decided they made a formidable pairing.

"Özlem is more a realizer of ideas, she sets goals and finds a way to meet them," he says. "Uğur is more imaginative and creative—in his head, his ideas are crystal clear, but out of his mouth they're not, unlike Özlem. Together, they complement each other."

Labmates understood that Şahin and Türeci were descendants of immigrants, and they were eager to hear how the couple felt about German immigration policies, Turkish politics, or other issues. The colleagues detected unease in the pair, though, and usually dropped the subject, sometimes reluctantly. Hengartner shared his own criticisms of some of Berlin's policies, but he couldn't get Şahin to offer an opinion. Their entire focus was their research.

"They just didn't want to be involved in national differences," says someone close to Şahin and Türeci. "I always hoped they would take a more vocal role, but they never wanted to speak about these issues."

In 2001, the couple decided to start a company to develop cancer therapies, to fulfill their long-term goals of turning research into therapeutic products. They named it Ganymed Pharmaceuticals, a derivation of the Turkish word "ganimet," which means trophy, usually the kind that results from some kind of difficult battle, as well as a nod to Ganymede, the handsome young Trojan of Greek mythology. The dot-com bubble had recently burst, big pharmaceutical companies weren't interested in their venture, and little money was available for German biotechnology start-ups. But Hengartner helped woo wealthy German families and others to invest in the new company, including a Swiss venture-capital firm called Nextech Invest, led by Alfred Scheidegger, who had a PhD in microbiology and biochemistry. The team had grand ambitions—Şahin spoke of building a German version of Genentech, the San Francisco biotech power that Bancel also was obsessed with—but their resources were puny. Nextech invested about 20 million euros, while Şahin, Türeci, and other employees chipped in a total of approximately 50,000 euro.

At that point, Türeci was thirty-four years old and Şahin was thirty-six. Neither had experience working in a biotech company, let alone running one, and they both wanted to continue their academic research. So Scheidegger installed professional managers to run Ganymed. The company worked on monoclonal-antibody drugs, or those designed in the lab to bind to and inhibit cancer cells or other proteins and mimic the function of natural antibodies. The company also targeted a variety of other diseases, including multiple sclerosis.

Türeci and Şahin wanted to use novel technologies, maybe even messenger RNA molecules, which they had studied while working with Huber. But those approaches didn't seem ready, nor was it clear the investors would have had patience for them to perfect novel therapeutic methods. Instead, Ganymed's scientists searched for antigens from various diseases capable of stirring the immune system as part of a drug or vaccine, a strategy that was a bit more mainstream.

Early progress was slow, and eventually Türeci assumed the position of chief executive while Şahin ran the company's research and development. They led the company as equal partners. With their backers and others, Türeci was the charmer, smoothly explaining the company's scientific activities while assuaging investor concerns. Şahin was the big-idea guy, describing Ganymed's ambitious goals while radiating confidence and determination. When Şahin's scientific spiels got too complex, Türeci would break them into pieces and explain them to the investors in simple terms.

The pair weren't traditional German pharmaceutical executives. Şahin wore T-shirts all summer, he liked lumberjack shirts in colder seasons, and he favored jeans and sneakers in almost every weather. He used a more informal form of the German language than usually was employed in businesses settings, and adopted a friendly style when interacting with employees, as if Ganymed were one big family.

Türeci and Şahin had difficulties relating to some staffers, though. The pair worked late into the night and they expected colleagues to match their work ethic. At scientific meetings, colleagues would head to dinner after the day's events, but Şahin would go back to his hotel room to read a pile of journals. His research kept him happy and energized; Şahin told staffers he felt more stress when he *wasn't* working. Once, he told a colleague that his goal was to "eradicate" everything in his life unrelated to his work.

One day, a senior researcher named Michael Koslowski tried to get Şahin to temper his expectations of his staffers.

"Uğur, you have to understand that some people see this as a job, they go home and don't think about it," Koslowski told him.

Şahin looked genuinely shocked.

"It was a concept he didn't understand," Koslowski says.

Later, when some employees grumbled that they weren't receiving enough Ganymed shares, Şahin was taken aback.

"Money shouldn't be their motivation," he told Koslowski.

When Şahin explained to a staffer that Ganymed's investors wouldn't allow more shares to be distributed to employees, a colleague responded: "You can give them some of yours, Uğur."

Şahin's stance didn't reflect any kind of hunger for fortune. Material items had little value to him and Türeci. They lived in a modest apartment in downtown Mainz and didn't own a television or car. Şahin didn't even have a driver's license. He relied on an aging Trek bicycle to get to work, or a regular taxi driver named Parviz if he had to go to the airport or elsewhere. Once, after colleagues saw moth holes in Şahin's shirts and rips in the elbows of his jackets, they urged him to buy some new clothing. He just smiled, as if to say clothing and other material goods were unimportant distractions from science.

Instead, Şahin and Türeci seemed to cling to Ganymed shares as a means to maintain control of the company, perhaps because they worried their investors might halt their cancer research or even remove them from the company if Ganymed's results proved disappointing.

One day in 2002, they did agree to take a short break from their lab bench. Around lunchtime that day, they headed to Mainz's city hall to get married. There were four people in the wedding party—Koslowski was the best man and the company's administrative assistant was a witness. After a fifteen-minute ceremony, the group headed back to the lab to resume their research.

"It felt exactly as it should have been," Koslowski says. "Anything else would have been a distraction."

Despite the hard work by the team, Ganymed missed milestone after milestone. There were indications they were making progress on an esophageal cancer drug and in other areas. But all their research was preclinical, meaning Ganymed hadn't even started testing its approaches in people, suggesting revenues were many years away.

By 2007, the sluggish pace had become a pressing problem, as was Ganymed's growing need for more capital. The company had already raised cash five times from various investors, at one point getting several million euros from Thomas and Andreas Strüngmann, German identical-twin brothers and billionaires. With each investment round, Türeci and Şahin saw their own stakes in Ganymed shrink, frustrating them. But still more money was needed, a drug was many years away, and Nextech needed to provide its own investors with a financial return.

"It was taking much longer than everyone anticipated," says Scheidegger.

The couple came under pressure to sell their company, and employees worried about their futures. The end of the road seemed in sight.

• • •

In late September 2007, Şahin and Türeci traveled over four hundred kilometers to Munich to meet Thomas Strüngmann. At that point, he and his brother owned about 3 percent of Ganymed, an investment they had made on the recommendation of a venture-capital friend, Michael Motschmann, who also held a small Ganymed stake. For the billionaire brothers, the Ganymed investment was a pittance, so they hadn't spent much time studying the company. Still, Strüngmann was eager to meet the young scientists.

As they approached Strüngmann's office in a tall office tower, Şahin and Türeci were hopeful that he might increase his investment in Ganymed or even buy Nextech out, removing a major thorn in their side. But ahead of the meeting, Motschmann had suggested they give Strüngmann a presentation that was about more than Ganymed. Now, they sat across from the businessman in his large conference room, Şahin in his usual T-shirt-and-sneakers outfit, Türeci dressed more formally in a smart blouse.

"What do you have in mind *after* this?" asked Strüngmann, who wasn't very excited about Ganymed's antibody research.

Şahin and Türeci handed a three-page printout to Strüngmann, Motschmann, and a few others in the room, and began discussing their true passion. What they *really* wanted to do was build a new kind of company, one that could unleash the immune system to fight cancer. Cancer is wily and adaptable, Türeci told Strüngmann, but so is the human immune system. Existing treatments were major disappointments. The breast-cancer drug Herceptin was a huge seller—but it only helped 20 percent of patients, Şahin said. Doctors could barely predict which 20 percent would be helped, he noted; each patient's cancer is a bit different.

Personalized cancer treatments were the answer, Şahin argued, referring to those targeted against the specific tumors of each individual. The two scientists, sharing the floor equally, said they wanted to build an immunotherapy company that would employ innovative drug-development approaches, such as using the mRNA molecule, to stir the immune system to combat cancer. The company would be called NT, short for New Technologies, and a hint at natural numbers, which are denoted by the symbol N. Şahin promised it would upend the pharmaceutical industry.

Strüngmann, who was in his late fifties, nearly six feet tall, and dressed in a crisp white dress shirt, listened attentively, growing more enthusiastic with each new point from the scientists. By the time they finished their pitch, he was visibly excited. Two years earlier, he and his brother had sold their generic-drug company, Hexal, to Swiss giant Novartis for more than $8 billion. Strüngmann dreamed of disrupting drug giants—that's what the generic business is all about. He had spent years listening to quips about his business. Generic companies were called pirates, copying machines, and worse by the health-care establishment. Strüngmann had heard it all. He wanted to be involved in true innovation. His father and brother were physicians, but he had chosen to go to business school; backing scientific efforts was his own opportunity to achieve medical advances.

Now, Strüngmann had two of the most ambitious and fascinating scientists he had ever met in his office, and they were offering him the chance to participate in likely medical breakthroughs. They didn't boast of their credentials or promise a Nobel Prize like those who sometimes came to Strüngmann asking for money, which also appealed to him. He didn't fully understand the details of Şahin and Türeci's potential approach. The whole mRNA thing was over his head. All he knew was he wanted to be part of it.

He smiled as he addressed his guests.

"Dr. Şahin and Dr. Türeci," Strüngmann said. "How much money would you need to fulfill your dreams?"

They weren't prepared for the question. Şahin knew German investors are usually reluctant to invest in biotech, so there was just so much he could ask. He looked at Türeci for a moment before responding.

"I think we can make it with one hundred fifty million euro," he said.

Strüngmann jumped from his seat and bolted to a nearby office to call his brother.

"In my conference room are two people who will change cancer," Strüngmann gushed to him.

A few minutes later, he returned. The Strüngmann brothers were in. Şahin and Türeci almost fell out of their chairs in disbelief.

"Is this guy serious?" Şahin asked Motschmann.

"I can assure you, he is," Motschmann said.

Finally, Şahin and Türeci had a chance to chase their dreams.*

• • •

Despite Strüngmann's support, Şahin and Türeci were still worried about Ganymed's future. Scheidegger and Nextech were breathing down their necks, pushing hard for a sale of the company. In the spring of 2008, Scheidegger met Ganymed's board of directors at the Hilton hotel in Mainz. It was time to put Ganymed up for sale, he said. Strüngmann understood that if Scheidegger couldn't find a buyer, new management would come in and Türeci and Şahin would be out.

Strüngmann didn't like what he was hearing about his new favorite scientists. Selling Ganymed was a mistake, he argued. If the company

---

* Motschmann also liked what he was hearing from Şahin and Türeci, so he insisted on kicking in 15 million euro as part of the Strüngmann investment.

wasn't even ready to test a product in humans, how much interest would there even be?

"If you want out, I'll buy you out," Strüngmann eventually told Scheidegger.

A bit later, he and his brother bought Nextech's controlling stake in Ganymed, and they also offered to purchase shares from other investors who wanted to bail on the company. It was decided that Türeci would continue to run Ganymed, while Şahin would lead the new company.*

Şahin wasn't yet ready to launch NT, though. He and Helmut Jeggle, who worked in Strüngmann's investment office, began difficult negotiations regarding the terms of their start-up. The talks dragged and Şahin and Jeggle eventually went on a walk through the city streets of Hamburg, debating what percentage of the new company Şahin and his wife would control. Memories of the Ganymed experience haunted Şahin. The couple's ownership had dwindled over time, leaving them at the mercy of Scheidegger and his firm. Şahin insisted on owning more of the new company. He wouldn't give in, and neither would Jeggle.

As they came to the end of their walk, Jeggle sensed an agreement was slipping away. He made one last offer.

"How about twenty percent of the company, but if Thomas is happy after a certain point, it goes up to twenty-five percent?" Jeggle proposed.

Şahin shook his head. He didn't look happy.

"No," he said. "Twenty-five percent and if Thomas isn't happy it drops to twenty."

They had a deal.

---

* In 2016, Ganymed was sold to Japan's Astellas Pharma for nearly a billion dollars, rewarding the Strüngmann brothers, though not Türeci and Şahin, who by then owned relatively few shares of the company.

• • •

In 2008, Şahin and his new backers launched their company, with Türeci lending a hand as she continued to run Ganymed. By then, the new venture's name had morphed into Biopharmaceutical New Technologies and then shortened to BioNTech. Şahin was set on developing personalized approaches to cancer to enable the body itself to destroy tumors.

The goal was to remove tumor samples and to design specific molecules on the basis of tumor markers from the samples, which were reintroduced into the body. The idea was to use cancer samples to train the immune system to attack tumors, much like the way viral proteins teach the body as part of some vaccines, including those developed by Gale Smith, the former MicroGeneSys scientist. Şahin and Türeci shared the concerns of others about traditional vaccine- and drug-development methods, which can be slow and are not always effective, so they searched for a better approach. Şahin examined the idea of creating genetic material to code for a desired molecule and then using an adenovirus to carry it into the body, much as Dan Barouch and Adrian Hill were doing with their viral vaccines, but Şahin was wary of relying on adenoviruses and decided against the approach.

He and Türeci remained fans of new technologies, so they decided to try to use mRNA molecules to instruct the body to create cancer-related proteins capable of activating the immune system—maybe the body could be told to destroy tumors, they wondered. At the time, most mainstream scientists dismissed the idea of using mRNA to treat or protect against disease or illness, even though Katalin Karikó and Drew Weissman were doing their groundbreaking research at the University of Pennsylvania. The concept was a bit more popular in Germany, however, giving Şahin and Türeci some company in their quest.

Back in 1996, the same year Eli Gilboa and his colleagues at Duke published their paper showing that messenger RNA could help shrink tumors in mice, a German immunologist named Hans-Georg

Rammensee at the University of Tübingen seized on the concept of using mRNA for a vaccine. He gave the project to a student named Ingmar Hoerr, who in 2000 helped start CureVac, the German biotechnology company. It directly injected mRNA in humans, much as Jon Wolff had earlier done in mice at the University of Wisconsin. One of CureVac's cofounders, Steve Pascolo, even injected himself with mRNA, successfully sending the genetic code of a firefly protein into his body, to see if the approach would work. Pascolo managed to avoid turning into the Fly or another superhero, an early mRNA accomplishment.

Still, Şahin and Türeci didn't feel they had many scientists to consult with as they began their mRNA research.

"It was a small community, and even within the small community, we were ignoring each other," Şahin says, referring to the few mRNA devotees at the time.[3]

Like Ganymed, Şahin's new company was set up in Mainz, which presented a bit of a recruiting challenge. The city was known for its Roman ruins, vineyards, top-notch wine, and Johannes Gutenberg, not innovative start-ups. Young researchers elsewhere in the country, such as Andreas Kuhn, were reluctant to come to work with Şahin. When Kuhn, who had spent several years working with mRNA in an institution in Göttingen, nearly three hundred kilometers away, interviewed for a position with Şahin's academic team, he couldn't mask his skepticism.

"How can you inject it in humans and expect it to do something?" Kuhn asked Şahin bluntly.

Şahin shared early data he had developed demonstrating how he and his colleagues were making progress using mRNA to tackle tumors in animals, winning Kuhn over.

"It didn't cross my mind that it could be therapeutic," says Kuhn, who assumed a senior role at BioNTech in 2008. "Three hours with Uğur had me convinced."

Over the next few years, Şahin's new company would emerge as a magnet for young, talented scientists.

• • •

Şahin and BioNTech wanted to be the first to develop a cancer vaccine. Although using mRNA wasn't the only strategy the company used, it was the one that excited many of its young scientists. The team's mRNA challenges were similar to those faced by the Moderna team in Cambridge, Massachusetts, such as how to keep mRNA stable and how to deliver it to cells consistently enough to create sufficient proteins to wipe out tumors. Şahin and his team developed ways to address some of their challenges, such as modifying its guanine nucleotide to "cap" the mRNA and make it less apt to break down, but their progress was slow. He tried to gather information about Moderna's activities, viewing the company as BioNTech's fiercest mRNA competitor, but was stymied by Moderna's secreticve approach.

Soon pressure began to build on Şahin once again. The Strüngmann brothers had promised about 150 million euros of financing, but their money wasn't going to last forever. And some of it was to be paid out over time, as certain milestones were hit. Just like at Ganymed, delays in the timeline for drug trials began to frustrate BioNTech's new backers, who were becoming concerned they had invested too much money in the biotech sector.

Thomas's brother, Andreas, in particular, voiced concerns. After all, Thomas had been wowed by Şahin and Türeci, not Andreas. Sure, the Strüngmann brothers were billionaires, but nearly 150 million euros was a lot, even for them. That was on top of about 50 million spent buying out the investors in Ganymed, which was also running into more delays. By now it was 2011 and neither company was even in phase 1, early-stage trials.

"Why did we put one hundred fifty million in this?" Andreas

asked in a meeting with his family's investment team. "Why do we believe in them?"

BioNTech hoped to challenge the world's drug powers, but in some ways it acted like a rank amateur. Şahin's laptop served as the company's backup server, and he walked around wearing a green string necklace holding a flash drive that some employees believed held all of BioNTech's key data.[4]

Hans Hengartner, the immunologist Şahin had worked with in Zurich who remained a trusted adviser, had to step in to defend Şahin and Türeci, urging the Strüngmanns and their representatives to have patience.

"They need time," Hengartner told them one time. "What they're doing is outstanding."

• • •

As Şahin and Türeci made slow progress using mRNA molecules, a pioneer in the field faced more serious setbacks.

In 2012, Katalin Karikó was still at the University of Pennsylvania, searching for ways to use mRNA molecules to develop therapeutics. She had yet to develop an effective drug or obtain research project grants from the National Institutes of Health.

Other members of her family were enjoying success, at least. That year, Karikó's daughter, Susan Francia, traveled to London to compete in the Summer Olympics as part of the U.S. women's eight rowing team, winning a gold medal, which she had also earned in 2008. Both times, Karikó and her husband cheered her on. Back home, though, Karikó's prospects were bleaker than ever. In 2013, she received $800,000 in research funding from Japan's Takeda Pharmaceutical Company, but the support wasn't enough for her bosses. She was asked to vacate her lab in Penn's neurosurgery department and move to a run-down lab next to an animal facility in Stemmler Hall, a twenty-year-old campus building. It was far from her old colleagues and close to no one doing interesting or important research. She had landed in a virtual gulag for serious researchers.

By 2013, Karikó had had enough. She found a job working for Şahin's company as a vice president. She retired from Penn after twenty-four years and moved to Mainz to work part of the year. Most everyone at the school was sure they had seen the last of Karikó, who was approaching the age of sixty. They'd no longer have to hear about the wonders of mRNA.

"When I said I was leaving, some of my colleagues laughed at me and said, 'BioNTech doesn't even have a website,'" Karikó says.

• • •

Uğur Şahin and his team were working on ways to defeat cancer using mRNA molecules and other methods. In Cambridge, Massachusetts, Stéphane Bancel and his researchers at Moderna were making their own headway employing mRNA to fight infectious disease.

Neither Şahin nor Bancel were particular fans of using adenoviruses to deliver genetic messages to the body for vaccines. Then again, they weren't following the progress being made by Dan Barouch in Boston and Adrian Hill in Oxford, or the controversies each was stirring.

11

2009–2017

Dan Barouch approached the podium, glanced at his notes, and began to speak.

It was late October 2009, and Barouch had flown to Paris to address nearly a thousand delegates at an annual meeting for scientists chasing an HIV vaccine. The virologist at Beth Israel Deaconess Medical Center in Boston was there to discuss the results of a clinical trial that had tested his lab's HIV vaccine in healthy, adult volunteers in the Boston area.

Barouch's shots, developed with the Dutch company Crucell, enlisted the rare human virus, adenovirus serotype 26, to carry synthesized genetic instructions for three HIV proteins into the body. Once deposited in human cells, Ad26's genetic payload produced harmless HIV proteins that spurred the immune system to produce antibodies and immune cells, preparing it to identify and destroy the awful virus in a future encounter.

Barouch's approach remained deeply controversial. Just two years earlier, Merck had crushed the hopes of AIDS researchers, members of the gay community, and others when it revealed that its own vaccine, which used a different adenovirus to shepherd similar genetic material into the body, had proved useless,

Few in the crowd had forgotten Merck's shocking and disturbing results. Earlier at the Paris meeting, the U.S. Army had unveiled surprisingly good results for a rival HIV vaccine using a canarypox virus, one that affects wild birds, suggesting their alternative vaccine strategy could be a winner. Now here came Barouch, a scientific boy wonder still in his thirties, to discuss early data from his group's own vaccine, which shared similarities with Merck's failed shots. The odds seemed stacked against him.

He looked out at the crowd and launched right in. The phase 1 trial showed his vaccine was safe. His group had determined an ideal dosage. Best of all, Barouch and his colleagues saw evidence that their vaccine was immunogenic, meaning that it stirred the immune system. The prime, or initial, shots produced a nice mix of antibodies from B cells in subjects, along with CD4+ and CD8+ T cells, with even more immune-system activity seen in subjects after they had received follow-up booster shots.

Barouch couldn't hide a slight grin. His vaccine still had a shot at success.

"These encouraging preliminary results pave the way for further development of this vaccine vector for HIV and other pathogens," he told the audience, some of whom nodded in approval.

Over the next two years, Barouch and his group worked with Crucell to improve their shots and give them to healthy volunteers in Africa. They also tested the vaccine in mice and monkeys, gathering additional evidence that it invigorated the immune system. These were initial, phase 1 trials, but Barouch was growing more optimistic.

Finally, his peers were beginning to appreciate the possibilities of the viral-vector vaccine approach and what the Ad26 virus could do, despite Merck's earlier disaster. Some of the same scientists were beginning to resent Barouch, however. Much of the carping appeared to be jealousy. Barouch was the kid in class who got straight As while making it all look so easy. He ran his seventy-person laboratory in Boston with precision, made time for his family, and regularly published academic papers, almost always in the best journals, turning his work around at a speed that made peers' heads turn.

"I never met anyone who works as fast as Dan," says Nelson Michael, the senior vaccine specialist at the Walter Reed Army Institute of Research. "He can write a paper in a weekend that would take most guys three days of day-and-night work. He doesn't need to walk around the block twenty times like the rest of us."

Barouch lived a disciplined life and had the self-control of a monk. He never watched television or slacked off. Barouch practiced violin for over an hour each day, even on weekends, a habit he had maintained since the age of four. It helped him stay mentally refreshed, he told friends. Many researchers keep their offices an absolute mess, with open, disheveled files and books piled high. Not Barouch. His desk and office were clean, tidy, and organized. He employed hundreds of yellow folders and colorful tabs to keep track of clinical trials, a systematic approach that allowed him to locate data at a moment's notice. He was so put together that colleagues sometimes felt compelled to walk into his office and disrupt his files just a bit, to get a rise out of him. Barouch would usually smile uncomfortably and immediately return his folders to their proper places.

No one accused Barouch of fabricating or embellishing his data. But there was something a bit too perfect about his work, rivals said. They coined a term for his academic papers: "Barouchian," by which they meant fast and nearly flawless.

"Dan gets these perfect statistics, they're all so neat and tidy," a senior immunologist said. "When we do monkey studies, they're messy. With Dan, not a hair is ever out of place."

Barouch largely enjoyed a squeaky clean image. Over time, though, some scientists became uncomfortable with some of his actions. In

2010, Hildegund Ertl, the adenovirus expert at the Wistar Institute in Philadelphia, helped write a paper in *Journal of Virology* that raised questions about Barouch's approach. Part of the reason Barouch believed Ad26 worked so well was its rarity; unlike the extremely common Ad5 virus that the Merck team had used, relatively few people around the world had been exposed to Ad26, which meant that few people had developed an immunity to it. But Ertl and her colleagues analyzed blood samples from people at seven sites around the world, concluding that the Ad26 wasn't rare, after all, at least in parts of Africa. As such, the adenovirus might not be an optimal vaccine carrier, the paper argued.

The critique was important. Prior exposure to human adenoviruses is what may have contributed to the failure in 2007 of Merck's Ad5 HIV vaccine. The reason: If the immune system previously encountered an adenovirus it would be trained to fight it off in the future, preventing the Ad26 virus from delivering its genetic cargo, effectively short-circuiting the vaccine before it could even begin its work.

"Despite previous reports to the contrary, we find that AdHu26 commonly infects people, particularly those in sub-Saharan Africa, the very people for whom the need for novel vaccine strategies is most dire," Ertl's study argued.

After the paper was published, Barouch became upset with Ertl, she says, approaching her at a conference to challenge the validity of her work. In an email in October 2010, Barouch told Ertl that her research represented "an aggressive attack on our program. . . . It has caused substantial problems that will take some time to resolve."

Barouch says Ertl was a competitor and that he never became angry with her or approached her at a conference. Later, Barouch published a paper showing that about half of the adults in some countries in Africa and Asia had preexisting immunity to Ad26, data that was similar to what Ertl had discovered. But follow-up work from

Barouch suggested that the exposure to Ad26 was unlikely to hurt its effectiveness as a vaccine vector, reassuring fans of his approach.

Barouch was experiencing more painful conflict closer to home. He and his former mentor, Harvard Medical School professor Norman Letvin, were squabbling and their rift was fast becoming the talk of a segment of the research community.

Letvin, a famed and influential AIDS specialist and concert-level clarinetist who was notoriously critical of the work of other scientists, told three people that he was concerned that Barouch was exaggerating the conclusions of some of his scientific papers, including work related to the Ad26 vaccine platform, criticism that was personally painful to Barouch.

But others close to Letvin say he resented the acclaim his thirty-nine-year old protégé was receiving. At one point, he demanded that Barouch delay publication of a scientific paper that overlapped with Letvin's own work, according to two people. Barouch agreed to hold off on the paper and they eventually published their research simultaneously, but it still burned Letvin that Barouch wrote his paper, according to someone close to both men.

The fractured friendship was difficult for both men, who once had been close and now were fierce competitors. It was especially awkward because the men had offices within feet of each other.

Around 2010, Letvin was diagnosed with pancreatic cancer. As he battled his disease, the five-foot-five professor amazed colleagues by continuing his life's work, flying to Washington, D.C., for a meeting of vaccine specialists even as his health deteriorated. One evening in May 2012, Letvin took members of his laboratory to a Red Sox game at Fenway Park. Exiting the stadium, Letvin felt unwell and headed to the hospital. He died soon thereafter at the age of sixty-two, a crushing blow to many in the AIDS research community. By then, his relationship with Barouch had improved.

Three months after Letvin's death, Barouch was chosen to lead a new center at Beth Israel Deaconess. It was a merger of the Division of Vaccine Research, which Barouch had been leading, and the Division of Viral Pathogenesis, which Letvin had been running. The powerful position was a new reason for peers to resent Barouch—even as he made progress with his vaccine.

• • •

There were still more unsettling developments in Barouch's life. In 2011, pharmaceutical giant Johnson & Johnson purchased Crucell for over $2 billion. The two companies had been working together to develop monoclonal antibodies, and executives said they now would join forces to tackle hepatitis, typhoid, cholera, yellow fever, tuberculosis, malaria, and influenza. As for the AIDS research Crucell was still doing with Barouch's lab, it barely merited a mention by the companies as they promoted their merger to Wall Street analysts, investors, and others.

It wasn't a good sign for Barouch. Neither was the fact that his key collaborator at Crucell, Jaap Goudsmit, had decided to shift to a new research area after the merger. Once again, it seemed, a major pharmaceutical company was pulling its support for AIDS research, hindering, or even crushing, Barouch's efforts.

It was hard to blame J&J. Barouch's lab had only conducted early clinical trials. It would be many more years before the team could be sure its Ad26 vaccine provided humans with protection, work that likely would drain hundreds of millions of dollars from J&J's coffers. Barouch couldn't develop a vaccine on his own. He was better than most at writing grant proposals and fundraising, which was how he managed to support the nearly one hundred scientists in his lab. But he needed a pharmaceutical partner to produce and test an actual vaccine.

In 2012, Barouch traveled to New Brunswick, New Jersey, for an afternoon meeting with top J&J executives. He was nervous as he approached the company's white, sixteen-story, ivory tower on Johnson Boulevard. Barouch barely knew Paul Stoffels, J&J's chief scientific officer and head of global scientific research and development. He wasn't sure how much Stoffels and other J&J executives even knew about his vaccine program, let alone whether they wanted to keep funding it. All Barouch knew was that Stoffels wanted to talk—a full year after they bought Crucell. It wasn't a great sign.

Inside a large, sparsely furnished conference room, Barouch and a few Crucell scientists updated Stoffels and a dozen or so senior executives of J&J's pharmaceutical division, called Janssen, on their AIDS work. Barouch shared the science behind the vaccine program and its plans, emphasizing why he thought the Ad26 approach could work, trying to sound positive and hopeful.

Then it was Stoffels's turn to speak. The J&J executives inched closer, eager to hear how their boss felt about the AIDS program. The fifty-year-old was an imposing figure. Heavyset, with a round face, thick, dark eyebrows, graying hair, and stylish, rounded glasses, Stoffels spoke with an accent, the result of his childhood in Belgium. He began by sharing some of his own history. As a student in medical school in the 1980s, he spent his vacations in central Africa helping to treat AIDS patients. He had worked with famed AIDS researcher and activist Peter Piot during some of the worst periods of the virus's outbreak. At one time, about one in three patients in the region's hospitals was HIV-positive and one in eight people in the streets carried the virus. Sometimes, Stoffels told the group, he went house to house in small townships, meeting twelve-year-olds struggling to care for younger siblings, the graves of their parents visible in their front yards. In 1987, Stoffels's best friend, a fellow physician named Jens Van Roey, contracted the disease while working with patients in Africa. Later, Van Roey battled AIDS-related ailments including a form of tuberculosis, Hodgkin's-like lymphoma, skin cancer, and spinocellular carcinoma of the tongue.[1]

Turning emotional, Stoffels told Barouch he couldn't shake images of his patients in Africa. They were why he had become a pharmaceutical executive. Drugs helped, but only a vaccine could put an end to the epidemic. An effective vaccine could be Stoffels's legacy.

"We're going to do this," he told Barouch and the others. "I don't know if it will work but it's worth trying. . . . There's nothing more important for us."

Barouch was elated. His vaccine program had new life.

• • •

Stoffels wasn't kidding about believing in the Ad26 approach. Two years later, in 2014, when West African nations suffered the worst-ever outbreak of Ebola, an infectious disease that kills at least half of those it infects, J&J hurried to act.[2] Working with government scientists, it developed a two-shot vaccine regimen relying on the Ad26 viral-vector technology and a second dose using a poxvirus. The shots proved safe and created an immune response, but the epidemic subsided—after killing more than eleven thousand people—well before efficacy data could be gathered.

Over the next few years, the company put shots in the arms of over one hundred thousand people, mostly in Congo and Rwanda. Eventually, J&J's Ebola vaccine received approval from the European Commission, though it was solely on the basis of its ability to generate an immune response. There still wasn't data proving the vaccine conferred sufficient protection.

Barouch hadn't spent much time focused on Ebola. He had his hands full perfecting his AIDS vaccine and running his Boston laboratory. But a new outbreak soon caught his attention. In early 2015, the mosquito-borne Zika virus, which began as a tropical malady afflicting Africa and several remote western Pacific islands, spread through the Americas. The results were frightening. Thousands of infants were born with horrifying birth defects, including a surge of babies in

Brazil diagnosed with microcephaly, a congenital condition that leaves babies' brains and heads abnormally small. For most people, the effects of the virus were mild, but many of the ailments were troubling, feeding anxiety. El Salvador's government even asked women to avoid getting pregnant until 2018. As the disease threatened to spread to the United States, public officials couldn't mask their growing fears.

"The level of alarm is extremely high," WHO director-general Margaret Chan told the public-health agency's executive board in early 2016. "We need to get some answers quickly."[3]

One early morning in late March of that year, Barouch picked up his office phone to call Nelson Michael, the physician-scientist at the Walter Reed Army Institute of Research. Barouch and Michael had spent the previous few years collaborating on the Ad26 HIV vaccine, but they didn't usually chat about other diseases.

"Have you guys been working on Zika?" Barouch asked.

Michael, who was speaking from his cell phone as he drove to his office, immediately pulled into a parking lot and stopped his car.

"Only every day," he responded.

"But you're an HIV guy," Barouch responded.

"So are *you*," Michael said.

"We have to talk," Barouch told him.[4]

By then, Michael and colleagues at Walter Reed had acquired a strain of the virus from a contact in Puerto Rico and were growing it in their Bethesda, Maryland, laboratory, the first step toward developing a vaccine. The Walter Reed shots would embrace a traditional approach, relying on an inactivated form of the Zika virus. Barouch's team was already set up to test HIV and other vaccines in mice and monkeys, so he offered to test the Walter Reed Zika vaccines on his lab's animals.

Over the course of several months, Barouch's laboratory tested two vaccines—Walter Reed's inactivated-virus vaccine and another that used an injection of genetically engineered plasmid containing the DNA sequence of a part of the Zika virus. Barouch's team decided to also build a vaccine using their Ad26 virus to carry a synthetic form of the Zika's surface proteins. It couldn't hurt to test that vaccine, too, Barouch and his colleagues figured.

Until then, Barouch hadn't thought about applying the Ad26 vaccine approach to inoculate against any viruses besides HIV. He and his colleagues were all in on AIDS. But that effort was proving a difficult slog, and Barouch wondered if the Ad26 viral-vector technology might prove more effective against a "well-behaved" virus that wasn't nearly as skilled at evading the immune system as HIV.

Barouch's researchers tested the various Zika vaccine shots in mice, as well as in a group of macaque monkeys, comparing the results with a control group of monkeys given empty shots. All the inoculated mice developed immunity. So did the monkeys. There was little evidence of Zika virus anywhere in their bodies after the animals were challenged with the virus. What was most surprising: The Ad26 vaccine, which was called Ad26-ZIKV, generated the most immune activity. The results gave Barouch an idea: Maybe the Ad26 vaccine could fight off other viruses.

A few months later, over beers in a Lisbon bar during a break at an AIDS conference, Barouch asked Johan Van Hoof, the senior vaccine executive at J&J's Janssen Pharmaceuticals unit, if his company might want to build a Zika vaccine.

Van Hoof grimaced.

"We want to wait, the science isn't well understood yet," he said.

That's when Barouch whipped out his laptop and shared his lab's data.

"We have the science," Barouch said.

Soon Van Hoof was on the phone with his boss, Stoffels. Within a year, J&J had produced Ad26 shots for Zika. They planned efficacy trials, but by 2017 the outbreak had mostly dissipated on its own, making it impossible to test the vaccine. Good for the world, bad for the scientists. Still, Barouch and the J&J team had learned a ton: They could build an Ad26 vaccine quickly, their approach seemed safe, and millions of doses could be produced in a short period. Working closely with government scientists had accelerated their work. And a single shot seemed enough to generate protective antibodies and a potentially durable immune response, more reason for optimism about the Ad26 method.

It had taken about a year to develop the vaccine. That was lightning-fast compared to most vaccines in history, but Barouch, Stoffels, and their colleagues knew they would have to move even faster to stop a future pandemic. Still, they were convinced they had an effective vaccine approach. They would have to wait for a new virus to be certain.

• • •

Adrian Hill was waiting for his own success.

For two decades, the molecular geneticist who founded and ran the Jenner Institute at Oxford University had been working with his colleague, Sarah Gilbert, to develop a malaria vaccine. The researchers still favored jabs that used a chimpanzee adenovirus to shepherd a malaria gene into the body. But they weren't close to declaring any kind of victory in their quest.

Hill and Gilbert were such believers in their chimp-adenovirus technology platform, which they called ChAdOx, that they also used it to build vaccines for hepatitis C, HIV, tuberculosis, influenza, and respiratory syncytial virus. The Oxford researchers took their chimp virus and inserted genetic material for each of those pathogens, hoping the immune system would react. They saw some signs of success, but these were challenging viruses and the Oxford team hadn't gained approval for a single one of these vaccines.

Limited results in the lab didn't stop Hill from assuming an outsize position in his field. By 2011, he had emerged as one of the most controversial and disliked men in the world of science, largely due to his sharp critiques of fellow researchers and caustic, even offensive, behavior.

At scientific meetings, Hill was usually the first to jump to his feet, grab a microphone, and challenge a point being made in a presentation. He often did it in degrading or insulting language. Here are snippets of quotes from Hill over the years, as related by various scientists:

"That's a really dumb idea."

"Your data sucks."

"That's the most ignorant thing I've ever heard."

Researchers came to meetings girded for Hill's blunt, even vicious, verbal lashings. If Hill merely cleared his throat, it likely meant some kind of savagery was on its way. Some learned to appreciate the remarks, realizing that Hill's punches were often packed with trenchant points. But younger or unprepared scientists were sometimes startled by the comments, which could be unnecessarily personal.

At times, the criticisms were made with such vehemence and intensity that Hill's face turned bright red, nearly matching his hair color. Hill's derisive comments hit hard because the self-worth of some researchers, not to mention their career prospects, were tied up in their scientific data and conclusions.

"It's like taking your kid out to play soccer and someone criticizing them, it can hurt," says Nelson Michael. "But they also shouldn't have taken it personally."

What bothered Hill's peers most was that he seemed far more critical of the work of others than he was of his own research. Hill had spent years developing a malaria vaccine and shots for other pathogens, and he had given endless speeches about the work of his institute. It seemed that almost every year, the BBC, CNN, or another media outlet profiled the progress he and Gilbert were making against some disease or other. Rivals thought he overstated his group's chances of success, while commending the team's persistence. Yet there was Hill, at one more medical conference, lecturing another scientist about why her approach was doomed. Gilbert was a quiet, restrained presence at the meetings, but Hill couldn't help sharing his critiques.

Once, at an annual meeting of experts in infectious tropical diseases, an academic named Chris Plowe corrected an answer Hill had given to the crowd. Plowe referenced work by Joana Carneiro da Silva, a younger colleague at the University of Maryland. Hearing her work mentioned, Silva approached a microphone in the audience to share her data and explain the mistake Hill had made. Hill waved off Silva's critique, exhibiting a disdain that researchers in the room had come to expect.

Silva was new to the field, though. She didn't appreciate being publicly disrespected. To the shock of the scientists, Silva walked right back to the microphone, her voice slightly trembling, to correct Hill again, providing detailed evidence to bolster her cause. Hill was dismissive once more. Silva stood up to challenge Hill again, this time even more forcefully, as the group privately cheered her on. It was like the new kid fighting back against a school bully accustomed to seeing his victims quiver.

"He was banking on his reputation to have his argument prevail, and that was infuriatingly abrasive," she says.

By then, the Jenner Institute had gained respect for conducting human trials for its own vaccines as well as for those developed by others, usually at a fast clip. It was a prowess that filled Hill with pride. In 2014, he gave an interview to a writer for the British scientific publication *The Lancet*. Sitting at his office desk with his shirt sleeves rolled up, Hill explained how vaccine power GlaxoSmithKline and the National Institutes of Health had turned to him for help testing their Ebola vaccine.

"They asked for the fastest conceivable timeline," Hill said, while sweeping back his disheveled red hair. "So I told them we could start vaccinating people by the middle of September, and funnily enough that's what happened."[5]

It was all too much, even for his fans.

"Adrian is a superb scientist, he truly believes in helping mankind and I like him," says Hildegund Ertl. "But a truly great scientist knows they don't know it all and are humble. Humble and Adrian Hill don't go together."

It didn't help Hill that he appeared a near-picture-perfect caricature of one of the most disliked of all British archetypes: the self-important Oxbridge academic. Hill was pompous, he had spent nearly four decades at Oxford, and he had floppy, unkempt hair. Hill loved tweed coats, and while he didn't wear bright red trousers, he probably had them at home, scientists joked, pressed and hanging in a closet.

Hill raised eyebrows for other reasons, too. When NIH researchers developed a vaccine during the Ebola pandemic, his group at Oxford began conducting phase 1 trials on the jabs. One day, he appeared on BBC television holding a vaccine vial featuring an Oxford label, speaking with pride of its promise to end the Ebola crisis. Hill neglected to mention that the vaccine had been developed at the NIH, two U.S. scientists recall. They felt Hill was claiming the vaccine as his own.

Behind his back, fellow scientists gave Hill nicknames, most of which poked fun at his perceived arrogance. Some called Hill, whose full name is Adrian Vivian Sinton Hill, "Lord Adrian VS Hill of Hillington," while others went with "Lord Adrian." Over a pint or dinner, Hill was more likable, researchers said. Scientists who weren't Hill's direct competitors noticed that he treated them with more respect. Within Oxford, Hill was supportive and helpful to younger scientists, gaining their loyalty. These researchers had more problems with his scientific partner, Sarah Gilbert, viewing her as cold and according to one colleague difficult to deal with. Gilbert was notorious for sending brusque emails to colleagues, while Hill had the affection of a number of colleagues.

"Adrian has a Marmite personality," says a senior colleague, referring to the odorous, brownish, vegetable spread beloved in the United Kingdom but detested most everywhere else. "You love him or hate him."

Even his critics praised Hill's perseverance. He and Gilbert were taking on difficult, intractable diseases and they were intent on making inexpensive vaccines to help those in poorer countries, all truly commendable goals.

"No other person has run so many phase one trials," Rino Rappuoli, a senior immunologist, says about Hill.

Rappuoli, a friend of Hill's, meant his comment as high praise: Scientists argue that there are no such things as failed drug trials—even those that don't lead anywhere teach important lessons. Investigators take pride in conducting phase 1 trials, which are crucial first steps toward an approved drug or vaccine. And Hill's peers were impressed by his institute's ability to quickly and efficiently get vaccines into arms, receiving results before most anyone in the world.

Still, saying someone is really good at running phase 1 trials is a bit like complimenting a soccer player for how many shots she's taken on goal. At some point, you have to score. Hill had never come close to an approved vaccine or drug.

• • •

By late 2017, Dan Barouch believed that just one shot of his Ad26 vaccine might provide sufficient protection against various pathogens. Hill and Gilbert were just as confident in their own vaccine approach, using the chimp adenovirus. But neither Barouch nor Hill had definitive, peer-reviewed data to prove their shots worked. They *thought* their vaccines would prove effective, and might even work if a novel, tricky disease arose. But they weren't sure.

What did seem clear was that a new, dangerous pathogen was on its way. Each year, humans were encroaching on nature, increasing the risks that animal-borne diseases would cross over to affect mankind, a key ingredient in every modern pandemic. Expanding global travel, especially international flights, made it easier than ever for new pathogens to spread. If one emerged, Barouch and Hill had technology with a chance of stopping it.

12

2005–2018

Rahul Singhvi was out of ideas.

In 2005, Singhvi became the chief executive officer of a publicly traded drug company called Novavax Inc. Singhvi's position sounded impressive, especially since he was barely forty years old, and it had only been a year or so since he had arrived at the health-care company in suburban Philadelphia. But Singhvi had the job because no one else wanted it. Novavax had barely any sales, just $5 million in the bank, and it was spending more than $2 million each month. Singhvi had to save the company, but he had no idea how to do it.

Just a few years earlier, Novavax had been rolling in cash. After nine years of development, it had introduced an estrogen-replacement cream called Estrasorb that alleviated the hot flashes experienced by many menopausal women. The lotion was generating rabid interest, but even the company's executives weren't entirely sure why. The cream wasn't *that* effective, after all. It turned out that some women were rubbing the lotion on their thighs, as directed, and then massaging the remainder on their faces. Somehow, the cream was evaporating the crow's feet around the women's eyes, almost overnight, like some kind of potion sold on late-night television, only this one actually worked. It was a true wonder drug—women were feeling better and looking younger. Novavax had never tested Estrasorb on wrinkles, so the Federal Drug Administration wouldn't let it advertise the lotion's bonus benefits, but word was getting out and Novavax shares were soaring.

Then, in the early 2000s, concerns emerged about estrogen-replacement therapies and other estrogen products, as studies indicated they might increase the risk of stroke and cancer. The fears quickly doused demand for Novavax's cream, though it hadn't been linked to any kind of illness. Wrinkles were a bummer, to be sure, but they were way better than cancer, customers concluded. Around the same time, interest in Novavax's other key product, a line of prenatal vitamins, shriveled amid competition from generic manufacturers. In the fiscal quarter before Singhvi took over as CEO in August 2005, Novavax recorded a measly $1 million in sales.

Singhvi had to find a way to stave off bankruptcy. He slashed the company's head count by more than half to thirty-eight staffers. But Novavax shares dropped to seventy cents, and it became clear he needed to do more. One day, Singhvi placed a call to a small laboratory Novavax ran in Gaithersburg, Maryland, asking to speak with Gale Smith, the same insect-virus and insect-cell pioneer who had worked with Frank Volvovitz on an AIDS vaccine a decade earlier. The previous year, Smith had joined Novavax after spending some time at MicroGeneSys's successor, Protein Sciences, where the tall, thin, and now balding researcher helped develop a successful flu vaccine relying on his baculovirus delivery system.

Novavax had long been trying to develop vaccines, even as it focused on women's health products; its name, in fact, derived from that early goal. Over the years, the company's scientists made a bit of progress, sometimes getting their shots to phase 2 clinical trials, but regulatory approval was elusive. It probably didn't help that Novavax's investigators dealt with more distractions than most rivals. At one point, its lab bordered a local golf course, and errant balls routinely crashed through the windows, startling researchers.

Why was a guy like Smith, who by then had made millions licensing his baculovirus system, working at an insignificant outfit on its last, wobbly legs? Mostly because his bosses let Smith run Novavax's vaccine division without interference, leaving him to pursue his unique vision for developing vaccines. To Smith, it didn't make sense that so many vaccines, including those for influenza, measles, and more, were still made in the cells of chicken eggs, an approach that had well-known limitations. He was sure the insect-vaccine strategy he had developed with colleagues in graduate school was a better option.

"Novavax was using my system and I still believed it had potential," Smith explains.

What Smith really wanted to do was create shots that could stop emerging diseases and pandemics. He was developing virus-like particles, or molecules intended to look like a virus and its key proteins, as a vaccine to teach the body's immune system to recognize and later repel these signs of danger. In some ways, his strategy was similar to those of traditional vaccine makers, because he was injecting viral proteins into the body. But his were recombinant proteins, or those created in his lab to *look* like the real thing but not be infectious. Recombinant proteins were being used to produce all kinds of drugs, and Merck had already used this approach to develop a vaccine for HPV. Smith was convinced he could produce similar shots for viruses.

Singhvi got Smith on the phone and shared his nervousness about the company's future. "What are we going to do?!" he asked Smith.

It turned out that Smith and his labmates had just published a paper detailing how a vaccine they had developed had protected ferrets from the lethal avian influenza virus. The results, which Smith's small team had generated in collaboration with the Centers for Disease Control and Prevention, suggested that Novavax's technology might produce efficacious influenza shots. Their vaccine was in preclinical stages, meaning it wasn't even close to being tested in humans, but Smith had already received a $200,000 grant from the National Institutes of Health and other government agencies to fund the research, which was more cash than most of the rest of the company was bringing in.

Singhvi decided to turn Novavax into a vaccine company. It wasn't a hard decision—it's not like he had other options, after all.

At least it's something, Singhvi thought.

It was a savvy move. Over the next several years, Novavax won a flu contract worth up to $170 million and announced a licensing agreement with a South Korean drugmaker.[1] Singhvi raised $70 million, Novavax stock jumped to six dollars a share, and he began appearing as a guest on business-television network CNBC to discuss the company's bright future. By then, Singhvi had fired Novavax's entire public relations staff in a cost-saving move, so he was writing his own press releases and publicity, but whatever he was doing seemed to be working.[2]

The strategy worked a bit too well, actually. By 2011, Singhvi was out at Novavax, as the company's board of directors embraced the vaccine strategy but decided someone with more experience was needed to run the company. The new chief executive was a sixty-two-year-old named Stanley Erck, who had seen his share of challenges. More than three decades earlier, Erck had fought in the Vietnam War, spending a year on the ground as a demolitions expert. During the war, he conducted regular patrols, detonating improvised explosive devices and surviving enemy fire. While on his tour of duty, Erck completed accounting correspondence courses, sometimes doing homework in trenches, while mailing assignments caked with blood and mud back to graders in the United States.

Returning home, Erck went to business school at the University of Chicago before working at a series of pharmaceutical companies, eventually running a company called Iomai Corporation, which was cofounded by Gregory Glenn, a former doctor at Walter Reed Army Institute of Research. At Iomai, Erck and Glenn developed skin patches to deliver vaccines, including one against traveler's diarrhea. The company was eventually sold, and Erck and Glenn made some money, but the patches never went anywhere.

Now that he was running Novavax, Erck quickly hired Glenn as the company's head of research and development, partly because he knew Glenn had a special passion for vaccines. Growing up poor in rural Indiana, he enlisted in the army and served as a pediatrician at a base in Germany and then as a resident in a Miami hospital. Over the years, he watched in awe as vaccines were introduced, including one for Hib disease, a bacterial illness that can lead to deadly brain infections in children. Suddenly, the shots were eliminating disease and the associated heartbreak he had seen inflicted on his patients and their parents. Glenn decided to change careers and try to develop vaccines of his own.

"They seemed like miracles," says Glenn.

Erck and Glenn loved Smith's approach, and the Novavax team spent the next few years developing vaccines for HIV, SARS, swine flu, Ebola, Middle East respiratory syndrome and others. Each time, the company, now based in suburban Washington, D.C., achieved early results that were promising enough to gain the backing of government bodies and nonprofits, including the Bill & Melinda Gates Foundation. Each time, though, the vaccines ran smack into imposing roadblocks and failed to win regulatory approvals. Either the epidemics ebbed or the shots didn't quite work, crippling the company's shares. Novavax was the little company that couldn't, it seemed.

Affable and encouraging, Erck walked Novavax's halls, wearing jeans and a golf shirt most days, trying to lift spirits. Around lunchtime each Friday, Erck led employees to a nearby bowling alley, where they competed over chicken wings and beer, occupying as many as thirty lanes. Erck liked to personally present trophies to the top teams. The staffers were amazed that he remembered each employee's first name, even as Novavax grew to over one hundred people. Erck handed out T-shirts when important milestones were hit and gave pats on the back when they were missed.

"Experiments fail," Erck liked to tell staffers. "Otherwise we wouldn't call them experiments."

Glenn had a harder time dealing with Novavax's setbacks, which forced him to find creative ways to keep the Novavax team together.

"Where else can you do something noble, interesting, and get paid for it?" he told his researchers.

The failures wore on Glenn. He tried to focus on each next step in the development process, treasuring the company's journey rather than concentrating on its destination. But science is a long, hard slog, and progress can take years, which can be difficult on those who are ambitious and impatient. Glenn lived on a farm in suburban Maryland, where he grew grapes and raised Plymouth roosters, Rhode Island reds, and other chickens, goats, and small animals. The more Novavax disappointed, the more time Glenn seemed to spend in the coop. Each evening and most weekends, he cleaned out the muck and worked on the cages. Tending to his animals became therapeutic. In the coop, Glenn's chicken eggs hatched in a matter of weeks, bringing him what felt like instant joy amid the frustrations in the office.

"It's very hard mentally waiting for results," Glenn says.

Most of all, Glenn enjoyed scattering stale bread and watching his chickens scamper to greet him at the end of a rough day. They didn't care about missed milestones or scientific stumbles, just that he had arrived home.

"The chickens like me, they're always excited to see me," Glenn says. "That felt really good."

Smith and others in the lab kept at it, learning lessons from all their mistakes and setbacks. One of those lessons was that their vaccine needed help. In 2014, Novavax purchased a Swedish company producing an agent that could boost the immune response generated by a vaccine. The agent, called an adjuvant, was derived from the bark of a Chilean tree primarily used for consumer products like soap and root beer foam.

Over time, the researchers discovered a better way to make vaccines. Their original strategy had been to take a baculovirus and insert DNA that encoded for a protein from a virus's outer coat. Now, they were producing a single, viral protein, mixing it with their Swedish adjuvant, and creating a nanoparticle to inject it all in the body. Instead of introducing genetic material to instruct the body to create a protein, as with an mRNA or adenovirus vaccine, Smith and his colleagues were injecting a version of the protein itself. Novavax's newly rejiggered vaccine was easier to produce than their earlier shots while doing a better job eliciting an immune response, encouraging Smith and the team.

By 2015, Novavax was working on shots to protect against respiratory syncytial virus, or RSV, the same pathogen that Barney Graham at the NIAID's Vaccine Research Center had long chased, a virus that was hospitalizing about 58,000 young children a year in the United States and nearly as many elderly people, and sometimes proved deadly. Glenn had passion for the project. As a pediatrician, he had treated two-month-olds struck by RSV. After experiencing infections in their lungs, some of the babies stopped breathing and died of respiratory failure, leaving him despondent. He wanted his company to be the one to stop the virus.

That year, Novavax shares doubled amid building excitement for its RSV shots. Erck encouraged the investor fervor, gushing to Reuters that the RSV vaccine had the potential to be "the largest selling vaccine in the history of vaccines in terms of revenue."[3]

As they raced toward clinical trials, some Novavax staffers believed

Erck and Glenn had become too confident in Smith and the vaccine group and were moving too quickly on the RSV shots, which didn't yet employ their new adjuvant. Employees heard rumors that larger pharmaceutical companies were interested in buying Novavax, but a takeover deal never emerged, which some attributed to Erck's unshakable and unjustified faith that Novavax could save the world from RSV.

"We're going to be the ones to do it," Erck once told colleagues.

In 2016, Erck, Glenn, and the team counted down to the results of a pivotal phase 3 trial of their RSV shots in nearly twelve thousand older adults. Early clinical trials had gone well, and the team was pumped, hiring over a hundred new employees to prepare for an eventual rollout of the vaccine. As Erck awaited the key trial result early on a Friday evening in mid-September, he couldn't find a way to relax. He paced his home office, waiting for Glenn to share the results.

Erck couldn't wait any longer. He picked up the phone and called Glenn.

"They're not good," Glenn told him.

Glenn said he had wanted to double-check the figures before calling Erck. He had just received confirmation, and the results were as bad as he first thought—a complete failure.

"Sorry, we missed," Glenn told Erck. "Not by a little, by a lot . . . I didn't think it was possible."

Complete silence. The men were stunned. Years of work were down the drain.

It turned out that the vaccine worked pretty well fighting off RSV's most severe symptoms, but an unusually tame RSV season had undermined the trial, reducing the "attack rate," or number of new cases that could be used to test the shots. The next day, Novavax shares plunged. Yes, a mild virus season had made it hard to know if the vaccine provided protection, but the investors were betting it would be a while, if ever, before Novavax could afford a new RSV trial.

Less than two months later, on the morning after Donald Trump beat Hillary Clinton to win the 2016 presidential election, Novavax's employees stumbled into the office. Many were Democratic voters who were still trying to come to grips with the surprise result. They were greeted with another shock: emails saying they were being laid off. That day, a third of Novavax's staffers lost their jobs. As employees carried their belongings out the door, remaining staffers were left shaken, and gloom enveloped the office.

Erck had never laid off any employees in his thirty years as an executive, and the move left him miserable. Glenn was overcome with his own sadness. He couldn't hold his emotions back. Driving home, he broke down in his car, crying.

Can we survive? Is it even worth it?

"I felt I let them down and had been overly enthusiastic," he says. "It was just hard to see people leave."

Smith and his colleagues still believed in their vaccine approach. So did Glenn and Erck. Friends who ran other biotech companies called the chief executive to try to boost his spirits, telling Erck that devastating drug-trial results were commonplace, especially for small companies.

"It's happened here, too," one told Erck.

By the end of 2018, the Novavax team was gearing up to test its RSV vaccine once again, this time in expectant mothers, hoping to show the shots could protect their babies from the virus. Erck, still an inveterate optimist, told investors that global sales of the RSV vaccine could top $1.5 billion and that Novavax was taking steps to prepare to market its shots, once they demonstrated efficacy and were approved, hopefully over the next year. Smith and his colleagues also became excited about a flu vaccine they were developing.

Few shared their optimism, however. JPMorgan Chase, Novavax's banking adviser, wouldn't invite the company to speak at its annual health-care investment conference in San Francisco, a serious diss. Erck did appear at other investor events, but sometimes as few as three people came to hear him. Looking out at those sparse crowds, Erck sometimes scrapped his prepared remarks. It just wasn't worth it, he decided.

"So, what would you guys like to talk about?" he would ask.

Moderna and BioNTech were making progress working with mRNA molecules. Dan Barouch and Adrian Hill had reason to believe their adenovirus vaccines would work. None of those vaccine specialists was even vaguely aware of Novavax, nor was most anyone else.

It was the little company that couldn't.

13

2017–2019

Stéphane Bancel was feeling optimistic.

For years, Moderna's scientists had struggled to use messenger RNA molecules to create potent and plentiful proteins. In late 2013, however, Eric Huang pushed the company to focus on vaccines. Now, Moderna was generating promising, albeit early, data from shots against a number of infectious diseases. An equally important advance came when Kerry Benenato tweaked the lipid packaging Moderna used to encase its mRNA, enabling the molecule's genetic instructions to reach cells while avoiding a toxic immune response.

By late 2017, Bancel had a team that was well suited for his combustible personality. Staffers often matched Bancel's drive and intensity, and most didn't seem to mind when he expressed frustrations about the pace of their work. He was so certain Moderna would be producing millions of vaccines, at least at some point, that he persuaded his board of directors to spend $110 million to refit a Polaroid film plant thirty minutes south of Moderna's office in Norwood,

Massachusetts, giving the company a manufacturing facility to manufacture vaccines in bulk.

Moderna's lead in the mRNA race seemed so insurmountable that Bancel finally encouraged his researchers to publish their work in scientific journals. He began opening up, too. In November, Bancel and Moderna's president, Stephen Hoge, traveled to Berlin for the International mRNA Health Conference, the most important annual gathering of mRNA specialists.

Scientists and executives at the event were still bitter about Bancel's appearance several years earlier, when he had warned the audience not to screw things up and blew off most everyone who wanted to chat. This time, though, Bancel took a different stance—he shared clinical-trial data and seemed to enjoy schmoozing with his peers, surprising some of them. Bancel even gave a speech sharing details of how his company was using lipid nanoparticles to deliver the mRNA, another shocker.

After Hoge gave his own presentation about Moderna's work on infectious-disease vaccines, Katalin Karikó, the mRNA pioneer who had joined BioNTech, approached him.

"That was fascinating," she said. "You know, we've started working in the space."

Hoge paused for a moment, digesting her comment. Until then, he and most others at Moderna had viewed BioNTech as nothing more than a cancer specialist. Sure, it had licensed the modified mRNA techniques Karikó and Drew Weissman had pioneered, just as Moderna managed to do a few years earlier. But BioNTech didn't even employ those modifications in its mRNA molecules, viewing them as unnecessary for its cancer vaccines. And BioNTech's shots weren't accompanied by any sort of updated LNP encasement like Moderna was employing, another reason Bancel, Hoge, and the others at Moderna barely thought about Uğur Şahin's company.

Now, Karikó had unintentionally tipped Hoge off that BioNTech aimed to be a direct competitor in the field of infectious diseases. Hoge wasn't too concerned, though. It seemed like nothing more than a stray comment, and he wasn't even sure how much influence she had at BioNTech. Later at the event, Hoge and Bancel even shared coffee with Şahin and Sean Marett, BioNTech's chief business and commercial officer, discussing ways their companies might work together.

On the last day of the conference, though, as Bancel and Hoge strolled through the hotel lobby, they noticed Şahin and Marett huddling with a top executive of a Canadian LNP company, the same one that had worked with Moderna on its first-generation delivery technology. Now Hoge was truly worried. It was all adding up—BioNTech was trying to catch up to Moderna in developing infectious-disease vaccines using mRNA, he warned Bancel.

Chill out, Bancel told him.

"They're so focused on cancer," he told Hoge. "And we have such a head start . . . there's no way they can catch us alone."

• • •

Bancel was newly confident, but others at Moderna were growing concerned.

Moderna's new factory, unveiled in 2018, came at an enormous expense for a company nowhere near recording profits. At the same time, research and other costs were also surging. Yes, Bancel was still finding investors willing to write enormous checks to cover their costs, another reason he was in such good spirits. In February 2018, he helped raise $500 million from Geneva-based Pictet Group, the sovereign wealth fund of Abu Dhabi, and New York hedge fund Viking Global Investors, among others. But many of Moderna's newest backers weren't health-care specialists. In corners of that world, skepticism of Bancel and Moderna had turned into outright derision, a shift in sentiment that was about to cause problems for the company.

In March 2018, the scientific publication STAT wrote that Moderna had "baffled its peers" by placing a value of $7.5 billion on itself during its most recent fundraising effort. The article shared marketing materials Moderna had used to excite the investors, some of which pointed to "billion-dollar futures" for drugs the company had only tested in mice, predictions that investors told STAT were "pretty absurd."[1]

The article suggested that Moderna was relying on naive or inexperienced backers who didn't know enough to question the company's rosy promises. It unleashed a new wave of ridicule aimed at Bancel and his company.

"They must be targeting the Theranos investors with slides like this," one person wrote on Twitter.

"Truly vi$ionary," was another mocking tweet.

By April, some biotech investors were becoming exasperated with Bancel's big talk. They remained unconvinced the mRNA molecule could consistently make it into cells and produce enough protein to be of much value. Skeptics seized on Moderna's decision to give up on shots to treat Crigler-Najjar syndrome, and they pointed to few obvious signs of progress on shots for methylmalonic acidemia and propionic acidemia, two illnesses that Moderna had told investors it was going to defeat just a year earlier.

On a panel discussion at a biotechnology event in New York, Adam Stone, a well-regarded chief investment officer at Perceptive Advisors, a hedge fund specializing in life-science companies, gave a blunt assessment of the likelihood mRNA could form the basis of a drug or a vaccine.

"It will never work," Stone told the crowd of over one hundred people, according to someone at the event. (Stone says he doesn't remember making the comment.)

By the end of 2018, Moderna had become a true battleground

company, with fans and foes equally adamant about its future. Enough mutual funds and other investors found Bancel's pitch persuasive, enabling Moderna to sell shares during the first week of December in the largest-ever biotech initial public offering. By the end of the year, however, its shares had fallen 34 percent and it was the most-shorted biotech stock in the market, meaning it was the company that bearish "short sellers" were most convinced was overpriced and overhyped. Moderna had raised $620 million in its IPO, but much more would be needed to keep it going until it could bring a product to market.

Soon Bancel would be wondering where the cash was going to come from.

• • •

BioNTech, meanwhile, was making scientific progress in 2018, as Şahin embraced an unorthodox management style that increasingly left his researchers shaking their heads in disbelief.

He and Özlem Türeci were still all work and very little play. Each evening they went home, brewed some coffee or tea, and began a night shift of more research and writing. They worked so hard that they only had time to sleep about four hours a night, they told members of their team. Fine, a lot of executives are workaholics. With Şahin and Türeci, though, it never was the *same* four hours—the couple only overlapped in bed about two hours each night, a staffer was told. It wasn't entirely clear why the couple had adopted the gonzo sleep habits. Some employees speculated they were trying to send a passive-aggressive message to their researchers, reminding them of the preeminence of the company's research.

"Uğur's attitude is, if you don't think you sleep enough, just look at me," says a former senior BioNTech scientist. "He expects you to dedicate your life to the company."

Employees traded stories about Şahin's quirks, most of which related to how consumed he was by his research. There was the running to-do list he supposedly kept of all the things he wished to accomplish, such as learning a new computer language, if he ever had ten free minutes. They buzzed that he sometimes pulled out a mat and placed it on the floor of his office to grab five-minute catnaps, but he didn't want anyone knowing that he needed the short breaks.

When Şahin and Türeci and their daughter, Delphine, went on a holiday, the family liked visiting all-inclusive resorts in the Canary Islands or elsewhere. These weren't traditional family vacations, though. They usually shipped three or four hulking computers to these hotels, along with twenty-seven-inch computer screens, and they packed six suitcases, at least one stuffed with scientific papers. Şahin spent most days reading and writing in their hotel room while Türeci and Delphine hit the swimming pool, accompanied by a nanny or two. Şahin sometimes joined the family, lugging his scientific papers to the pool.

In 2018, the couple still lived in the same apartment in Mainz, even as their ownership stakes in BioNTech surged in value as the company raised money from new investors. Wealth and signs of affluence barely crossed Şahin's mind, however. In a town hall meeting with employees after Türeci became BioNTech's chief medical officer, she said she had purchased herself a necklace as a treat.

"I bought it myself because he would never buy it," she said about Şahin. Türeci wasn't leveling criticism—she was just teasing Şahin for how little he valued luxuries and material rewards.

Asked about his motivations, Şahin told a colleague: "You do it for the altruism, for the patients, for the glory."

In some ways, he had become the Michael Scott of the biotech world. Like the boss in the fictional television series, *The Office*, Şahin wanted BioNTech to be one big, happy family. For years, he had been on a first-name basis with staffers, many of whom were quite young, and he showed unusual patience when the researchers shared family, relationship, or other problems. Şahin and Türeci hosted extravagant Christmas parties featuring chocolate fountains, an assortment of expensive and exotic meats, and loud, local bands. As staffers danced and chowed down, the couple stood at the front of the room, beaming with pride and pleasure.

But Şahin demanded that his team prioritize the company and their work as much as he and Türeci did. Those not deemed dedicated enough were often let go, or sometimes Şahin froze them out.

"It was like the mafia, either you're in the family or you're nothing," says Björn Kloke, a scientist who worked at BioNTech in 2018. "I like the guy . . . his heart is usually in the right place, but he's dedicated his life to the company. That's not for everyone."

• • •

For years, Şahin and BioNTech had been focused on cancer vaccines, but that was changing, as Hoge had discovered. In the spring of 2018, Şahin welcomed two visitors to BioNTech's headquarters in Mainz: Kathrin Jansen, who ran vaccine research and development at U.S. drug giant Pfizer, and her colleague, Philip Dormitzer, who led Pfizer's viral vaccine R&D. The Pfizer executives were facing pressure to identify the next big thing in the pharmaceutical world. The company remained a global power, but revenues had been declining for several years, huge brands were losing their patent protections, and new-drug development was lagging. Pfizer's popular chief executive, Ian Read, was preparing to step down, and his replacement, a Greek-born veterinarian named Albert Bourla, was pushing the company to become more innovative.

Jansen and Dormitzer were eager for Pfizer to become involved in mRNA drugs or vaccines, but Pfizer had shuttered its infectious-disease unit years earlier and it hadn't done much mRNA work, making it difficult to catch up to Moderna or others, so Jansen and

Dormitzer began looking for a partner. The Pfizer executives had some initial conversations with Şahin before flying to meet him and his team.

As they toured BioNTech, they were impressed, but also taken aback. Pfizer was packed with tens of thousands of veteran scientists. It was hard to walk the company's hallways without spotting gray hair. But everyone at BioNTech seemed right out of school, making the executives nervous.

"Where are the adults?" Dormitzer asked one of his hosts, only half jokingly.

Over several months, though, he and Jansen became more comfortable with Şahin and his colleagues. They appreciated that Şahin obsessed over new scientific articles, just like they did, and they loved his passion for using mRNA molecules to build effective vaccines. In August 2018, the companies agreed to work together on mRNA shots for influenza, betting they could build a technology that was more protective than existing vaccines. Teaming up on flu also raised the possibility that the two companies might find a way to use mRNA to take on other pathogens, at least down the road.

For years, Stéphane Bancel dreaded competition in the field of mRNA. Now, just when he thought Moderna had built a comfortable lead, he had a fierce rival. Bancel didn't realize it, but Şahin was feeling his own pressures. BioNTech was still years away from an approved vaccine or drug and serious revenues weren't even on the horizon. The company would need a lot of money to pay for research if it wanted the chance to advance its work, no matter that it now had a partner in Pfizer. BioNTech could no longer solely rely on cash from the Strüngmann brothers or other private investors. The company would have to offer shares to public investors as part of an IPO, Şahin and his team decided, just like Moderna had done a year earlier.

During the summer of 2019, he and several colleagues spent two weeks traveling throughout Europe and New York to drum up interest in BioNTech's IPO, planned for October of that year. The executives visited the offices of dozens of hedge funds, mutual funds, and other investors, visiting twenty-four cities in total, detailing their plans to introduce vaccines and treatments to combat cancer and infectious diseases. Soft-spoken and understated, Şahin impressed audiences with his breadth of knowledge, the creative ways he and his scientists were enabling the immune system to fight disease, and his outsize ambition for his company.

Then the investors dug into the data. By then, BioNTech had been around for nine years, but only one drug was in a medium-stage phase 2 trial. That was a melanoma treatment BioNTech was developing with Genentech, meaning Şahin's company would have to split future revenues, if any ever resulted. Just 250 patients had even been treated with BioNTech's vaccines. It only *hoped* to start its first study of an influenza vaccine by the end of 2020.

As Jeffrey Jay, a Greenwich, Connecticut, health-care investment investor, listened to Şahin's pitch, he liked what he heard. Nonetheless, he decided to pass on the shares. The idea of developing another flu vaccine was "boring," and he wanted to see more evidence of progress on BioNTech's cancer research before buying shares.

"I like to see more data," Jay says.

Şahin and his colleagues kept hearing the same thing: Their company was "too complex." BioNTech was working on more than twenty-five different vaccines and drugs in total and it was using three different approaches in addition to mRNA molecules, including so-called CAR-T treatments, which are ways to enable the body's immune system to attack cancer. It was all too much for some investors.

"There was skepticism about our vision," Şahin says.

As the date of their early October share sale approached, Şahin and his colleagues experienced bad luck. Office-rental company WeWork was collapsing, a trade dispute between the United States and China was heating up, and other biotech shares were falling, including those of Moderna. On October 2, days before BioNTech's market debut, ADC Therapeutics, a Switzerland-based cancer drug start-up, decided to postpone its own IPO, startling Şahin and his team.

On Friday night, October 4, Sean Marett met with some senior colleagues for drinks in New York. They all knew the difficult position they were in, but they were so glum they avoided discussing the IPO and its problems.

Marett, who had just been told by a big investor that his firm wouldn't be buying shares due to the market's meltdown, was particularly dejected.

"I felt sick to my stomach," Marett says.

Şahin and the BioNTech team met with their bankers at JPMorgan to make a tough decision: scrap the company's IPO and maybe try it again in the future, or slash the price and size of the sale to try to entice investors. Şahin wanted to go forward.

"We can't go home without doing this," Marett agreed.

The team realized they didn't really have much of a choice—BioNTech needed the money. And an IPO, even a smaller one, would make it easier to raise money in the future by selling additional shares. BioNTech cut the price and the size of the deal, raising $150 million, just over half what they had hoped for.

Şahin believed in his company and his approach. It wasn't clear how many others did.

• • •

Dan Barouch and Adrian Hill still had faith in their own vaccine approaches.

By the fall of 2019, Barouch's partner, Johnson & Johnson's Janssen division, had put adenovirus vaccines, including its Ebola, HIV, and Zika vaccines, in over 110,000 people. The side effects were minimal and each of the shots appeared to generate impressive immune-system responses, training both B cells and T cells to fend off the pathogens.

Small doses of the vaccines seemed enough to jump-start the immune system. Using adenoviruses to deliver a genetic payload appeared safer than relying on traditional vaccines made from killed or weakened viruses. And the J&J technology seemed the kind that could be used to tackle future pathogens. The outside of future vaccines would look the same, always featuring the Ad26 common cold virus. On the inside, J&J scientists would simply insert genetic material coding for the key protein of whatever new virus they were trying to combat.

But the earlier studies hadn't aimed to prove efficacy—they hadn't compared whether subjects receiving the vaccines had lower rates of disease caused by Ebola or Zika than unvaccinated people who received a placebo, for example. J&J had decided it wasn't feasible to run placebo-controlled trials during deadly outbreaks of those diseases. In all its years of effort, Barouch and J&J still hadn't proven they could protect anyone with a vaccine, but they remained hopeful about their appraoch.

Over at Oxford University, Hill, Sarah Gilbert, and their team were equally optimistic about their own adenoviruses-based vaccine strategy. Their jabs seemed easy and inexpensive to produce and could be kept at standard, refrigerated temperatures for long periods, much like the Barouch and J&J shots, making them ideal for poorer nations without cold-storage capabilities. In total, though, the Oxford group had given their chimp-adenovirus shots to just 336 people, with another 1,500 or so receiving similar versions of the shots. The results that were insufficient to prove very much.

The Oxford researchers had begun a trial to test how their chimp-adenovirus vaccine delivery strategy might fare against MERS, to finally determine if their vaccine approach worked. But there still wasn't a single adenovirus vaccine for humans with proof of efficacy, and none appeared close to regulatory approval, at least in the West.

In late November 2019, Hill flew to National Harbor, Maryland, just south of Washington, D.C., for a meeting of global infectious-disease experts. At the conference, Hill was cocksure, as usual, weighing in on various pathogens and ideal vaccine approaches. He didn't realize it, but as he spoke, the threat of his lifetime was emerging thousands of miles away.

• • •

As 2019 began, Gale Smith and Novavax were taking one more shot at success with their own vaccine strategy.

It was only three years earlier that a clinical trial for Novavax's RSV vaccine had been such a crushing failure that Stan Erck and Gregory Glenn had been forced to fire a third of their staffers in a cost-cutting move. It had barely kept the company alive.

Somehow, Erck had subsequently managed to raise over $90 million from the Bill & Melinda Gates Foundation, enabling Novavax to complete a four-year study testing whether inoculating pregnant mothers with the company's shots could protect their babies from the vicious RSV virus.

In early 2019, Novavax shares were climbing once again as the company awaited results of its study, the latest shots from Smith's lab outside Washington, D.C. On February 28, 2019, the trial results were released: The vaccine protected just 39.4 percent of infants against lower respiratory tract infections (LRTI) compared with those who had received a placebo. It was another shocking and embarrassing failure for a company that by now had a long history of these flubs.

There was disbelief within Novavax. Some staffers cried in their offices, aware that jobs would again be shed and that the company might not survive. The researchers had dedicated years of their lives to protecting people from serious illness. Once again, clinical results had proven all the sweat and tears had been for naught.

Glenn was so despondent that he found it difficult to get out of bed. Even his favorite chickens couldn't soothe him.

"I had to face investors, my own staff, my own family, my own board," Glenn says. "I'm in the field of RSV, I had created conferences. . . . To stand up and say, you know, we just failed. That was very hard."[2]

Smith's colleagues were morose, but in many ways, he and his labmates viewed the new results as *good* news. Well, maybe not good news, but surely not as awful as most presumed. Their vaccine had protected 44 percent of babies against hospitalizations due to LRTI, providing better protection against RSV-related hospitalizations than anything available on the market. The Novavax shots had also reduced severe hypoxemia related to RSV—a serious condition in which too little oxygen makes it to the body's cells and tissues—by 60 percent.

Even the 39.4 percent primary-endpoint result was close to the 40 percent lower-end figure viewed by regulators as a success. They had missed their primary endpoint by a single case, it turned out. And in South Africa, which saw many more RSV cases than the United States, the vaccine achieved an efficacy rate as high as 76 percent. This wasn't the time to give up, Smith argued to colleagues.

Smith and the other researchers returned to the lab, discovering better ways to elicit immune response. They determined an ideal amount of adjuvant to use and how much protein from the targeted virus was necessary to get protection. The scientists also found ways to expose segments of the virus that usually are hidden to the immune system.

Investors didn't care. By May 2019, Novavax traded for a measly thirty-six cents a share and the company was in danger of getting tossed off the Nasdaq market. Novavax resorted to a one-for-twenty reverse stock split, meaning that employees and other investors holding one hundred shares now owned just five shares, though they were worth over six dollars a share. The move didn't help—by the end of 2019, Novavax's shares had plunged another 39 percent as most investors left the company for dead.

Desperate for cash, Novavax sold manufacturing assets. From that point on, the company would have to depend on others to produce its shots. Executives figured they'd worry about that issue if they ever got a vaccine approved. Erck also let one hundred employees go, about a quarter of its workforce, another painful step.

Some outsiders weren't quite sure why Novavax wasn't just throwing in the towel already.

"They weren't viewed as crooks or incompetent, but after the first attempt with RSV failed, folks were surprised they kept trying," says Rod Wong, managing partner of New York health-care investment firm RTW Investments. "Over time, investors lost interest."

In December 2019, Erck and Glenn made plans to host a company holiday party, hoping to bolster lagging spirits. In the past, Novavax staffers had been treated to elaborate parties. They also once had their rollicking bowling leagues and shiny trophies. Now, there was little left in Novavax's coffers to pay for the fun and games. Instead, the group gathered in a conference room over pizza slices and a few measly bottles of Coca-Cola. It was like a grade-school birthday party without the presents or sense of joy.

A few weeks later, employees met in a nearby Rockville bar, this time without any executives around. They wanted to discuss how they might salvage their careers. Over beers and other alcoholic drinks, somber staffers shared job leads and debated Novavax's future. They knew the company only had enough cash to survive a few months, and the stock traded under four dollars a share. In total, Novavax was worth $127 million, less than the cost of a superyacht.

A few employees said they still believed in the company's vaccine technology and vowed to stick around. Others said they also would be staying, but only because they had stock options that soon would vest. Then they were outta there.

Later, when some staffers handed in their resignations, Erck told them he understood their decisions and didn't harbor any ill will. Erck knew they needed a more stable place of work than he could provide.

As 2020 began, Novavax was conducting late-stage trials for yet another vaccine from Smith and his research team, which was now down to fewer than twenty people. This time, they were tackling the flu. Early data was impressive, but existing flu shots were largely effective, and no one was willing to fund Novavax's program.

"We were down to not a lot of people, no facilities, no money, no confidence," Glenn says.[3]

The flu vaccine was the company's last chance. Erck had managed to keep Novavax going for over a decade, pulling his team off the mat after each failure and frustration. Even he was getting gloomy, though.

"There were dark clouds hanging over us."

• • •

Things were also turning grimmer for Bancel and Moderna in late 2019. By then, cash from investors had stopped pouring in, partnerships with Merck and some others had been discontinued, and the company was resorting to cutting its research budget and other costs. In executive meetings, Bancel emphasized the need to stretch each dollar, and employees were told to reduce travel and other expenses, a frugality they were advised would last several years.

"We were freaked out about money," Hoge says.

Bancel, Hoge, and other top executives tried to shield staffers from the money worries so they could focus on their research, but there was only so much they could do. Employees knew the company had enough cash to last a couple years. They were relieved Moderna hadn't begun firing people, but they were also concerned about their futures.

Bancel and his colleagues were still convinced that injecting mRNA molecules packed with genetic instructions could get the body to produce proteins capable of teaching the immune system to protect against disease. At that point, Moderna's six hundred scientists and other staffers were running clinical trials or planned to for shots they had developed against Zika, chikungunya, flu, and other viruses and diseases, and Moderna had backing from the Bill & Melinda Gates Foundation.

Perhaps most important, Moderna had a big fan in Barney Graham. The senior scientist at the Vaccine Research Center didn't know about Moderna's cash concerns and he wasn't bothered by the continuing suspicions surrounding Bancel and his company. Graham was intrigued by Moderna's mRNA approach, and he wanted to see if it might be able to fend off the next threatening virus.

Back in 2017, Moderna and the government scientists had developed a MERS vaccine that had produced impressive levels of antibodies in mice and monkeys. A year later, they made progress on a vaccine for Nipah, a virus with a high mortality rate. In September 2019, Moderna produced its best results yet from a phase 1 study of a vaccine against cytomegalovirus, or CMV, and the company made plans for its first phase 2 study.

Later that fall, Graham and John Mascola, director of the VRC, toured the Norwood manufacturing plant and came away impressed. Moderna and the government scientists decided to run a drill in early 2020, to test how fast they could work together to build a vaccine in the event of a new viral infection. It would just be an exercise in pandemic preparedness, but it would help determine if the mRNA approach actually worked.

Years of sniping from critics had taken a toll on Moderna, however. At the end of 2019, the company's shares were 15 percent below their IPO price, making it hard for Bancel to raise new money to keep the business going. Even former fans, including Viking Global Investors, were dumping the stock. The $29 billion New York hedge fund had owned over 5 percent of the stock at the end of 2018, but it now owned almost no Moderna shares, a sign of the enduring skepticism about Bancel and Moderna.

• • •

In late 2019, Bancel flew with his family to their home in southern France for the holiday season.

Waking up early with a cup of tea nearby, Bancel read about the lung disease that was spreading in southern China.

Bancel began emailing Graham, the VRC scientist.

"Do you know what it is?" Bancel asked.

Graham said he and his team were aware of the outbreak. Rumors on Twitter and China's Weibo social-media platform pointed to a cluster of pneumonia cases around the city of Wuhan, in southern China. Graham had already emailed a younger scientist in his lab, Kizzmekia Corbett, saying they needed to prepare for whatever was emerging in that country. Details were scant, though—Graham didn't even know if a virus or bacteria was causing the infections.

Bancel couldn't stop thinking about the spreading illness.

He sent more messages to Graham, who promised to let Bancel know as soon as he learned the cause of the sickness. A few days later, Bancel and his family flew back to Boston, but he couldn't get the outbreak out of his mind.

Bancel's scientists had no experience with bacterial infections, so if that was the problem, Moderna couldn't be of much help. But if a new virus was in fact emerging, maybe his team could do something about it, he thought. Perhaps they could finally show that mRNA worked, proving the skeptics wrong. Maybe Bancel and Moderna could help stop the new virus.

14

January–February 2020

The single biggest threat to man's continued dominance on the planet is the virus.

—JOSHUA LEDERBERG, WINNER OF THE NOBEL PRIZE FOR MEDICINE, 1958

Wuhan is a beautiful place. It's also full of danger.

The capital of central China's Hubei province, Wuhan is an enormous city of eleven million, about as many as the combined populations of New York City and Chicago. Full of spectacular lakes and lush parks, Wuhan is divided by the magnificent Yangtze River and historically important Han River. The city boasts high-speed trains to various cities around China and flights to the rest of the world, with three train stations and a major international airport ferrying a steady stream of visitors.

Wuhan is known for a variety of fish dishes, thanks to its proximity to fresh water, and a hot noodle dish known as reganmian. Like some other big Chinese cities, Wuhan is also home to dozens of sprawling markets that sell a variety of fresh meat, fruits, seafood, and vegetables. Some also slaughter live animals on-site for their customers. Animals for sale include raccoon dogs, civets, mink, badgers, rabbits, hedgehogs, baby crocodiles, and bats, which sometimes are the size of chickens and are used for food, ceremonial, and medicinal purposes.[1] Much of the wildlife trade is illegal, and though a third of the species sold in Wuhan's markets are protected by the government, there's been precious little enforcement.[2]

Many of the animals butchered in the Wuhan markets are susceptible to infection and can transmit viruses. And they're often stored in cramped, unhygienic conditions, making it easy for pathogens to jump species. The storage and handling of the animals has long been a matter of concern, partly because similar conditions led to serious problems elsewhere in the country. In 2002, the SARS-CoV coronavirus first appeared in and around a similar market in the southern Chinese city of Foshan, about one thousand kilometers from Wuhan. Nearly half of the early patients who developed the SARS disease were food handlers who likely had close contact with some of these same animals.[3]

In December 2019, word began to emerge about a mysterious sickness spreading in the Wuhan area. Reports on social media and elsewhere described dozens of people sick from some kind of respiratory virus. No one knew the cause of the ailments—in early January, *The Wall Street Journal* described it as "a mystery viral pneumonia" that was causing "fever and breathing difficulties."[4] Some of the infections were linked to vendors at the Huanan Seafood Wholesale Market, one of the city's bigger markets, featuring a set of complex stalls and alleyways. It wasn't clear if the sickness originated in the market or if it was merely spreading there, but Chinese authorities, who already were battling an outbreak of African swine fever in the country, ordered it shut down.

Around midday on Friday, January 3, Zhang Yongzhen, a fifty-eight-year-old infectious disease expert at the Shanghai Public Health Clinical Center, which is part of Fudan University, received a package he had been eagerly awaiting: a metal box containing a test tube, packed in dry ice, with lung-washing swabs from seven patients suffering from the new virus in a Wuhan hospital. They had all been in the Wuhan market or lived nearby. Zhang and his colleagues got right to work and didn't stop for the next forty hours, spending two straight nights in the lab. By two a.m. on Sunday, January 5, the team had mapped the virus's genome, or its complete set of genetic instructions, declaring the pathogen to be "very similar to SARS-type coronavirus."[5] They also noticed a gene producing a spike protein on the pathogen's surface, one that resembled the one used by SARS-CoV to bind to human cells.

This was truly bad news—SARS had inflicted enormous damage on China, sparking the kind of social unrest that kept authorities up at night. If the new pathogen was anything like that one, the country was in some trouble. Local scientists knew it and so did Chinese officials. Over the next week, though, Chinese authorities went out of their way to reassure the public and others. Wuhan health officials said they hadn't seen new cases in the previous week, which was encouraging, and they hadn't found "significant" human-to-human transmission, though they didn't elaborate on what "significant" meant.[6]

The World Health Organization, a United Nations agency specializing in global health, issued statements complimenting China's public-health resources as well as its system for monitoring illness outbreaks, providing more reason for comfort. Wuhan itself was the home of China's first Biosafety Level 4 laboratory, a specialized research laboratory dealing with potentially deadly infectious agents, a sign the city was no scientific backwater. Experts said that even if a new coronavirus had in fact emerged, it was unlikely to have the impact of the virus that led to SARS. Health authorities had learned so much since 2002 and the Chinese government was better prepared to respond, they said.

For all the calm and confidence displayed by health authorities and others, Zhang and other Chinese scientists were becoming alarmed about what was happening in Wuhan. They were especially worried about a family of six who lived in a different and even larger city, Shenzhen, over one thousand kilometers away. Just before the New Year, the family had traveled to Wuhan for a weeklong visit. Now, five members of the family were infected with Wuhan's new virus, each suffering from a variety of maladies, including fever, upper or lower respiratory tract symptoms, and diarrhea.

People get sick while traveling; it happens. But what was especially troubling about this case was that one of the family members hadn't made the trip to Wuhan, yet had still become infected with the new virus after several days of contact with family members. It was a clear sign the virus was potentially transmittable between people. Just as chilling: One family member—a ten-year-old who was later described in the medical journal *The Lancet* as being "non-compliant to parental guidance," seemingly because she didn't wear a surgical mask during the Wuhan vacation like another child on the trip—had become infected yet didn't demonstrate any symptoms of the virus.[7] That was great for her, but awful for everyone else. To Zhang and others, it meant many more asymptomatic people in the country and elsewhere could already be carrying and spreading the new virus, without anyone knowing they had been infected.

Zhang, who also worked for the Chinese Center for Disease Control and Prevention, had to figure out what to do. A few days earlier, the National Health Commission (NHC), a cabinet-level agency overseeing the Chinese CDC, had issued an internal notice ordering laboratories that had tested samples of the new virus to destroy them or hand them to the government, while forbidding anyone from publishing research on the virus.[8]

Zhang looked at his phone and saw another email from Eddie Holmes. He had been emailing for days but Zhang mostly ignored him. Holmes, an infectious disease specialist at the University of Sydney, had written a number of scientific papers with Zhang about the evolution of various new and emerging viruses. They were even working on a paper about respiratory disease in Wuhan, of all places. Now, Holmes was hearing chatter about an emerging virus in the city and he was desperate to learn what Zhang knew about the new pathogen.

"Are you working on it?" Holmes asked in yet another email.

Zhang didn't share any details about his work or the new virus. Early on Sunday, January 5, though, a few hours after he finished sequencing of the virus genome, Zhang sent an email to Holmes, who read it as his wife drove their car to a Sydney beach for an outing with family members visiting from the United Kingdom.

"Please call me immediately!!!" Zhang wrote.

Holmes excused himself from his guests and phoned Zhang. They began discussing details of the new pathogen and its similarities with previous deadly viruses. Almost simultaneously, they reached the same conclusion.

"It's SARS, it's SARS!" Zhang said.

Shit, it's back, Holmes thought, referring to another pernicious coronavirus.

Zhang and his colleagues in China began cautioning authorities in the country. After sending a warning to the NHC, Zhang boarded a flight to Wuhan, where he told senior public-health officials in the city that they needed to take emergency measures to protect against spread of the pathogen ahead of the busy Lunar New Year holiday season later that month.[9]

That wasn't enough, Holmes told Zhang. Cases were growing in Wuhan, Hong Kong, and elsewhere. You need to share the genetic details of the virus with the world, Holmes said. If a SARS-like pathogen is spreading, testing kits would be needed within days. A vaccine might even be required. But no test kits or vaccines could be produced without knowledge of the virus's genetic makeup.

Zhang was torn. He was a serious scientist who had sequenced thousands of virus genomes in his career. Like Holmes, Zhang was sure the genetic data he had would make a well-read paper in a high-profile journal, a goal of every researcher. The two researchers had received interest in their paper from the prestigious journal *Nature*. The information would be helpful to scientists around the world. Yet Zhang also knew Chinese authorities wanted to control information about the new virus. Other government labs had decoded the same genetic material, and on January 8, Chinese leaders confirmed they were dealing with a new coronavirus.[10] But they still sat on the genetic information. It was a warning sign to Zhang—the Chinese government didn't want the information released, possibly because it would invite scrutiny of the country's handling of the new virus.

Zhang had already dealt with his share of recent personal trauma. Several months earlier, Zhang's wife had died of cancer, and he was still mourning her loss. He already led a stressful life, even apart from that tragedy. Zhang was so busy chasing viruses that he sometimes slept two or three nights a week in his office. The last thing he wanted was to add more tension to his life. He already had done a lot to help stop the virus. It seemed wise to avoid crossing his superiors and to do nothing more with the genetic information.

Now Holmes was getting frustrated. Each day without the genetic information meant another day before tests could be developed, potentially jeopardizing global health. Besides, he and Zhang had a huge scoop they were bound to lose to some other researcher. Word was getting out that the sequence data was available, and that a scientific paper had been written, but someone was refusing to release it. On January 10, Jeremy Farrar, the director of the huge Wellcome Trust in the U.K., one of the largest foundations in the world, tweeted that if the rumors are true and someone wasn't releasing this crucial information, "something is very wrong."

Oh God, that's me! Holmes thought.

Holmes called Farrar, asking if he might be able to get the Chinese CDC to share the sequence and try to persuade Zhang. Then Holmes called Zhang, trying to convince him once again.

"We really, really need it," he told Zhang.

On the morning of Saturday, January 11, Zhang sat on a plane on the runway at Shanghai Hongqiao International Airport. He was about to take off for Beijing so he could warn additional authorities about the virus, when he got another call from Holmes.

"Can you release it?" Holmes asked.

"I need to call you back," Zhang said.

The cabin crew saw Zhang speaking on his mobile phone and ordered him to turn it off.

"You need to release it to me," Holmes said.

Silence.

"Okay," Zhang said softly.

Zhang made a quick call to a staffer in his lab. A few minutes later, Holmes saw an email with an attachment in his in-box. He did a quick calculation and realized it was after midnight in Edinburgh, Scotland, the home of Andrew Rambaut, an academic who ran a website called virological.org. He and Holmes had agreed to publish the sequence on his open site if Zhang ever released the information. Rambaut, a night owl, picked up the phone right away. Holmes told him the sequence was on its way. Holmes hadn't even read Zhang's attachment—there wasn't any time.

"It could have been DNA from a blowfly," Holmes says. "I didn't even check."

Fifty-two minutes later, during the evening of Friday, January 10, on the East Coast of the United States, the information was available and scientists around the world were furiously downloading the sequence of the virus, which later would be named SARS-CoV-2. A day later, the Chinese CDC officially released the virus's genetic information and Holmes felt enormous relief. Finally, the world could start defending itself against the virus.

"It was a weight off my shoulders," Holmes says.

Zhang was just as thrilled, at least at first. A day later, though, he began to come under pressure from Chinese authorities. They were unhappy that the nation was receiving criticism for its handling of the emerging virus, and that he had released the sequence without their permission. Holmes sent emails to senior officials saying Zhang's act had benefited global science and health. It was a great moment for China. Don't punish Zhang, he urged the officials.

Soon, though, Zhang's lab was temporarily closed for "recertification," and funding for his research was suspended, according to someone close to him.

• • •

Barney Graham wanted to act quickly.

On January 6, Graham, the deputy director of the Vaccine Research Center at the National Institutes of Health, phoned his former collaborator, Jason McLellan, who now ran his own lab at the University of Texas at Austin. He caught McLellan at a good time—he was in a ski lodge in Park City, Utah, and had a few minutes to chat while waiting for his snowboarding boots to be heat molded. Graham and McLellan had worked together on two previous coronaviruses, HKU1 and MERS. Now, Graham wanted to know if McLellan had interest in collaborating on a vaccine against the new virus and its resulting disease, which would be named 2019 novel coronavirus, or Covid-19.

"Are you ready to get back in the saddle?" Graham asked McLellan.

Graham sounded more excited than nervous. At that point, the virus was worrisome, but it was far away and he didn't fear it would cause tremendous damage. Instead, he saw the perfect chance to take on a new pathogen and show his group could quickly build an effective vaccine.

McLellan expressed immediate interest in the new project, but he was even less concerned about the new virus. All around him, skiers and snowboarders were enjoying the sunny winter day, sharing warm embraces and relishing the closeness of friends and family. If anyone in the Utah lodge had health concerns, they were about the ongoing flu season or a possible injury on the slopes. The new virus felt a million miles away.

Still, Graham and McLellan wanted to be fast—to protect people in China and maybe elsewhere, to write a potentially important academic paper, and to prove they could quickly develop effective shots using messenger RNA molecules. And they needed to do it before others had a chance. Right away, McLellan sent WhatsApp messages to Nianshuang Wang, the Chinese-born scientist in his lab, and a graduate student named Daniel Wrapp, relaying details of Graham's call and saying their team was going to move quickly to build a new vaccine.

"We're going to race," McLellan said.

A few days later, on the Saturday morning that Zhang and Holmes shared the new pathogen's genome with the world, Wang got into his Subaru Forester and drove fifteen minutes to McLellan's campus lab to begin designing a vaccine candidate. Wang didn't need a sample of the actual virus, just its molecular backbone: the genetic sequence Zhang had shared featuring four bonded chemicals—adenine (A), thymine (T), guanine (G), and cytosine (C).

Wang, Graham, and McLellan had already developed vaccine candidates for SARS, MERS, and other coronaviruses, so they were pretty certain their new vaccine would need to teach the body's immune system to recognize and attack SARS-CoV-2's spike protein, the key spot on the virus that grabbed on to the host cells, just like their previous antigens. With some simple software, Wang identified a nucleotide sequence producing the 1,273 amino acids that composed the new virus's full-length spike protein.

Then came the hard part. Wang set out to alter the genetic code of the protein, to make it an ideal target for the immune system. Four years earlier, he and McLellan had added two prolines to the stem of the MERS-CoV spike protein, holding the protein in the shape it took just before it infected host cells. For the new vaccine, Wang once again adjusted the amino acid sequence of the spike protein to include these rigid amino acids, so the body could generate a protein matching the shape of the virus's spike protein before it fused with the body's cells. Wang tweaked the protein's genetic sequence in other ways as well, such as making it soluble and removing its furin cleavage site, or the spot where the protein is split in two.

Wang kept going and going, spending Friday night into Saturday morning on his genetic modifications, then working all day Sunday. He mostly subsisted on instant noodles, which he mixed together with water and fresh eggs, all warmed in a nearby microwave. There was hardly anyone around, making it easier for Wang to concentrate on creating the perfect vaccine. He had developed similar genetic constructs for various molecules hundreds of times, but he still felt pressure to finish quickly with no errors.

It will be a disaster if I make a mistake, he thought.

By Monday morning, Wang had succeeded in designing genetic sequences for over a dozen different constructs, or versions, of the spike protein. Looking at his work, Wang realized his DNA sequences, based on the viral RNA sequence, would be too long and complicated for companies to quickly produce, so he designed a way to slice them into shorter, easily synthesizable fragments. Wang sent his sequences to a gene-synthesis company to turn them into DNA. A few days later, he received a delivery of tubes full of his custom-made genetic material. He spent the next week working with Wrapp to place the DNA in plasmids, and then put them in human cells, creating ten different versions of the spike protein, which he called nCoV 1–10.

Wang was so caught up in his work, which sometimes lasted until four a.m., that he wasn't aware that on January 21, the U.S. CDC had confirmed the nation's first case of the novel coronavirus in Washington State, worrisome evidence the virus was spreading. At one point, he grabbed a few minutes to call his parents in their village, far from Wuhan. Earlier, Wang had sent them face masks, just in case the pathogen reached their area in China. Now, he mentioned to them that he was working on a possible vaccine for the new virus. That wasn't a great idea—Wang's folks didn't understand his work and immediately became worried about their son's health, certain that he was handling a version of the dangerous virus. Wang was too busy to explain how modern vaccines worked. He also didn't have time to reflect on the fact that it was he, a Chinese native waiting impatiently for an American green card, who was racing to protect the world against a pathogen that seemed to have originated in his home country.

On Thursday, January 23, Wang packed his material in a container, trying hard to ensure it didn't leak, and shipped it all to Kizzmekia Corbett, the government scientist who was doing similar work with others in Graham's lab. Corbett, Graham, and John Mascola chose an ideal spike-protein design and sent it to Moderna. The company's scientists, relying on McLellan and Wang's earlier work, had built their own spike-protein design. It matched the one from the government scientists, confirming they made the right choice. Moderna took their chosen sequence, employed some sophisticated computer software, and built an mRNA molecule capable of producing the stabilized spike protein. This would be Moderna's vaccine antigen.

McLellan's and Graham's labs also sent the plasmids to scientists in over two hundred other labs around the world, jump-starting the global scientific community's work on tests, vaccines, and drugs for the new virus. Wang's hustle meant tests and treatments could be produced several weeks faster than otherwise would have been possible. It still wasn't clear how necessary they would be, though, or if any of them would actually work.

• • •

Stéphane Bancel kept tracking the new illness. There was just so much he was going to worry about it, though.

Over the previous two decades, Bancel had seen two coronaviruses, SARS-CoV and MERS-CoV, emerge and then largely disappear, at least in the West. Bancel continued to email Graham about the new pathogen, and he kept an eye on Moderna's work with the government scientists to build a vaccine. But Moderna had its hands full with other work, so Bancel was happy the NIH team were leading an early clinical trial of their shots. As intrigued as he was, Bancel decided that he had more pressing concerns than a coronavirus half a world away.

By early 2020, Moderna was burning through a half a billion dollars each year. Two years earlier, the company had raised over $600 million in its initial public offering, but Bancel knew he'd soon have to raise cash from investors once again. With Moderna's shares at $19, still down sharply from their IPO price, some executives at the company weren't sure how he was going to do it.

On January 12, Bancel flew to San Francisco to attend JPMorgan Chase's annual health-care conference, hoping to impress attendees with a speech about Moderna's progress on its shots to protect against cytomegalovirus, a common virus affecting babies, two cancer vaccines, and one for a rare childhood disease.

During his speech and his conversations with investors and others,

Bancel didn't mention the new pathogen circulating in China. The topic was shockingly irrelevant to the thousands of health-care specialists who had trekked to San Francisco for the conference. They were mainly searching for the next hot drug. Indeed, for three days, drug-industry pros mingled and glad-handed.

Bancel's pitch received a lukewarm response. Some at the event remained unsure why Moderna had pivoted to vaccines from drug research. Others were growing impatient that the company still didn't have a vaccine approaching late-stage, phase 3 clinical trials, let alone in the market.

"People weren't thrilled with us," Bancel says.

By the time Bancel boarded a red-eye flight on Friday, January 17, to Davos, Switzerland, to join thousands of global leaders at the annual meeting of the World Economic Forum, he was becoming more concerned about the novel coronavirus. At the event, attendees debated economic, political, and environmental topics, and Bancel spent some time trying to understand why investors were so discouraged about his company.

At one point, Bancel spotted Andreas Halvorsen and Brian Kaufmann, two top executives at Viking Global, the hedge fund that had dumped almost all its Moderna shares in previous months.

"Why did you guys sell everything?" Bancel asked them.

The stock had barely moved since its debut, they told him. A Viking executive who wasn't at the JPMorgan Chase event gave an additional reason the hedge fund had qualms about Moderna: Bancel was "superpromotional and a little expansive," code words for someone apt to exaggerate his company's potential.

But Bancel spent most of his time at the event in the back of various conference rooms, away from the investors and politicians. There, he huddled with Jeremy Farrar, the director of the Wellcome Trust, and Richard Hatchett, an epidemiologist who ran the Coalition for Epidemic Preparedness Innovations (CEPI), a foundation that funds vaccine development. Farrar and Hatchett were glued to their phones, receiving running updates on new infections in China. Bancel sat close by, eager to hear the latest news.

Farrar and Hatchett grabbed napkins from nearby tables and began calculating the pathogen's reproduction number, or its R0 (pronounced "R naught"), which is the number of new infections caused, on average, by a single contagious person. They reached a quick consensus: This was going to be the mother of all coronaviruses.

Now Bancel was truly worried. He took out his iPad and began reading about the city of Wuhan, realizing it was an enormous place. Flights from the city's airport reached every Asian capital, all of Europe, and West Coast cities including Seattle, San Francisco, and Los Angeles. Things were starting to look grim.

"It's everywhere isn't it?" Bancel asked.

"It's everywhere," Farrar said.

Shit, this will be 1918, Bancel thought.

On January 23, the third day of the forum, Chinese leaders locked down Wuhan and three other cities, in the biggest quarantine in history. The Chinese must know it's bad and they're not telling anyone, Bancel concluded. He looked around—heated discussions were under way about the future of work, blockchain traceability, and inclusivity. A tsunami was just beyond the horizon, yet everyone was frolicking on the beach.

On Saturday morning, January 25, Bancel woke up scared. A pandemic was coming but his company wasn't ready. The NIH planned to test Moderna's vaccine but he didn't know if the government agency could move quickly enough or if it was as frightened of the new virus as he had become. His company had never come close to producing a vaccine, but hundreds of millions of doses might be needed. Bancel had personal worries, too—his mother was battling blood cancer and her immune system wasn't strong. She'd be in potential jeopardy if the powerful virus swept the world.

Bancel set up conference calls with his team back in Cambridge, telling them the coronavirus vaccine would need to be their priority.

"It's not an outbreak, it's a pandemic," he told them, his voice rising.

Bancel canceled plans to attend a board meeting in Germany and bought a one-way flight to Washington, D.C. At eight a.m. on Monday morning, January 27, Bancel walked into a conference room on the seventh floor of the National Institute of Allergy and Infectious Disease's headquarters. He pulled up a leather chair at a long, faux-wooden table, across from Graham, Mascola, and Anthony Fauci, the NIAID's director.

Within minutes, Fauci and his colleagues said they were just as intent on swiftly starting a phase 1 clinical trial for their vaccine. The whole reason the NIH had started working with Moderna was because mRNA shots can be designed and produced faster than those based on older technologies, which usually require growing a virus in eggs or a protein in enormous vats of cells, processes that can take months. In fact, Fauci needed to be convinced that Moderna wasn't going to drag its feet.

"How quickly can you get into clinic?" Fauci asked, referring to a phase 1 trial, the first step to testing a vaccine.

"Sixty days," Bancel replied confidently.

The meeting ended on an optimistic note. The NIH and Moderna would do everything they could to prevent impending horror. Bancel said he just needed to confirm the plans with his executive team.

• • •

Back in the office, Bancel told Stephen Hoge, Moderna's president, and others at the company that they had a lot of work ahead. The team would need to prepare doses for phase 2 and 3 trials so they could prove their vaccine's efficacy. They also had to buy bioreactors, add capacity in the Norwood site and elsewhere, and take other steps to scale up their manufacturing process to somehow make a billion vaccine doses, which Bancel was sure would be needed over the next year.

Not so fast, Hoge told him. Moderna had only eight hundred employees, including all its scientists and manufacturing personnel. The company had never run a late-stage trial, let alone had an approved vaccine or drug. And now Bancel was promising the U.S. government a vaccine in record time?

Moderna was making progress on its other vaccines and work on a Covid-19 vaccine would be a huge distraction, Hoge and others told Bancel. What if the virus fizzled out? Most important, it would cost as much as $2 billion to produce all those vaccines, money Moderna just didn't have. If it built a Covid-19 vaccine and it failed, Moderna was likely doomed—investors would never forgive the company if they dropped everything to build a vaccine that wasn't effective or was beaten to the market by a rival.

"Should we really be doing this?" Hoge asked Bancel. "We're betting the company."

Bancel was insistent. A pandemic was around the bend. They had a historic opportunity: Moderna could be the one to develop an effective vaccine. All their hard work over the past decade would finally pay off.

He eventually wore his colleagues down. Moderna would go all out to develop a vaccine that could stop the new virus.

• • •

In late February, Bancel convened a meeting with about thirty top Moderna executives in a ninth-floor conference room. By then, the company had shipped its first batch of Covid-19 vaccines, called mRNA-1273, to Corbett, the NIH scientist, to begin testing in mice. Within weeks, early results showed it elicited antibodies to the coronavirus, a promising, albeit early, sign.

Moderna staffers were accustomed to self-confidence, even boasts, from Bancel. When he met with Fauci and the others, he had oozed confidence. Now, they noticed, he was unusually serious and measured.

"We've been asked to make a vaccine," Bancel said in the meeting. "It will be a big test for us, but we've been preparing for this."

Staffers listened somberly, many understanding the virus's seriousness for the first time. They thought of their own health, the imminent threat to their families, and the challenge ahead.

"We have to try," Bancel said.

• • •

Uğur Şahin and Özlem Türeci sat down for a meal that would change their lives.

On Saturday morning, January 25, they headed for the farmer's market in the historic center of the German city of Mainz. Each week, the couple came with their daughter for breakfast. When the weather allowed, they grabbed an outdoor table near a pedestrian walkway and the Mainz Cathedral, a majestic, one-thousand-year-old Romanesque structure. The outing gave the family an opportunity to chat about the week, and discuss topics of interest.

Soon after ordering tea and toast, along with some jam and butter, Şahin told his family he had read something disturbing the previous evening. An article in the latest issue of *The Lancet* gave details of the family from Shenzhen that had traveled to Wuhan in late December and had become infected with the new coronavirus. What was worrisome, Şahin said, was that members of the family had tested positive for the virus without exhibiting any symptoms. How can quarantine measures work if it's not clear who is infected? he asked.

Just a few weeks earlier, Şahin had largely dismissed the significance of the new pathogen. Now he appeared unnerved.

"I think this is going to be a pandemic," he said.

Really? A pandemic? Türeci didn't buy it. Yes, Şahin responded.

Wuhan is one of China's best-connected cities, he told her. He was sure Chinese authorities wouldn't be able to contain the virus. He began doing some math in his head—current cases, potential exposure, likely spread; the results were ugly.

Before long, Türeci became convinced. And nervous, too. BioNTech was going to have to scrap its plans for the year; so would the rest of the world.

Now Şahin was energized—he had an idea.

"I think we can build a vaccine quickly," he said. "We have to contribute."

They headed back to their apartment where Şahin planted himself in front of his computer and downloaded the virus's genetic sequence. He needed to move fast, to help stop the coming plague and to catch up to the scientists he knew had two-week head starts working on vaccines and drugs. The rest of that day and all day Sunday he barely budged from his computer, using the same methods Wang, the NIH scientists, and the Moderna team employed days earlier to design ten possible coronavirus-vaccine designs. Each was a little different, but they all included the coronavirus's spike protein, like Moderna. And they all used the same two-proline modification to the protein's sequence that McLellan and his colleagues had developed.

Early Monday morning, Şahin convened a meeting of five of his most senior executives. He told them about the *Lancet* paper and shared his concerns. Trouble was coming. The company was going to drop everything to develop a vaccine.

"We don't have much time, maybe a few weeks," he said.

Şahin was somber. But he looked around the room and no one seemed very worried. The BioNTech executives remembered how SARS and MERS had both died out. Wasn't this outbreak far away in Wuhan? Şahin described the city's major airport and said he was certain the pathogen was already circulating in their midst. He outlined his mathematical calculations, the same ones he had shared with Türeci in the farmer's market.

"This is going to come," he said. "It will kill up to three million people."

Finally, he had everyone's attention.

"We're going to need a vaccine," he said. "I think we can do something about it with our mRNA."

Later, Şahin spent two hours on the phone with Thomas Strüngmann, convincing BioNTech's most important investor that calamity was coming and securing his support for BioNTech to try to tackle the new virus.

Two days later, though, Şahin came to a disturbing conclusion. Walking the office, he heard chatter about the Mainz Carnival, known as Fastnacht, a season of festivity and merrymaking culminating in late February. His team wasn't taking his directive seriously. It drove Şahin nuts.

"I told you we're going to run into the worst pandemic in fifty years, but I don't think you understood," he told one staffer. "If you did, you wouldn't behave like this."

He told another: "I'm *serious* about this."

Şahin told employees to cancel holiday plans and to stop taking public transportation, to avoid infection. He divided staffers into shifts; that way if someone from one group became infected with the coronavirus he'd have a better chance protecting the other group.[11] Now his researchers got the message.

He called Philip Dormitzer, the senior Pfizer executive, to tell him about BioNTech's plan to go after a Covid-19 vaccine. Dormitzer wasn't thrilled with the idea. Before joining Pfizer, he had worked at Novartis and had seen the drug company lose money developing a coronavirus vaccine that proved unnecessary. He had high hopes for the joint effort with BioNTech to develop a new flu vaccine.

Coronavirus research seemed like a distraction. Go for it, Uğur, but try not to get too caught up, Dormitzer said.

"Remember, SARS was contained," Dormitzer told him, "MERS, too."

"No, this is *big*," Şahin told him. "We really want to pursue this."

In February, Şahin's worries began to appear justified. Scientists at Imperial College in London estimated that two-thirds of Covid-19 cases in travelers from China had not yet been detected, and that it was "highly likely" that these undetected cases "will have started chains of transmission" in countries around the world.[12] The U.S. Centers for Disease Control and Prevention had said it was preparing for a possible pandemic,[13] though Secretary of Health and Human Services Alex Azar was confident the virus was "contained." The CDC had started sending out test kits, another sign of the building concern, though they were quickly recalled because they were flawed.[14]

By the end of February, Şahin had given their effort a name: Project Lightspeed. They were going to push to make a vaccine before the end of the year, faster than any vaccine had ever been made. But BioNTech only had about $300 million on its balance sheet, even less cash than Moderna. Şahin's company would need to develop, test, manufacture, and distribute shots, all of which would be hugely expensive.

It became clear to Şahin: His company would need help.

• • •

Back in Boston, Juan Andres was freaking out.

The fifty-three-year-old Madrid native ran Moderna's huge manufacturing site in Norwood, Massachusetts. Andres had a pharmacy degree and he knew a ton about making vaccines and drugs for various infectious diseases, but he was no expert in the diseases themselves. Still, he couldn't shake awful memories of living in Europe during 2009's swine flu pandemic, which was caused by the H1N1 virus. That illness left thirty thousand people sick across seventy-four countries, killing several individuals in New York City, Australia, and elsewhere, while forcing the government in Hong Kong to close schools for weeks.[15]

Sure, in hindsight, political and health leaders of various countries had been overly cautious, even alarmist, in declaring the first pandemic in forty-one years. But Andres recalled the experience differently—he remembered a run on goods in some countries that left people scrambling for basic needs. He was a supply specialist, lifesaving equipment was what he thought about all day, so the earlier experience had left a distinct memory.

In late January, Andres started reading articles about the new virus in China. He already knew Moderna was shifting to produce a potential vaccine. Quickly, he became anxious. Andres had been in the pharmaceutical industry over three decades, previously running drug manufacturing at Novartis, so he knew how quickly respiratory disease can spread. Increased global travel since the 2009 swine flu outbreak only increased the dangers of the new virus, he figured.

At his home in the Boston suburb of Newton, Andres started warning his twenty-four-year-old daughter, Enesta, that something bad was coming. She rolled her eyes. People will be hoarding things soon, he promised his wife, Marina. She told him he was crazy.

Andres didn't care. He went on a shopping spree, purchasing dozens of cans of disinfectant and enough paper towels and tissue paper to last his family a full year. Now they were outright laughing at him. Piles of toilet paper in their home were among the funniest things they had ever seen.

He went on Amazon to order face masks. Not the regular surgical kind, they wouldn't help much, he decided. Andres bought boxes of N95 masks, the type that filter 95 percent of airborne particles. Now he was getting giggles.

"What's thc big deal?" he asked his wife and daughter, sounding a tad defensive.

One day in early February, Andres walked into his kitchen and told Marina he had ordered a new refrigerator from Costco. We'll need to store a lot of food if there's a lockdown, he told her.

Marina was no longer laughing.

"Where are you going to put it?!"

"In the basement," he replied.

"You've lost it," she told him, flashing him an unhappy look. "We already *have* a refrigerator down there!"

A week or so later, Marina traveled to Madrid to visit her mother. At the time, their other daughter, Sylvia, was studying in London. Andres kept hearing reports of new infections. For days, he dreaded picking up the phone, but he finally had to call Marina.

"Tomorrow, you're coming home," he told her. "And you need to bring Sylvia back. The world may be closed for a year."

Marina bristled. "What is this, a command?" She told Andres, "No, I just got here. I'll stay another week with my mother."

Andres apologized for his tone but said there was good reason for his insistence.

"Marina, in thirty years, I've never told you anything." Andres pleaded. "I'm telling you now—you're taking the plane tomorrow."

Sylvia came home. So did Marina. Two months later, Covid-19 claimed the life of her mother.

15

February–March 2020

There are decades where nothing happens; and there are weeks where decades happen.

—Vladimir Ilyich Lenin

It started as a slight cough.

During the weekend of February 22, Lawrence Garbuz visited a synagogue for a funeral, before attending both a bar mitzvah as well as a bat mitzvah. The fifty-year-old father of four in New Rochelle, New York, a suburb of New York City, thought he might be developing a cold, so he mostly kept to himself and left each event shortly after arriving. Garbuz had read that a coronavirus was circulating in China, and he knew there had been outbreaks in parts of Italy and other areas in Europe, but he wasn't too concerned.

Within a few days, however, Garbuz was dealing with a dry, persistent cough. He was also feverish. His body ached and he was too weak to speak. Before long, he felt like he was drowning. As his doctor rushed him to a local hospital, Garbuz wrote him a note: "Am I going to die?"

Garbuz's lungs were full of fluid and his X-rays suggested he was getting shockingly little air. His doctors said they didn't know what was wrong, disturbing his family. Soon Garbuz was placed on a ventilator in a medically induced coma and transported to the intensive care unit at New York–Presbyterian/Columbia University Irving Medical Center.

On March 2, doctors shocked Garbuz's wife, Adina Lewis, who was also his partner in their trusts and estates law firm in Manhattan. They said they had a diagnosis: Covid-19. Garbuz's children raced to be near him, some flying in from Europe. As they landed in New York, Lewis called, calmly asking that they not react out loud to what she was about to say, in case someone overheard.

"Daddy has corona," she told them.

Word quickly spread, despite the Garbuz family's attempts to keep the illness private. Soon camera crews were in front of the family's home and New York governor Andrew Cuomo had imposed a containment zone around their town, hoping to halt the virus's spread. Before long, more than one hundred cases had emerged in their area, Westchester County. Cuomo described Garbuz as the region's "Patient Zero," even though others had similar symptoms at the time and a New York woman had earlier been diagnosed with the virus. Garbuz's sickness was baffling—he hadn't traveled outside the country or interacted with anyone who had been abroad.

He was fighting for his life, and Lewis desperately wanted someone to be there for him. Though Lewis was quarantined in the family's home, she obtained permission from New York's Department of Health for two of her children, who had been carefully avoiding potential exposure to the coronavirus, to visit Garbuz's hospital, in case he emerged from the coma. When they walked into the building and made it clear whom they were visiting, a nurse recoiled, retreating to a wall and then crawling away. Most everyone on the hospital staff was caring and professional, but another nurse told the children their father was responsible for the developing outbreak in the region.

Late at night on March 13, Garbuz woke up, after nearly two weeks on a ventilator. He had no idea what had happened to him or that fear was now gripping the region. Lewis spoke to her husband on a video call, advising him not to Google himself or read the news. He didn't need to go online to know something had changed. He saw it on the faces of the doctors and nurses around him. The United States, like the rest of the world, had awoken to a nightmare of its own.

"I wake up and there's a pandemic. There's fear in people's eyes," Garbuz says.[1]

A few weeks later, Garbuz was asked to be on the *Today* show. He didn't want to make the appearance. He still felt weak and unwell, and he didn't want additional publicity. The show's representatives told Garbuz he could play a role calming the public, so he reluctantly agreed. He walked the long path of his home as the cameras filmed, an uplifting image for television viewers of a resilient, recovering patient. What they couldn't see was that members of the crew were off-camera, prepared to catch Garbuz if he fell.

It was more important to allay the public's concerns than to face the new reality.

• • •

As the new coronavirus spread, it seemed similar to most other respiratory illnesses, at least at first. Patients suffered from fever, coughs, and shortness of breath. Soon, though, it became clear this one was uniquely treacherous. The novel coronavirus could affect the kidneys, heart, and liver, and the circulatory and gastrointestinal systems. Sometimes patients' lungs filled with so much fluid they weren't able to breathe, as Garbuz experienced. Many of those infected with the virus lost their senses of smell and taste. Few children were getting sick, but the elderly and those with compromised immune systems faced more acute danger. The virus had a unique ability to inhibit the body's virus-fighting T cells and B cells. The immune systems of some patients overreacted, resulting in dangerous "cytokine storms," as the body starts to attack its own cells.[2]

It soon became apparent that SARS-CoV-2 was spreading through droplets transmitted into the air, likely from coughing and sneezing. Respiratory diseases are dangerous because they infect so easily. This one was proving especially lethal. Measures that had tamed past viral epidemics, such as isolation and proper hygiene, failed to help, partly because infected people could spread the disease without exhibiting symptoms of illness.

Health authorities were stunned—few had seen such significant escalation of a disease in such a short span of time. Merely being in the vicinity of an infected person could be dangerous. Viral particles traveled to the backs of nasal passages and to mucous membranes in the throat. Soon the virus was spreading all over the body. Coronavirus particles, with their trademark spiked proteins protruding from their spherical surfaces, hooked on to the cell membranes, enabling the virus's genetic material to enter human cells. The particles then multiplied by hijacking the cell's metabolism.[3]

Much like the early days of the AIDS pandemic more than two decades earlier, the very people trained to combat serious illness were among the most overwhelmed and uncertain. There was no standard treatment, no medicine, and no cure, and the course of each patient's viral infection appeared to differ dramatically.

As patients streamed into the surgical intensive-care unit at Boston Medical Center in March, Tracey Dechert felt powerless. A fifty-three-year-old trauma surgeon, Dechert was the director of the twenty-eight-bed unit, which had become one of several dedicated Covid-19 wards in the hospital. All day and night, Dechert hustled between dozens of severely ill patients. She and her colleagues did everything they could to help, but the ward was soon filled with despair. She nursed several patients back to health but watched many more succumb to the cruel illness. She and her colleagues took solace in the few patients with a chance of recovery.

"When you would find one where there was hope, you'd be holding on to it for dear life,'" she says.[4]

Doctors repurposed old medicines and turned to unproved ones. Early on, Dechert and her colleagues put their patients on the antibiotic azithromycin and an anti-malaria drug, hydroxychloroquine, though she and others later would drop the experimental treatments when their benefits were questioned. Ventilators proved helpful to some, insufficient for others. Dechert hardly had a break, working days, nights, and weekends.

Authorities were struggling to understand SARS-CoV-2 and how to best protect against infection. Masks and testing kits were hard to find, as was protective gear, even for health-care workers like Dechert. She and her colleagues at the hospital were limited to one N95 mask each day, even as they came into close contact with hundreds of infected patients. American authorities barely attempted measures that seemed to be helping elsewhere, such as test-and-trace strategies employed in countries in East Asia. Coordination from federal officials was almost nonexistent as President Donald Trump and members of his administration sought to downplay the virus's danger.

On March 11, global confirmed cases reached 124,663, with more than 4,500 people dead. That day, the World Health Organization declared a pandemic, the first since HIV/AIDS, saying the novel coronavirus had reached 112 countries and regions. Italy ordered the nationwide closure of all restaurants, bars, and most stores, racing to contain the worst outbreak outside China. In the United States, the stock market tumbled, marquee events were canceled, including New York City's St. Patrick's Day parade and the Coachella music festival, and the National Basketball Association suspended its season.

By late March, much of the world was in lockdown, morgues were filling in major cities, and millions were gripped with fear.

• • •

Even those who took precautions found they were at risk of the new disease.

Jessamyn Smyth was an avid athlete who suffered a martial-arts injury in 2005 that left her with limited mobility. Eventually, her spine collapsed, and she underwent spinal reconstruction. She spent years regaining her strength and endurance, thanks in part to regular swimming sessions. She completed a one-mile swimming race in Boston Harbor, and then an eight-mile race, accomplishments that filled her with a renewed sense of confidence and hope.

But Smyth's body had difficulty producing immunoglobulin, an antibody that helps ward off infection. Fearing the new coronavirus, she began to self-isolate in late February. The forty-seven-year-old was relieved that the humanities class she taught at a college in Holyoke, Massachusetts, was among the first at the liberal arts school to shift online. Nonetheless, in March 2020, Smyth contracted Covid-19, likely from those in her life who weren't as cautious.

"I got it in spite of having done my best to prevent it," she says.

Smyth developed a fever that didn't seem to go away for weeks. Her heartbeat raced and her oxygen levels dropped so low she lost consciousness. Her organs were swollen, causing tremendous pain. She was unpredictably exhausted some days and unable to work. Over the next four months, she would be hospitalized three times.

Her health eventually stabilized, thanks in part to steroids that reduced her body's inflammation, but her illness never fully went away. Her long-term symptoms eventually would be described by scientists as "long Covid."

Will I ever feel healthy again?

• • •

In March, many medical experts said it was folly to count on a vaccine to stem the pandemic. Most vaccines take years to develop, they noted, and a protective vaccine had never been found for some of the most challenging viruses, including HIV.

"A coronavirus vaccine will take at least 18 months—if it works at all," said an early March article in the *MIT Technology Review*. "A vaccine won't save us."[5]

At the end of March, Paul Offit, among the world's foremost vaccine specialists, said expecting a vaccine in the next twelve to fifteen months was "ridiculously optimistic."[6]

Early hope centered on the possibility that drugs might prove effective at treating sick patients, or maybe even help people to avoid the virus. Scientists began employing techniques they had developed to fight previous viruses and diseases, including AIDS, to slow the new coronavirus.

It had taken years, but by early 2020, researchers at companies like Gilead Sciences, outside San Mateo, California, had introduced cocktails of antiretroviral pills to prevent HIV from replicating, usually by inhibiting the body from copying the virus's genetic material. A few years earlier, Gilead had applied those same techniques to produce a drug called remdesivir, which it developed to thwart the Ebola outbreak of 2014. As the new coronavirus raged, Gilead decided to see if remdesivir might be effective in dealing with the new enemy. Within a few months, they saw evidence that the drug sped the recovery of hospitalized Covid-19 patients.

Other scientists who previously had worked on AIDS treatments also shifted to Covid-19, attempting to genetically engineer antibodies in the laboratory that could form the basis of drugs capable of attacking the invading virus. These researchers knew that some patients carry antibodies in their blood that could neutralize viruses. Over time, they had learned to identify these antibodies and to develop laboratory versions to use as drugs.

In early 2020, Eli Lilly and Regeneron Pharmaceuticals began producing these kinds of drugs, called monoclonal antibodies, to help some patients dealing with the new coronavirus. A cheap steroid called dexamethasone also proved capable of decreasing mortality, providing doctors with still another way to fend off Covid-19.

It soon became clear these drugs were far from perfect, however. Doubts would emerge about how much remdesivir impacted survival, for example. And some monoclonal antibodies didn't work well if they were administered after a patient showed symptoms lasting longer than ten days. Others proved ideal only for those with mild cases of Covid-19. Later, these drugs would pile up unused in hospital pharmacies as some physicians grew hesitant about relying on them.

By late winter, it was clear that effective vaccines would be needed to halt a pandemic that was only getting more terrifying. Scientists in countries including China and Russia raced to produce vaccines that they promised to share with the world, but health-care experts worried that any data supporting the efficacy of those nations' vaccines might not be reliable. Instead, they pinned their hopes on Western vaccine powers, such as Merck.

• • •

As news of the new coronavirus emerged, Merck's executives gathered at the company's West Point, Pennsylvania, research and manufacturing site and elsewhere, debating whether to participate in what they knew might emerge as the most important vaccine chase in modern history.

A split quickly emerged. Michael Nally, the company's chief marketing officer, and John Markels, president of global vaccines, pushed to develop a Covid-19 vaccine, as did some other executives and researchers. Merck was perfectly placed to focus on the emerging virus, they argued. The company had been the first to develop shots to prevent chickenpox, rubella, shingles, and other diseases. Staffers still spoke proudly of the accomplishments of Maurice Hilleman, the legendary Merck vaccinologist. The company's mumps vaccine, introduced in 1967 after four years of work, was the fastest turnaround in history at the time. Someone needs to solve this emerging global health crisis, the Merck scientists said. It should be us.

Their bosses were more reluctant to get involved in the vaccine effort. Chief Executive Ken Frazier and R&D chief Roger Perlmutter argued that shots take years to develop. A concerted Covid-19 effort would divert resources from thriving and vital areas at the company, including cancer research. The executives weren't sure the virus would keep spreading. They concluded that there wasn't reason to pour everything into fighting the new coronavirus. Some of the company's researchers mined Merck's library of chemical compounds for potential Covid-19 drugs or vaccines, but the company decided against an all-out effort.

The decision rankled some in the company. Merck, with its rich history of vaccine development, should be at the forefront of the vaccine race, the researchers insisted.

"*This isn't Merck*," one scientist complained to a friend at another pharmaceutical company.

Merck's decision reflected a cool and understandable logic. Vaccine development is difficult. The failure of Merck's HIV adenovirus vaccine back in 2007 continued to haunt the company, as did a more recent attempt to develop an Ebola vaccine. Merck had reacted quickly to a deadly outbreak of the disease in late 2014, spending over five years developing a vaccine, shifting top scientists to help in the effort. But the emergency ebbed before the company could even introduce its shots. In December 2019, it won approval for its Ebola vaccine, but some executives griped that, after all the years of hard work and good intentions, the shots weren't needed and almost certainly would be money losers. It cost the company about $50 million each year just to maintain its vaccine supplies, in case they were needed for a new outbreak.

Merck wasn't the only vaccine giant having a hard time getting going on Covid-19. Sanofi of France and GlaxoSmithKline of the United Kingdom jumped in quickly, teaming up in early 2020 to develop their own Covid-19 shots. But a miscalculation in the manufacturing process resulted in volunteers being given lower doses than intended in initial clinical trials, an embarrassing flub.

The virus was spreading, the world was panicking, and civilization's most likely saviors would be of little assistance.

16

February–April 2020

Early in 2020, Adrian Hill and his longtime collaborator at Oxford University, Sarah Gilbert, paid little heed to the new pathogen. Hill spent much of the first two months of the year traveling to Senegal, New York, and elsewhere, busy with his malaria research. Emerging pathogens weren't Hill's thing. Besides, for all his negativity toward his peers, Hill was an optimist by nature, and he doubted the new coronavirus would emerge as a global threat.

Gilbert wasn't much more concerned. After the new virus's sequence was released in January, she began building a vaccine based on their ChAdOx vaccine technology, much like Moderna and BioNTech's researchers were doing. But for Gilbert and her colleagues, it was largely an academic exercise. She hoped clinical trials of her vaccine might begin in July or so, a timetable that she deemed sufficiently ambitious. There didn't seem a need to rush.

Jabs that Gilbert and Hill had developed a few years earlier to protect against Middle East respiratory syndrome had trained the body's immune system to recognize that coronavirus's key spike protein, so it didn't take long for Gilbert to design a similar vaccine for the new coronavirus. First, she and others at Oxford's Jenner Institute took the genetic sequence of the coronavirus's full-length spike protein and used it to clone a gene for the protein. Then they inserted the gene into the genome of their chimpanzee adenovirus, which was modified to ensure that it wouldn't replicate. Oxford's chimp-adeno was then charged with delivering genetic instructions to the body's cells. The idea was to get the cells to produce the spike protein in the body, stirring an immune response and thereby priming the immune system to attack the virus if it later infected the body.

On February 17, Gilbert began injecting mice with her shots. The Jenner Institute had its own small vaccine manufacturing facility, giving it the capacity to produce batches of vaccine if it wished. But the facility was busy making Ebola shots for a different project Gilbert was leading. She resisted the idea of putting that work on hold to allow the facility to produce coronavirus vaccines. Gilbert was partial to her Ebola research and rushing to make a coronavirus vaccine just didn't seem necessary.

There was little urgency elsewhere at Oxford as well. When senior members of Oxford's Nuffield Department of Medicine met to discuss the new virus, there were more yawns than attendees, with just three or four researchers showing up. Emerging pathogens always get people scared but peter out on their own, don't they? London's Imperial College got an early start on their own vaccine and many in the United Kingdom assumed that school's effort would be the nation's best chance at developing protective jabs.

But some younger scientists at Oxford were growing anxious. Alexander Douglas, who goes by Sandy, read some disturbuing articles about the virus, and the underlying data seemed to point to trouble. Douglas called and texted Hill, hoping to engage him in the developing crisis. Douglas also tried to convince Gilbert to go faster, but he wasn't getting anywhere.

With each news article and fresh data point, Douglas became more agitated. A thirty-seven-year-old physician, Douglas had first-hand experience with Britain's tightly funded National Health Service, unlike most of the researchers he worked with. He knew the health service could become overwhelmed in a crisis. Douglas flashed back to lessons from a mentor who had spoken of the damage flu pandemics can bring, which only added to his fears. Around the same time, Douglas's father, who had cancer and was on chemotherapy treatments, went on a trip to Rome, even as the virus was rapidly spreading in Italy, stirring Douglas's fears.

"I was going nuts," he says.

Slowly, Hill began to shift his focus to the emerging virus, thanks in part to Douglas's nudges. By late February, he was telling colleagues they needed to go superfast and that their vaccine needed to be ready for testing as soon as April—"No later," he said. Gilbert initially resisted the idea of rushing to test and introduce a vaccine, but she, too, got on board. Soon she was leading the group's effort.

Gilbert woke most days around four a.m., mulling ways to improve her vaccine approach, before biking to the Jenner Institute, where she worked into the evening.[1] For weeks, she and her colleagues pushed forward on their jabs, working on a shoestring budget, desperate for funding. At one point, Jenner researchers joked about sending a professor on a train to 10 Downing Street to impress upon Prime Minister Boris Johnson the importance of supporting their efforts. By the end of March, though, Gilbert had lined up more than enough backing from U.K. bodies and others to push the program ahead.

The Oxford team had a clear advantage over other Covid-19 efforts. By then, Gilbert and Hill had developed vaccines for MERS, the flu, Zika, the tropical disease chikungunya, and others, all based on their chimp-adenovirus approach. They had given their jabs to enough people to demonstrate that they stirred the immune system and appeared safe.[2]

But the Oxford group had never produced more than a few thousand doses of any of its vaccines. The prospect of manufacturing hundreds of thousands of vaccines, or even more, was daunting. A few young scientists, including a postdoc named Carina Joe, decided to study how J&J, Merck, and others had previously manufactured their adenovirus vaccines. Joe discovered ways to grow cells in culture and remove contaminants and impurities from the vaccine, making it easier to produce their shots, buoying the team.

In February, the scientists received early evidence their shots might work. Researchers at the National Institutes of Health's Rocky Mountain Laboratories in Montana inoculated six rhesus macaque monkeys with single doses of the Oxford vaccine. Then, the researchers exposed the monkeys to a huge amount of the coronavirus. Twenty-eight days later, the monkeys, which are as close to humans as lab animals get, all appeared to be healthy. The study also suggested the vaccine was safe, alleviating a concern many had about so-called vaccine-associated enhanced disease, which is when someone develops a more severe form of an illness after being inoculated.

Some outsiders who scrutinized the early tests noted that Oxford's shots didn't produce high levels of neutralizing antibodies, which can be crucial for protection. Nonetheless, the results were reason for Hill, confident as always, to let out a cheer.

"It wasn't promising—it was fantastic," Hill said a bit later.

The Oxford scientists' goals were admirable. Gilbert and Hill built their shots to be inexpensive and easy to manufacture, store, and transport, making them ideal for developing countries and other parts of the globe that didn't have sophisticated health-care systems. Those were among the reasons the British government now seemed to be pulling hard for their homegrown candidate.

But Gilbert and her colleagues made early choices that raised eyebrows. For one thing, they left out the two-proline modification that Jason McLellan and his team had developed to stabilize the coronavirus's spike protein. The Oxford researchers hadn't used the two-proline tweak in their earlier MERS vaccine, and it wasn't clear how valuable it would be for adenovirus-based shots against SARS-CoV-2, so the decision wasn't without justification. Still, most every other group working on a vaccine took the time to make this change in the spike-protein's gene, determining that adding the prolines would likely induce better-quality antibodies. Some senior scientists in the field wondered whether Hill and Gilbert had been too proud to rely on an innovation developed by other scientists, while others asked whether they and their colleagues had made a mistake in their rush to produce a vaccine.

As the Oxford group began preparing for human trials of their vaccine, they made another decision that would be questioned. As the researchers screened healthy volunteers in the Thames Valley Region, they focused on those aged eighteen to fifty-five years old, even though older people were most in need of a Covid-19 vaccine. The virus was disrupting daily life and spreading panic around the world, so the Oxford team was rushing and they wanted to see if their vaccine worked. Trial results from older volunteers can sometimes be confusing, slowing an efficacy determination. It also wasn't clear any vaccine would work for older people, and Oxford faced limited resources for large trials.

Gilbert, Hill, and their colleagues were eager to get ahead in the vaccine race and pass Moderna and BioNTech. But another competitor was making rapid progress with a similar approach.

• • •

On Friday afternoon, January 10, Dan Barouch hosted an annual retreat for the sixty members of his laboratory at Beth Israel Deaconess Medical Center. In an expansive meeting room at the Boston Museum of Science, the researchers discussed progress they were making on their long-running work to develop vaccines for HIV, Zika, and tuberculosis.

They also made plans for the year ahead. Through floor-to-ceiling windows, the group enjoyed a panoramic view of the nearby Charles River, admiring a spectacular sunset that evening.

A postdoc in Barouch's lab had just returned from his home in Wuhan, and the scientists soon were discussing the mysterious cases of pneumonia in the city. They kept coming back to the same concern: The virus had never been seen in humans before, so no one had antibodies conferring immunity, and it was much more contagious than SARS-CoV-1 and MERS. Severe illness, even death, seemed likely.

Later that evening, when a researcher told Barouch the new virus's sequence had been released, he decided the team should build a vaccine. His lab often engaged in pilot programs to develop shots for new pathogens, exercises that sometimes led to academic papers or insights that helped their existing research. Barouch emailed four of his researchers, asking if they could begin cloning a gene for the new virus's spike protein.

Like Adrian Hill and his colleagues at Oxford, Barouch's team wanted to insert the gene into the genome of an adenovirus. It would ferry the DNA into the body's cells, creating the spike protein that would prompt an immune response. Rather than Hill's chimp adenovirus, Barouch went with his own favorite, the cold virus Adenovirus26, or Ad26, the same one he had used to build vaccines for HIV and Zika.

On Saturday, January 25, Barouch decided to email Johan Van Hoof, the head of global vaccines at Johnson & Johnson's Janssen Pharmaceuticals division, his partner on the HIV and Zika vaccines.

"The coronavirus outbreak in China is looking bad," Barouch wrote. "Human-to-human transmission appears quite efficient, including from asymptomatic individuals without fevers, which may make epidemic control by standard public-health measures difficult. . . . Are you interested in making a rapid Ad-based vaccine like we did for Zika?"

Van Hoof replied almost immediately: "Would a call work now?"

Within days, they had an agreement to collaborate on a Covid-19 vaccine. Barouch and his team put their HIV work on hold and got to work designing a vaccine antigen for the new pathogen.

The Oxford scientists had acted swiftly, choosing a design identical to their previous MERS vaccine. Barouch and his colleagues chose to be slower and more methodical. They designed a dozen versions of their vaccine antigen, some that produced the full spike protein, others that generated a portion of the protein, and still others that encoded variations of the protein, including the proline modifications Jason McLellan and his colleagues had introduced to stabilize the protein. Barouch didn't think it made sense to hurry; he wanted to see which design sparked the highest immune response before deciding on a final version.

The group spent over a month testing their various potential antigens, first in mice and then in monkeys. In February, Barouch's group, working with J&J's scientists, identified several potential vaccine candidates they believed could elicit the best immune response. The lead contender was a version of the gene that directed the body's cells to create the virus's full-length spike protein.

By late March, the city of Boston was all but closed, with many people working from home, fearful of Covid-19. But Barouch and his researchers came to the lab to do their work, battling their own fears of contracting the disease.

They soon had reason for hope: Their vaccine was stimulating production of antibodies in the animals against the new coronavirus. The team didn't know whether the antibodies were sufficient to stop Covid-19, or if their vaccine would prove as safe and effective as those rival labs were developing. Their methodical approach meant it would be an uphill battle to produce the first Covid-19 vaccine, but they had a chance. Barouch and J&J had a contender.

• • •

By the end of February, Şahin and his team at BioNTech had developed twenty different vaccine candidates. They wanted to introduce a vaccine by the end of the year, but there was so much work ahead: They needed to test their candidates around the world, win approval from regulators, manufacture huge numbers of doses, and put them in arms. Şahin knew it would be a difficult challenge for his 1,500 employees to pull off on their own. He decided it was time to ask for some help.

Earlier, Şahin had spoken with Phil Dormitzer, the Pfizer scientist who advised him not to chase a coronavirus vaccine. Şahin decided to speak with someone else at the company. On March 1, Şahin called Kathrin Jansen, the senior scientist at Pfizer.

By then, the two companies already had spent two years working together on an mRNA flu vaccine, so he and Jansen were having regular conversations about the progress of their research. On this call, though, Şahin said he had another topic to discuss. He told Jansen about the early Covid-19 work he and BioNTech had done and their optimism that they could develop effective shots.

"Do you want to collaborate on Covid?" Şahin asked her.

Jansen barely hesitated.

"Uğur, you are asking?" she replied. "Of course we are interested."[3]

Over the previous month, Jansen and her colleagues at Pfizer had debated whether they could develop a drug or shots to help stop the pandemic. Building an mRNA vaccine directing the body to produce the coronavirus's spike protein seemed the fastest and most straightforward way to produce effective shots. So much was still unknown about the virus that scientists still weren't sure what parts of the immune system would need to be stirred to provide protection. But mRNA vaccines seemed to trigger both neutralizing antibodies and

T cell activity, which the Pfizer researchers viewed as another advantage of that approach.

BioNTech and Pfizer quickly forged an agreement to split the remaining development costs and all potential profits. The effort wasn't a top priority for Pfizer, though. The company had dozens of drug and vaccine programs that demanded attention, and many Pfizer scientists were unconvinced the new virus would remain a threat long enough to justify an allocation of huge amounts of time and resources.

Just a day after Şahin's call to Jansen, Pfizer's urgency about the coronavirus would change.

• • •

On March 2, some of the world's most prominent drug executives flew to Washington, D.C., to meet President Trump, members of his administration, Tony Fauci of the NIAID, and others. Representatives from J&J, GlaxoSmithKline, Sanofi, and others were there, as were Bancel of Moderna and Stan Erck of Novavax. Pfizer chose Mikael Dolsten, its top scientist, to make the trip and represent the company.

The executives lined up and made their way through layers of security to enter the West Wing. So many people had been invited for the meeting that, at the last moment, it was moved to a large conference room next to the Oval Office. As the executives found spots around the room, even that space began to feel cramped, however.

Trump went around the room, asking for updates on the progress the various companies were making on vaccines and drugs. Bancel didn't disappoint his host. Sitting across from Trump and Vice President Mike Pence, Bancel spoke with confidence, saying Moderna would move its vaccine into phase 2 trials in the coming few months, before beginning a phase 3 trial shortly thereafter.

Bancel promised such a lightning-fast pace that some around the table became uncomfortable, viewing the timetable as unrealistic and overoptimistic. Trump became visibly excited, however, as he tried pinning Bancel down on a date when he could expect Moderna to deliver a vaccine.

"So you're talking within a year—" Trump began, before Fauci stepped in. He seemed worried Bancel was exaggerating the likely speed of his vaccine program, which was being run with the NIH.

"A year to a year and a half," Fauci told the president, something he didn't seem thrilled to hear.

When it came time for Dolsten to speak, the Pfizer executive didn't say a word to Trump about a Covid-19 vaccine, despite his company's new collaboration with BioNTech. Instead, he said that Pfizer hoped to develop drugs that might slow the new virus. He mentioned a possible vaccine in private conversations with others in the White House, but dwelling on a vaccine didn't seem appropriate when so many of Dolsten's colleagues back in New York still presumed the virus would prove a dud, like so many others had in the past.

On his flight home from Washington, D.C., though, Dolsten began to reflect on the meeting's significance and the seriousness of the emerging threat facing mankind. Listening to the executives and scientists in the room, and fielding questions from the president, left an impression on Dolsten.

"You sit in the [White House] cabinet room, it's where war and peace agreements are signed," he says. "It started to be clearer to me that we were in a global war against an invisible enemy."

As the flight continued and he considered the potential course of the virus, Dolsten started to become nervous.

This could be another 1918, he thought.

After landing in New York, Dolsten called Albert Bourla, Pfizer's chief executive officer, recommending an all-out attempt to build a vaccine. Bourla was arriving at the same conclusion, as were others at the company, including those who previously had dragged their feet, like Philip Dormitzer. Just a month or so earlier, the Pfizer scientist had warned Şahin not to become distracted with the coronavirus. Now that the infections were mounting, Dormitzer was urging his company to go full speed ahead.

"I had the zeal of the converted," he says.

Some of the Pfizer executives were witnessing coronavirus's impact firsthand. Jansen and some others continued coming into the company's Midtown Manhattan office, sometimes passing refrigerated trucks that stored victims who had not yet been buried. These chilling images reinforced their determination to act.[4]

"Whatever it takes," Bourla told some of his senior executives, "just get it done."

If Pfizer was going to have an impact, the company would need to move quickly, Bourla told his team. He wanted a vaccine by October, a timetable that startled some of the scientists.

Bourla had an idea to speed up their work: What if the various steps necessary to develop a vaccine could be done simultaneously, rather than sequentially? In other words, the research, trials, manufacturing, and distribution of a Covid-19 vaccine would be done in parallel, instead of waiting to see success after each phase. Perhaps that would allow Pfizer and BioNTech to produce a vaccine in months, rather than years? The cost would be high, but he said it was worth it.[5]

"If we go in, we go all in," Bourla told them.

• • •

Moderna was moving quickly, just as Bancel had promised the president. The day after the White House meeting, the Food and Drug Administration gave the company a green light to begin testing their shots in humans, eager to see if they worked. Jennifer Haller wanted to help.

In January, Haller had become concerned. A forty-three-year-old operations manager at a machine-learning company in Seattle and the mother of two teenagers, Haller had read about the damage the novel coronavirus was inflicting in China, Italy, and elsewhere. In late January, the first-known infection in the United States was reported, a man in nearby north Seattle who had traveled to China. Over a month later, the state's second infection was recorded. In late February, a long-term care facility in Kirkland, Washington, about ten miles from Haller's home, experienced an outbreak of Covid-19, with 27 of its 108 residents contracting the disease.

Haller worried about her parents, who lived near the nursing home. Her stepfather was at risk for a couple of reasons: He had asthma, meaning he likely would have a tougher time handling a respiratory disease like Covid-19, and he had a habit of making daily runs to a Taco Bell close to the facility at the center of the outbreak.

"Can't you stay home for a week?" Haller asked her stepfather, who reluctantly complied with her request.

As cases mounted in her area, Haller thought of the sacrifices health-care workers and others were making and became frustrated that there was nothing she could do to help. She worked from home and felt she was in a position of relative privilege. When a friend posted a link on Facebook to a registration form for an upcoming Covid-19 vaccine study to be conducted by nearby Kaiser Permanente Washington Health Research Institute, Haller decided to sign up. She figured the odds were slim she'd actually be chosen for the trial, but it felt good to volunteer.

A few weeks later, Haller was having dinner with a friend when she received a call on her cell phone from a number she didn't recognize. Usually, she ignored those kinds of calls. This time, for some reason, she felt compelled to answer. Haller had been selected for the trial; without much hesitation, she agreed to participate.

There was risk involved. By then, Moderna had produced mRNA vaccines for various viruses that had been tested in thousands of people and were deemed safe. But the company had yet to release the full results of the tests the NIH had conducted on animals for the new SARS-CoV-2 shots. Now, Haller would be inoculated with those shots.

Her husband asked if she was sure about her decision. A friend suggested she wait.

"Why do you need to be the first one?" the friend asked.

Haller was sure she wanted to be part of the trial, even grateful for the opportunity.

"It felt like a gift," she says. "It was a chance to protect my family, have some control over my situation, and do something to help."

On the evening of March 15, 2020, Haller read a breaking story from the Associated Press: The next morning, the first person was going to receive a Covid-19 vaccine as part of a Moderna trial. Haller checked her calendar and saw her appointment was slated for eight a.m. the next day.

Wow, that might be me.

On the morning of March 16, just sixty-six days after the virus's RNA had been sequenced by the scientists, Haller drove to Kaiser. She walked into the hospital without a face mask. Inside, hardly anyone was wearing a mask. It didn't seem necessary at the time. And there was guidance from some health officials that masks might increase risk from the new virus.

Haller saw she was the first of three people scheduled for a Covid-19 shot that day. In the clinic, she signed a stack of documents acknowledging the risks she was about to assume. When it was time, she removed a heavy sweatshirt and sat on the edge of an examination table in a gray tank top. As an AP photographer snapped away, a pharmacist took a syringe filled with colorless liquid and injected Haller in her left arm. She stared straight ahead, expressionless. It was quick and painless. She sensed a positive energy in the room and smiled.

"It was a ray of hope," Haller says.

• • •

When he spoke to Trump and Fauci in early March, Bancel seemed full of confidence. He believed in his company's vaccine approach and was sure mRNA vaccines would prove efficacious.

Privately, however, Bancel and his colleagues were becoming disheartened, even despondent. The Moderna team was certain they had a winning formula for a vaccine, but they had a huge problem on their hands: The company didn't have money to manufacture many doses.

Moderna had begun the year with money pressures that had only become more pressing. In February, the company raised $500 million by selling new shares at a price of nineteen dollars a piece. That sum sounded like a lot of money, but in many ways the sale was an embarrassment. Back in late 2018, Moderna had gone public at twenty three dollars a share. Over the following year or so, the company made substantial progress on a number of vaccines, including one against CMV. Now it was making headway on a vaccine to halt a virus that had the world in its grip. Yet its stock price had gone down, suggesting that Moderna was *less* valuable than before.

"It was humbling," says Stephen Hoge.

The worst part about the stock sale: The Moderna executives didn't feel they could use the new cash for their Covid-19 work. Some of the big investors who had purchased the shares told Hoge and others they didn't want the company to become distracted with a coronavirus vaccine, which had an uncertain likelihood of success.

Juan Andres, who headed Moderna's manufacturing effort—the executive who a month or so earlier had purchased the extra refrigerator for his basement over his wife's protests—was desperate to start making tens of millions of doses of the company's vaccines, or even hundreds of millions of doses. Moderna needed to get ready so it could distribute its shots as soon as they were authorized by regulators.

But Andres couldn't get the process going because he didn't have enough money to buy the essential ingredients for the shots. Moderna needed hundreds of millions of dollars, perhaps even a billion dollars. Bancel and Hoge didn't know where the money was going to come from. Time was ticking, rivals were acting, people were dying, and Moderna was sitting on its hands. It was eating the team up.

Throughout February, March, and April, Bancel begged for money. He asked Trevor Mundel, a top leader of the Gates Foundation. He reached out to an arm of the World Health Organization called Covax. He phoned or went on Zoom calls with representatives of other government bodies and charitable foundations. Each time, he presented reasons why Moderna deserved financial assistance. As Bancel became frustrated by the rejections, his requests became more plaintive.

"Look, if you don't help us, and this [vaccine] works, it will cost hundreds of thousands of lives, if not hundreds of millions," Bancel told one person, a colleague recalls. "It's a tragedy . . . we need help."

Each time, Bancel came up empty. Sometimes he swallowed his pride and asked an organization more than once, hoping for a change of heart. Still, the answer was no. Some of the potential funders deemed mRNA too risky. Others were committed to helping other vaccine efforts. Still others didn't have the free cash. Moderna managed to get some money from the Biomedical Advanced Research and Development Authority, or BARDA, an arm of the U.S. government, but that cash was earmarked to fund the company's vaccine trials, not for Andres and his team to manufacture any doses.

At one point, Bancel called Roger Perlmutter, the Merck R&D chief, suggesting that the companies team up on a Covid-19 vaccine, just like Pfizer and BioNTech were doing. With a deep-pocketed partner, Bancel was sure he could make enough shots to inoculate hundreds of millions of people around the world. Initially, Perlmutter expressed enthusiasm about the idea. A few years earlier, Merck had worked with Moderna on shots against various infectious diseases, so it made sense that they would join forces against SARS-CoV-2.

Merck never followed through on Bancel's pitch, however. Some at Moderna got the sense that Merck executives, including the company's head of infectious disease discovery, Daria Hazuda, viewed mRNA-based vaccines as unproven, a stumbling block for an alliance.

Bancel was upset with himself, convinced that he had failed his company, his shareholders, and the world. He was a master fundraiser but when it truly counted, he had come up short. Lives were at stake and he had blown it. He was overcome with sadness.

"I wasn't good enough to get it done," he says.

17

Spring–Summer 2020

BioNTech and Pfizer were racing to develop effective Covid-19 vaccines, Moderna was searching for money to stay ahead of the pack, and Johnson & Johnson was running hard to keep up. Before they knew it, however, Adrian Hill and his colleagues at Oxford University had raced past them all.

In March, Hill and others at the Jenner Institute and the Oxford Vaccine Group discovered a way to speed up their vaccine program. They still didn't have an approved vaccine, of course, but the Oxford scientists were sure their approach was safe, at least. Their earlier progress gave the researchers an idea: Maybe they could accelerate the usual testing schedule for their shots?

Vaccines, like drugs, need to be proven both safe and effective. After regulators sign off on a new-vaccine application, which can include preclinical animal studies, human trials begin—phase 1 trials to demonstrate safety, and phase 2 and phase 3 trials, involving a higher number of participants and randomized control groups, to prove effectiveness and that side effects are manageable. But international regulatory agencies, including the U.S. Food and Drug

Administration, generally give companies and other sponsors a degree of latitude in designing clinical trials.

Since the Oxford group was pretty certain its vaccine was safe, they proposed plans to combine phases 1 and 2 to speed things up, a schedule British regulators approved. The scientists also made plans to accelerate phase 3 human trials. Their trial design meant that they could quickly collect data on their Covid-19 vaccine's safety, side effects, and the ideal dosage, and then see if their shots could trigger an immune-system response and were efficacious, all in a record-breaking length of time. That would enable an emergency distribution of their shots, including injections in the arms of health-care workers and high-risk people, as soon as September, well before any of the Covid-19 competitors in the West.

Before long, Oxford had leapfrogged its competitors. Sarah Gilbert, who had designed the vaccine, could hardly contain her optimism. As her team made plans to start a 1,100-person trial in April and a subsequent 10,000-participant trial in the U.K., Gilbert told *The Times* (London) that she was "80 per cent confident" the Oxford vaccine would work.[1] Gilbert's own three children, twenty-one-year-old triplets all studying biochemistry, signed up to take part in the early human trials, with their mother's approval, a true sign of Gilbert's confidence in the jabs.[2]

In late April, Oxford's leaders forged an agreement with AstraZeneca, a British drug giant based in Cambridge, U.K., to help test, manufacture, and distribute the group's Covid-19 shots. AstraZeneca had little vaccine experience, but the company enjoyed a long history of producing drugs, which promised to be useful. AstraZeneca even agreed to produce the Covid-19 vaccines without making a profit for as long as the pandemic lasted, and to try to manufacture shots in low-income countries, satisfying one of the university's requirements for a partnership.

By April, the virus had reached almost every corner of the world, overwhelming the health-care systems of many countries. On April 15 alone, the United States saw 2,752 deaths from the virus, a new high. On April 28, the United States recorded its one millionth Covid-19 case. By the end of April, the world was seeing an average of about 80,000 new cases of Covid-19 a day, up from 1,500 in early March. Authorities were desperate to slow the virus's spread. That month, the U.S. Centers for Disease Control changed its previous guidance, advising all Americans above the age of two to wear face masks outside the home.

As the situation turned grim, health authorities and others began to see Oxford's jabs as the most likely means for the world to escape the virus's grip. The WHO's chief scientist said the Oxford team had the most advanced vaccine, *The Economist* called the Oxford team "the likeliest candidate to produce the world's first vaccine against covid-19," and *The New York Times* said Hill and Gilbert's effort was "a bellwether."[3]

Soon a rivalry seemed to develop between the two scientists over who could exhibit more confidence, or even arrogance, about their vaccine while finding flaws in their rivals' approaches. Hill started things off in May, telling Reuters that the Oxford/AstraZeneca shots were "almost certainly the best single dose rapid-response vaccine," and that rival mRNA shots were "total unknowns" and "wild cards."

"Why would you take a vaccine technology that is new, unproven, maybe quick to manufacture, but expensive to manufacture and has never been scaled up—and has never been shown to protect against anything in humans, and prioritize that in a global emergency?" Hill asked. "It's very odd."[4]

Gilbert mounted an impressive comeback, though, saying in July: "We know the adverse event profile and we know the dose to use, because we've done this so many times before. . . . Obviously we're doing safety testing, but we're not concerned."[5]

Gilbert shared some additional thoughts about the Oxford/AstraZeneca shots with the Royal Society of Biology's website in July: "If this doesn't work, I don't think anything will work."[6]

By then, the cockiness of the Oxford researchers appeared well deserved. Early tests demonstrated that Oxford's shots had produced two kinds of immune response to defend against Covid-19, while not causing serious side effects, encouraging the team to begin a phase 3 trial of thirty thousand volunteers in the U.K., Brazil, and South Africa.

Watching from across the Atlantic, Moderna executives conceded the Oxford team was likely to receive the first regulatory approval of a vaccine. They had the most advanced vaccine, enjoyed ample funding, and seemed to have the full support of the British government. The Oxford/AstraZeneca team committed to making two billion doses, helping people around the world protect against the new plague.

Gilbert and a colleague focused on producing the Covid-19 shots, while Andrew Pollard, the Oxford scientist who ran the Oxford Vaccine Group, worked with AstraZeneca to test the shots. Hill was happy to provide guidance and help.

When a friend called asking Hill about his team's progress and the help it was getting from AstraZeneca, Hill sounded optimistic, even relieved. Finally, it seemed, he had an undisputed winner.

• • •

By May, Moderna still couldn't produce much of its vaccine. AstraZeneca, Pfizer, and J&J were all bulking up their own manufacturing capacities, preparing to produce tens of millions of doses as soon as regulators authorized their shots. Moderna was sitting still. Each day without progress, Juan Andres, the company's manufacturing chief, became more frustrated. He wanted to begin buying the supplies his team needed to build vaccines, but he didn't have access to the cash. People were dying all over the world and Andres was in a position to help, yet he couldn't do a thing to pitch in. His hands were tied.

"We need to place the orders if we want vaccines," he told a colleague in the spring. "We need to do it *now*!"

In the spring, Stéphane Bancel became hopeful his company might finally get some help. On May 15, President Trump stood on the White House lawn to announce the official formation of Operation Warp Speed, an effort to hasten the development of coronavirus vaccine candidates, with the goal of rolling out 300 million safe and effective doses by January 2021. Some administration officials had tried to talk Trump and others out of the idea, saying it would be harmful to raise expectations and to set an unreasonably short deadline, but he went ahead, picking pharmaceutical veteran Moncef Slaoui to run the effort.[7] Gustave Perna, a four-star Army general who had been responsible for overseeing efforts to supply U.S. forces around the world, was placed in charge of the production and distribution of eventual vaccines.

Slaoui, a Moroccan-born Belgian American who once led GlaxoSmithKline's vaccine division, had been a member of Moderna's board of directors since 2017. Slaoui had long been skeptical of using mRNA molecules. His expertise was in vaccines that injected synthesized proteins into the body, the approach that Gale Smith and Novavax were working on. While on Moderna's board, Slaoui routinely questioned the company's focus on mRNA vaccines. But impressive data in 2019 for Moderna's CMV shots had convinced him that mRNA could work, suggesting that he now might be open to helping Moderna's Covid-19 effort.

Right away, though, Operation Warp Speed pledged up to $1.2 billion to help the Oxford/AstraZeneca team develop, produce, and manufacture their vaccine, securing at least 300 million doses of the shots, which were expected to be ready as soon as October. The British effort was furthest along—they'd already planned a thirty-thousand-person trial of adults in the United Kingdom and elsewhere, as well as a trial for younger people, so the decision made sense, even if it brought more disappointment to the Moderna team.

Moderna's executives decided to turn to the one place they were feeling love: Wall Street. By then, the company's shares were absolutely soaring. After starting 2020 below twenty dollars a share, the stock topped sixty-six dollars on May 15, as investors became hopeful that the company's Covid-19 vaccine could be a big seller. Moderna hired investment banking firm Morgan Stanley to sell new shares to investors, this time specifically to pay for the manufacturing of the vaccines.

On the morning of Monday, May 18, Moderna reported results from its first human study: Eight subjects in the phase 1 study who had been inoculated with the company's Covid-19 vaccine had developed neutralizing antibodies comparable to those seen in patients who were infected by the virus and subsequently recovered, and the shots were generally safe and well tolerated.

The data—which came from patients including Jennifer Haller from Seattle—were early and based on a small number of subjects, of course. But investors were so excited about the prospect of an effective vaccine that they sent the Dow Jones Industrial Average up 899 points that day, or 3.8 percent, while Moderna's shares jumped 20 percent, past seventy-five dollars. The company immediately announced it would begin a phase 2 study and then a larger, late-stage study as soon as July, with plans to have a vaccine available for emergency use by the fall.

The trial results were good news for the vaccine, less so for Morgan Stanley's bankers. The stock's climb made it harder to sell a big batch of new shares—who wanted to buy a stock that has already jumped in price? Nonetheless, Morgan Stanley agreed to purchase $1.34 billion of Moderna's newly issued shares, betting it could sell them to the bank's customers.

The money meant everything to Bancel and his team—they finally had a genuine chance to produce huge numbers of doses. Right away, they told Andres to start spending it all on lipids, glass, steel, and every other kind of material and piece of equipment he needed. *Go, go, go.* Bancel and Hoge breathed deep sighs of relief. They had hope.

Then came the backlash. Members of the scientific and investment communities were incensed. Moderna's study hadn't been peer reviewed, yet the company shared the preliminary results publicly, in a press release, no less. Moderna had sold a ton of shares, taking advantage of its bright news, but the company hadn't shared crucial details of the trial, such as the durability of the vaccine's protection, or the level of antibodies that had been generated.

"My guess is that their numbers are marginal or they would say more," John Rose, a vaccine researcher from Yale University, told STAT, in an article that sent Moderna shares tumbling and put a damper on the entire stock market. Rose noted that antibody levels among people who had recovered from Covid-19 vary dramatically, so simply saying a vaccine induced antibody levels as high as those generated by infection, as Moderna had done, wasn't saying much.[8]

"It seemed like they might be grasping at straws for some silver lining out of the data," Peter Hotez, a professor at the Baylor College of Medicine who was developing his own Covid-19 vaccine, told the *Financial Times.*

It didn't help that Bancel and other Moderna executives were selling bushelfuls of their personal shares, even as they were expressing optimism about their vaccine's prospects. Yes, most of the sales were part of plans established by the executives months earlier. But it wasn't a good look for the executives to be dumping stock while the team was developing a vaccine that some in the public already were suggesting they'd be hesitant to put into their arms. Some asked: If their shots were so safe and protective, why were the executives selling their shares?

"You can turn those off if you're actually bullish" about a company's prospects, noted *Bloomberg News* columnist Matt Levine, referring to the automated stock-sale plans.[9]

Scientists had spent years doubting Bancel and Moderna. Now they had a new reason to be dubious. Senior researchers got in touch with Moderna's founders, including Noubar Afeyan and Robert Langer, and scientists at the company itself, griping about the company's behavior. Afeyan and Langer tried to defend Bancel and his team, but they didn't make much headway.

"You're doing science by press release," one researcher told Langer.

The Moderna team was incensed. The NIAID was running the trials for its vaccine. There wasn't much the company could disclose if the government scientists weren't going to say more. At the same time, Moderna hadn't felt comfortable sitting on the trial data—the results were so crucial that not revealing them would likely be considered a violation of rules dictating financial disclosure, they believed. Morale ebbed in the Moderna labs and Afeyan and others worried it would interfere with the company's research.

"We're desperately trying to make vaccines and we're getting *lectured*?" an exasperated Hoge asked a colleague.

• • •

Uğur Şahin and BioNTech wanted to introduce their Covid-19 vaccine as swiftly as possible. So did his new partner, Albert Bourla, the chief executive of Pfizer. Early results of their vaccine were just as impressive as Moderna's had been, encouraging Şahin and his colleagues to pick up their pace.

Bourla wanted their vaccine to be ready for distribution by October and to produce 100 million doses by the end of 2020, enough for 50 million people. To reach that goal, Pfizer and BioNTech decided to combine the second and third stages of their trials, much like the Oxford/AstraZeneca team was doing.

Bourla was so intent on developing and distributing the team's vaccine quickly that he made a surprising decision: The companies wouldn't ask for help from Operation Warp Speed. Yes, they would sell their vaccines to the U.S. government, but Bourla didn't want to take money from the government to develop or manufacture the Pfizer/BioNTech shots, fearing bureaucratic red tape that might slow his team.

The Pfizer team began building a global manufacturing network, to be ready when its vaccine won regulatory approval. Their pace wasn't fast enough for Bourla, though. On a warm June day, working from his suburban New York home, Bourla got on a Webex conference call, telling his team that he wanted to increase Pfizer's commercial production potential at least tenfold from what they were promising.

"Why can't we make more and why can't we make it sooner?" Bourla demanded.

The call turned tense as Mike McDermott, Pfizer's head of manufacturing, pushed back on his boss, saying he and his colleagues were already working furiously.

"What we're doing already is a miracle," he said. "You're asking for too much."[10]

Eventually, McDermott and his team arrived at a timetable that satisfied Bourla. For all their focus on speed, though, Pfizer and BioNTech's top scientists became stalled as they tried to make an enormous decision: which vaccine design to use. Pfizer's research and manufacturing teams needed to start planning a crucial phase 3 trial, slated for late July, to test their vaccine's efficacy. But they hadn't even settled on what their vaccine should look like, a fundamental decision they knew could mean the difference between effective and disappointing shots.

Back in January, when Şahin first had begun to develop his company's Covid-19 vaccine, he had selected a number of attractive candidates. They all used mRNA molecules to ferry instructions to the body's cells to create the coronavirus's spike protein, or fragments of the protein, but some were more elaborate than others, including one that made modifications to the molecule's chemical backbone, to avoid a hostile reaction from the immune system. These modifications were improvements on those Katalin Karikó and Drew Weissman had invented, the kinds that Moderna had adopted years earlier. Şahin wasn't sure the modifications were necessary, however, so he also built a vaccine that used a self-replicating mRNA molecule, which didn't have those modifications.

Another of Şahin's mRNA candidates told the body to make the full spike protein. Still another directed cells to produce just a part of the protein, the portion that first attaches to the cell's surface, which is called the receptor-binding domain. In all, Şahin and his colleagues developed twenty potential vaccines, each a bit different than the next. In some ways, it was one giant science experiment for Şahin, who was curious to see which candidate might work best.

Pfizer and BioNTech researchers tested them all in animals and then in humans, dismissing some because they caused uncomfortable side effects, like chills and fever. By July, they were down to two candidates, both of which employed nucleoside modifications, but one that generated the partial-spike protein and the other that produced the full protein. The results weren't clear-cut, but one design was favored by Şahin and a few other senior scientists: the vaccine producing just the small, receptor-binding area of the spike protein.

There was good reason Şahin favored this choice: A vaccine using only a small piece of the spike seemed likely to be easier to manufacture, among other advantages. The receptor-binding domain was the most active part of the protein, and there was reason to think it was all the body needed to generate sufficient antibody protection against SARS-CoV-2. Şahin and BioNTech's researchers had already published scientific literature showing the value of this approach.

Some researchers also liked that they weren't going with the full spike protein, the design that all the rival vaccine efforts had chosen. It felt good to choose a different approach. Impressive data received on July 1 confirmed that the partial-spike choice generated substantial protection against SARS-CoV-2, another reason Şahin and the others were fans.

By mid-July, McDermott and his team needed a decision so they could begin cranking up production. Şahin, Bourla, and their top executives scheduled a video call to settle the issue. The slice of the spike protein seemed the consensus choice, but they still needed to make a final decision.

Ahead of the meeting, Mikael Dolsten, the senior Pfizer scientist, began worrying they were about to make a huge mistake. There were good reasons Moderna, J&J, and others were creating a full spike protein in the body. That kind of molecule was likely to stir the immune system to generate a large variety of neutralizing antibodies, for one thing. The full spike version also seemed likely to provide more protection if the virus were to develop dangerous variants. And there was reason to think the full spike would elicit milder reactions upon inoculation, an important consideration given that many in the public were expressing hesitation about getting vaccinated.

A bit before the meeting, Dolsten shared his concerns with Bourla, who said he also was having second thoughts. A few years earlier, Pfizer had hired Daniel Kahneman, the psychologist and economist, to give a seminar to its top executives. Kahneman, who is famous for his research on decision-making, discussed the dangers of embracing a choice solely because others favored it, what Kahneman called the "bandwagon effect." He also explained the "ostrich bias," which is when decision-makers make a choice and bury their heads in the sand, unwilling to reconsider their choice and examine new data.

Now, Dolsten and Bourla were concerned the companies' scientists were making the same mistakes Kahneman had warned them to avoid. Just because the team had a long-running fondness for using a piece of the spike protein didn't mean it was the best choice.

"We're getting too affectionate" for the receptor-binding-domain design, Dolsten told Bourla, who agreed.

During the meeting, Bourla and Dolsten persuaded Şahin and others to shift to the full-spike design. Jansen and some others wanted to keep debating the choice, and Şahin said he was working on still more design possibilities, but Bourla said they needed to make a choice. They would keep testing the two designs, but he signaled to McDermott that he could get moving on ramping up production capacity for the full-spike candidate.

For days following the meeting, Dolsten had difficulty sleeping, worried that he had made a mistake helping to push for the new design. They didn't have nearly as much data to back this candidate, he realized. Dolsten began hounding Jansen, asking if she had received the results of the tests on their full-spike design.

Finally, on July 22, Jansen said the data were in—the full-spike candidate generated a strong immune response, just like the partial-spike shots. But the full protein vaccine was more tolerable than their original choice, with fewer cases of side effects such as fever and chills.

Both Dolsten and Jansen could relax for the first time in weeks. Pfizer and BioNTech told the Food and Drug Administration they had decided on a vaccine. They could start a crucial phase 3 efficacy trial.

• • •

Dan Barouch and Johnson & Johnson's researchers were also making progress.

Back in January, Barouch and his team had worked with J&J scientists to design and test a coronavirus vaccine based on Ad26. It would be up to J&J's enormous team to produce and distribute the shots after they were authorized by health authorities.

First, though, they had to decide how potent their shots should be. For several months, the team tested a version of the vaccine that induced high antibody levels, an approach favored by Hanneke Schuitemaker, J&J's global head of viral vaccine discovery. Schuitemaker had a lot in common with Barouch, which had helped smooth their partnership. She was an AIDS expert and former academic who had transitioned to become an executive, first working at Crucell, the Netherlands biotech company that developed the Ad26 technology with Barouch, before climbing the ranks at J&J.

Over the years, she had emerged as the company's most vocal advocate of its vaccine work.

"Treatments save lives," Schuitemaker liked to tell colleagues in Crucell's offices in the Dutch city of Leiden. "But vaccines save populations."

When the coronavirus crisis worsened in the early spring, however, some senior J&J executives were having second thoughts about Schuitemaker's idea of using high-potency shots. Over a series of Zoom meetings, the J&J executives, including the company's chief scientific officer, Paul Stoffels, pointed to recent data suggesting that a lower-strength version of the vaccine would provide sufficient protection while generating fewer and milder side effects. This approach seemed the best of all worlds, the executives argued.

The debate raged on, time ticked away, and Schuitemaker grew frustrated. She understood why a lower-dose vaccine was attractive. A key reason many people were expressing hesitancy about taking potential Covid-19 vaccines was their fear of painful or even harmful side effects. But switching to a new version of the vaccine would set the J&J program back at least three weeks, a delay Schuitemaker argued wasn't worthwhile.

She tried to hide her unhappiness in video meetings, but with each new video meeting to discuss the potency issue, Schuitemaker became more irritated. Now, her blood pressure was really rising. The pandemic was killing people, rivals were accelerating their own vaccine programs, and J&J was contemplating slowing its own effort to switch to lower-potency shots? It didn't make sense to her.

Let's get going already, she thought.

J&J decided to go with the lower-potent shots. The Oxford/AstraZeneca effort was sprinting past them, and both Pfizer/BioNTech and Moderna were close behind, leaving J&J in the dust. The company's top executives didn't seem to mind—they were betting that J&J, which had a one-and-done regimen featuring just one shot, would make its vaccine unique and attractive, as would the fact that they didn't need to be kept at supercold temperatures, like the mRNA shots.

In July, J&J, working with Barouch and his colleagues, showed that a single dose of their Ad26 vaccine had protected, or nearly protected, six rhesus monkeys from SARS-CoV-2. The results were from a small sample of the animals, but they looked promising. By then, Janssen's researchers in the Netherlands had already begun producing vaccines for clinical trials. That month, they planned to study the safety and immune response of their shots and move into a phase 3 efficacy trial of sixty thousand subjects in September.

Barouch and J&J knew they might not have the first vaccine, but their shots had a chance to be the most protective and convenient.

• • •

As the coronavirus spread, thousands of scientists around the world raced to build vaccines capable of protecting people from what increasingly seemed like a modern-day new plague. It was clear to all that a number of different vaccines would be needed to stem the pandemic. By the summer of 2020, over one hundred groups were developing shots, some using slower, traditional methods, such as injecting a weakened version of the actual virus, and others employing more questionable approaches, including DNA-based shots.

It made little sense for Gale Smith and his colleagues at Novavax to join the chase. By early 2020, the tiny Maryland outfit had never developed an approved vaccine, it had only a few months of cash, and most employees had a foot out the door. At the time, it was conducting late-stage trials for a flu vaccine, the company's last chance for success. Executives knew any distractions from their work could prove perilous.

By this time, Smith had just a dozen or so researchers working with him. Pfizer and other drug giants had thousands of pedigreed scientists on staff. Heck, most of those companies had more *lobbyists* in Washington, D.C., than Smith had colleagues in his lab. Yet he couldn't help tracking the virus as it spread from Wuhan. He had spent years perfecting his "protein subunit" approach, which involved producing a virus's protein and injecting it into the body. Smith and his colleagues had helped build vaccines for the most serious recent coronaviruses, including SARS-CoV-1 and MERS-CoV, among other pathogens. They were skilled at targeting spike proteins. Smith didn't see a reason why the team couldn't develop an effective vaccine targeting the new coronavirus.

Smith tried to persuade his bosses to shift gears. After weeks of debate, Stan Erck and Gregory Glenn agreed—they would wager the company on shots to stop SARS-CoV-2. The opportunity seemed too great to ignore, even if it meant risking Novavax's future.

"We have to work on this," Glenn told Erck.

The Novavax scientists stumbled right out of the gate. They ordered the gene for the spike protein from a supplier in Shanghai, but it never came—flights from China had been frozen due to the outbreak. Fortunately, the supplier's New Jersey office was able to produce another version of the gene and agreed to drive it, in a red-capped vial, overnight to Novavax's offices.

Smith and his team got to work. They inserted the gene, with its DNA instructions to create the spike protein, into the DNA of an insect virus. Then they took this newly infused baculovirus and used it to infect cells that originally came from an insect called a fall armyworm. The cells were grown in large bioreactors holding up to six thousand liters of liquid—vats that looked like they came from breweries—to cook up a batch of spike protein. The protein antigen was isolated, purified, embedded in a lipid nanoparticle, and blended with its adjuvant compound and—ta-da—they had a vaccine.

Erck began telling investors and nonprofit bodies that Novavax was building a Covid-19 vaccine, and he was able to raise some money to help the effort. Novavax was tiny and unproven, but its protein-subunit approach was more traditional than the newer techniques of leaders in the vaccine race, part of why some charitable foundations and others proved helpful. Their shots weren't telling the body to create the spike protein, like Moderna and BioNTech's mRNA vaccines or the shots from J&J and the Oxford groups. Erck emphasized that their vaccine didn't need to be kept at supercold temperatures, unlike the mRNA shots, an advantage for hospitals, clinics, and pharmacies lacking freezer capacity, especially those in developing countries.

Novavax's vaccine injected a synthesized, slightly modified version of the spike protein, using Jason McLellan's two prolines to keep it stable. Novavax's shots simply asked the body's immune system to recognize the protein as a foreign invader and attack it if the protein were to be encountered down the line as part of an actual virus. The same approach had produced effective shots for shingles and hepatitis B, which also reassured backers.

The company needed a lot more cash, though. And all those extra production steps meant it was slower off the mark than those developing mRNA and viral vector vaccines that simply delivered genetic instructions.

In March, when Erck joined Bancel, Dolsten, and the others at the White House meeting with Trump, he sat at the end of the long table of pharmaceutical executives, far from the president. Nonetheless, he was thrilled just to be included with the industry's heavyweights. When it was his time to speak, Erck decided to swallow his pride and plea for help.

"Frankly, we need money," Erck told Trump. "We're a biotech company, and not one of the larger pharma companies. And so we need money to get scale."

Trump hadn't expected anyone to plead for cash at the meeting. He mostly wanted to hear the execs promise to deliver a vaccine in a few months, at most. But Erck knew it was no time to be coy. Over the next couple of months, he reached out to Operation Warp Speed, a Norway-based nonprofit called the Coalition for Epidemic Preparedness Innovations, and other organizations. Former Novavax executives worked for some of these institutions, opening doors for Erck. He also pitched a Boston health-care hedge fund called RA Capital Management.

Glenn sought a different kind of support. In March, his Presbyterian congregation in rural Maryland stopped meeting in person, as churches and other religious institutions shuttered in many places around the world. Now, they met each Sunday on Zoom.

Word spread within the church that Glenn and his colleagues were working on a vaccine. Soon he was receiving words of support and encouragement from neighbors, friends, and others, many of whom said they appreciated the health risks Glenn and his team were accepting by continuing to go to work each day. The company was cleaning every door handle, window, desk, and surface in its labs many times throughout the day, but its researchers still felt nervous about their own health.

"We're praying for you," congregants told Glenn.

The words were uplifting. But Glenn sensed the congregants were anxious. It wasn't clear if anyone could develop effective and safe shots or how long they would take. They were scared about the damage the virus was wreaking.

Glenn felt he had a God-given ability to potentially halt the new plague. But rather than providing him with a sense of confidence, the responsibility felt like a crushing burden. By late spring, the pandemic was getting worse, Fauci was warning that the nation could soon see one hundred thousand new infections daily, and experts were still skeptical that Glenn and others would produce protective vaccines.

"I just don't see a vaccine coming anytime soon," Nevan Krogan, a molecular biologist and director of University of California, San Francisco's Quantitative Biosciences Institute, which worked with one hundred research laboratories.[11]

Seeking divine assurance and guidance, Glenn met with his pastor, who pointed him to Psalms 91:14–16:

I will protect him, for he acknowledges my name.
He will call on me, and I will answer him.

By June, Erck had lined up over $2 billion in funding so Novavax could pursue its Covid-19 vaccine. To begin testing it, Glenn called researchers at the University of Oklahoma, who offered fifteen baboons especially bred for medical research. The subsequent trial, along with other animal studies and early human trials, demonstrated that Novavax's shots produced remarkable amounts of neutralizing antibodies, stirring buzz in the industry that sent its shares to $170 from about $4 at the beginning of 2020.[12] Novavax couldn't produce its own vaccines, because it had been forced to sell its manufacturing facilities the previous year, but had an agreement with Emergent BioSolutions to make its shots, and that company's nearby Baltimore factory had already produced vaccines for Novavax's early clinical trials.

But Erck received crushing news. Moncef Slaoui and others directing Operation Warp Speed called to say they were kicking Novavax out of the Emergent facility. Novavax was taking too long to produce a vaccine and J&J and Oxford/AstraZeneca's shots were making faster progress, so Novavax was going to have to make way for its larger rivals. The Warp Speed officials arranged for a second manufacturer, Fujifilm Diosynth Biotechnologies, to make the Novavax vaccine in its plants in North Carolina and Texas, but Erck and Glenn knew the move would set the company's effort back weeks, if not months. They tried to convince Slaoui to change his mind, but he wouldn't budge.

Gloom set in around Novavax's offices. Staffers had been planning huge clinical trials in South Africa, the United Kingdom, Mexico, and the United States to prove their vaccine was effective. Now they'd have to transfer their technology to the Fujifilm plant and start the process all over, even as competitors raced ahead with their own trials. With the finish line in sight, the government had tripped Novavax up, sending it sprawling.

Erck walked the halls at the company, telling colleagues they'd yet find a way to rebound, as they always had in the past. At home, Glenn joined his church for their regular Sunday Zoom meetings. Friends and other congregants chatted with him about golf, soccer, and their kids' activities, hoping to keep his spirits up.

They knew enough not to ask for an update on Novavax's vaccine.

18

Summer–Fall 2020

Juan Andres was getting nervous once again.

Earlier in 2020, Andres's family had poked fun at the Madrid native when he'd expressed fears about the emerging virus. At the time, the toilet paper and other supplies the Moderna executive had accumulated seemed over the top, as had Andres's insistence on purchasing a third refrigerator to store food for a potential lockdown. By the summer, though, as a wave of infections swept parts of the United States, including areas of the South and West that had escaped the brunt of earlier Covid-19 spikes, no one was mocking Andres.

By then, Andres was largely running Moderna's vaccine-manufacturing operation from a dining-room table in his home in suburban Boston to reduce the risk of contracting the disease, though he sometimes traveled to nearby Norwood, Massachusetts, to oversee work at the facility. Andres had a second-floor office in his home, but it was full of boxes and storage items and he didn't have a free moment to clear it all, so he mostly stayed in the dining room. It was a decision that didn't thrill his family; most of the day, they scattered to other floors, trying to avoid him.

"I was working eighteen hours a day and they got tired of listening to it all," he says.

In the first few months of the year, Andres and his team made a couple of hundred vaccine doses, enabling Moderna to complete its early clinical studies. In May, he took the $1.3 billion from Moderna's stock sale and spent it on supplies to begin preparing many more doses. He began to realize how hard it was going to be, though. In its ten-year history, Moderna had produced only about one hundred thousand vaccine doses. Now, in the middle of the summer, Andres and his colleagues were gearing up to make hundreds of millions. There were about six hundred components needed for a single vaccine, including filters, connectors, labels, vials, stoppers, and more. And Andres needed to find the necessary equipment and raw materials at a time when supply shortages were emerging throughout the country.

Each vaccine had to be identical. Its potency, stability, and every other characteristic couldn't vary, so Andres and his colleagues needed to produce the vaccines in the exact same way—the same temperature ranges, same equipment, and same raw materials.

They had to do it all quickly, too. The company wanted to start rolling out shots in the fall; Andres and his colleagues would need to move fast to make it happen. It was a bit like a chef at a fine restaurant being asked to make the same top-notch meal for thousands of people from his existing kitchen, and to do it overnight.

With his team, Andres projected confidence, exhorting them with a series of inspirational maxims.

"A moment of fear is a moment lost."

"This is our chance to help mankind."

Often, Andres, a huge Real Madrid fan, relied on soccer adages, while emphasizing the need to work together.

"Play your position and trust your teammate," he often said.

The exhortations seemed to work. Soon Andres's staffers were volunteering to work weekends and organizing themselves into shifts that allowed them to avoid wasted time. The team still wasn't sure if their vaccine was going to work, or if so many effective shots would be produced by others that theirs might not be needed, but they wanted to do everything they could to try to help protect people from the devastating disease. One employee on Andres's team with stage 4 cancer was so moved by their mission that she insisted on coming to work, amid grueling treatments.

What Andres didn't tell his team was that he was up nights, worried about potential complications in the manufacturing process and if they could pull it all off.

Is this really going to be possible?

• • •

In a matter of months, the Oxford/AstraZeneca team lost its lead in the vaccine chase.

In May, Operation Warp Speed had given them $1.2 billion to test and manufacture their coronavirus vaccine, in exchange for 300 million doses. A month later, the effort had begun—a combined phase 2 and 3 trial, aiming to recruit one hundred thousand participants by midsummer and have final efficacy data and regulatory approvals by September.

But U.S. officials soon became concerned. Some at Oxford, including Sarah Gilbert, Adrian Hill, and clinical-trials specialist Andy Pollard, didn't seem to communicate well with AstraZeneca's own scientists, Warp Speed officials noticed. American authorities sometimes waited weeks for important trial data—such as details about various vaccine batches—that other vaccine companies were delivering overnight.

American federal health authorities told the Oxford/AstraZeneca team and other vaccine efforts that the FDA would likely need late-stage data from trials with at least thirty thousand participants before the agency would consider authorizing a vaccine. By early summer, however, AstraZeneca had enrolled far fewer people in its trials in Britain and Brazil. And the company hadn't even begun a larger trial in the United States, suggesting the effort's shots wouldn't be authorized any time soon, at least not in America.

In the summer, even worse news emerged for Hill and his colleagues: Two trial volunteers developed troubling neurological symptoms, forcing a trial halt of several weeks until officials could determine that the shots likely hadn't caused dangerous side effects. Trial pauses of this sort are not uncommon. But the FDA was concerned that some of its officials had been blindsided by news of the neurological issues and the resulting trial pause, another communication gaffe that raised questions about the Oxford/AstraZeneca alliance.[1]

• • •

Moderna was dealing with its own tensions with U.S. officials.

In early summer, spirits were running high as the company's executives counted down to the start of Moderna's phase 3 trial during the first week of July. This would be the last step to prove their vaccine was effective. Even better, the company's study was set to begin a few weeks before Pfizer's own phase 3 study, giving Moderna the inside track at producing the first Covid-19 vaccine.

That all changed in early June when Stephen Hoge, Moderna's president, received an early-morning call from Moncef Slaoui, the head of Operation Warp Speed. He had bad news: Moderna would need to collect more data during the upcoming phase 3 trial than the company had planned on gathering. Scientists around the country needed additional data from Moderna's trial subjects for their own studies, Slaoui said, so Moderna would have to make sure to collect it as part of its clinical trial. When someone in the trial was diagnosed with Covid-19, for example, Moderna would now have to perform a daily test on the subject, using swabs provided by the company, for up to twenty-eight straight days, to help track their level of infection. Kits that Moderna had assembled for those conducting its trial, which included vaccines for some subjects, placebos for others, and more, would have to include additional supplies to regularly test the volunteers for Covid-19.

Hoge couldn't believe what he was hearing. The new data had nothing to do with Moderna's vaccine or its potential efficacy; it was to help outside scientists better understand the disease and its duration, and maybe allow them to build medicines. Sure, that kind of information could be helpful. But a pandemic was killing people and the change was going to delay Moderna's final-stage efficacy study. Not only that, but Pfizer wasn't subject to the same data-gathering requirement, because it wasn't taking money from Operation Warp Speed and didn't have to answer to its officials.

"It's going to take us weeks to rebuild these kits!" Hoge told Slaoui. "We just don't think it's necessary."

Slaoui, who was feeling his own pressures from the scientists and others, said there was no getting around the change. He was right. Operation Warp Speed officials were negotiating with Moderna for the purchase of 100 million shots, a deal that would be worth about $1.5 billion, or sixteen dollars a dose. Moderna continued to work closely with Tony Fauci, Barney Graham, and other government scientists. If the company dug in its heels and rejected a request from the government after getting all that help, the resulting publicity would surely be ugly.

"You're going to have to accept it," Slaoui told Hoge. "Find a way to minimize the impact."

Moderna rebuilt the kits so its subjects could receive the regular tests and the information could be accumulated, though it ultimately didn't prove very useful. The effort set the company's late-stage trial back a few weeks: On July 27, the first volunteer in Moderna's final-stage efficacy trial in the United States received an injection of the company's shot. Thirty thousand people participated in the study, all of whom had a good chance of becoming exposed to the virus. Some received the actual vaccine while others got a placebo, allowing the Moderna researchers to see if their vaccine reduced rates of infection and disease. That same day, BioNTech and Pfizer began their own, similar phase 3 trial in the United States, Brazil, and a few other countries. Moderna's lead over Pfizer/BioNTech had evaporated.

About a month later, the U.S. government asked Moderna to slow its trial once again, this time to include more minority subjects in its final-stage study. It was a request the company better understood and one that also was requested of Pfizer. But Moderna had a tougher time than Pfizer recruiting thousands of new minority subjects, delaying the company's study. Going into the final lap, the Pfizer/BioNTech team had grabbed the leader position in the vaccine race.

• • •

During the summer of 2020, BioNTech staffers grew frustrated.

The company was making progress on its vaccine, but the company's executives were becoming irritated that Pfizer was hogging the limelight. It was BioNTech that had spent years perfecting its mRNA technologies, not Pfizer, and it had been Şahin and his team who had developed the original constructs for the vaccine. Yet the giant American company was garnering most of the international publicity. Pfizer executives were courting the media and leaving the impression that their company had created the shots, BioNTech employees griped to one another.

"We're up against the Pfizer media machine," a BioNTech executive complained to a colleague, explaining the company's predicament.

Uğur Şahin was too busy to be very upset, though. He was working on early trials for the Pfizer/BioNTech Covid-19 vaccine, helping to solve manufacturing issues and leading negotiations on agreements to distribute the vaccine in various countries.

In late summer, though, as Şahin awaited the critical results of the vaccine's phase 3 clinical trial, he became more anxious. He knew that an effective vaccine could help bring an end to the pandemic while giving his company a prime opportunity to produce future drugs and vaccines. Failure would likely mean a lengthier pandemic and more global misery. Covid-19 vaccines developed by researchers in China and Russia had already been given to people in those and other nations, but there still wasn't enough data to determine their effectiveness.

Thomas Strüngmann, BioNTech's billionaire backer, stayed in regular contact with Şahin and saw that he was exhausted and in need of a distraction. During weekly Sunday night calls, Strüngmann began chatting with him about books, movies, and other lighter topics—anything but Covid-19 and his shots—succeeding in brightening Şahin's mood.

Bancel and his colleagues at Moderna needed a way to calm their own nerves ahead of their own phase 3 results. As they conducted daily video calls during the summer, Bancel, Hoge, Andres, and other executives decided to loosen things up and share a drink during their daily deliberations; some sipped glasses of wine, while others drank beer.

"We needed to keep our sanity," Andres says.

After a few weeks, though, the group realized they were inviting trouble with their nightly drinking sessions, so they returned to alcohol-free meetings. For a healthier escape, Bancel turned elsewhere. As difficult as he had been on early employees, Bancel showed a tender side with others in his life, including a group of long-standing friends. Over the years, he sent them handwritten notes, sharing how much their friendships meant to him.

Ahead of the key late-stage data, Bancel joined regular Zoom calls with these close friends. He looked exhausted, sometimes joining the calls after getting three hours of sleep the previous night. He didn't want sessions to end, though, as if he were clinging to the fleeting moments of calm amid the building tensions.

• • •

During the first weekend of November, just after Americans voted in a contested presidential election between Donald Trump and Joseph Biden, Pfizer and BioNTech executives were informed that early results from their vaccine's phase 3 trial were ready to be revealed. The study had been designed to deliver an interim analysis after a significant number of its 44,000 subjects had become infected with SARS-CoV-2. By early November, 94 subjects had developed Covid-19 symptoms, a figure deemed large enough to deliver an early determination of the vaccine's efficacy. If the bulk of those infected had been inoculated with the Pfizer/BioNTech vaccine, it would be a crushing disappointment; but if a high number of the infections came from the placebo group, the shots would be proven protective. An outside panel of independent experts, known as a data-safety monitoring committee, was ready to share the key figures.

At eleven a.m. on Sunday, November 8, the committee members began a video meeting to discuss the results. Kathrin Jansen, the senior Pfizer scientist, and Bill Gruber, who ran Pfizer's clinical trials, were selected to receive the information on behalf of the company. Jansen would then relay it to Albert Bourla, the Pfizer chief executive; Mikael Dolsten, the company's chief scientist; and three other senior Pfizer executives, who had gathered in a conference room in the company's research office in Cos Cob, Connecticut. In the room, the group gathered around a long, wooden conference room, each Pfizer executive wearing a black face mask adorned with the phrase: "Science Will Win." They looked bleary-eyed; few in the room had slept much the night before.

Around noon, a lunch was served featuring salads and sandwiches—

but barely anyone touched it. Instead, they mostly sipped coffee from mustard-colored paper cups.

The group sensed the pressure of the moment. Disappointing results would mean Pfizer/BioNTech's shots couldn't help protect people from Covid-19. Failure would also likely mean other vaccine efforts were doomed, since so many shared common elements with Pfizer/BioNTech's approach, such as targeting the coronavirus's spike protein.

Some at Pfizer had intensely personal reasons to explain why they were praying for good news. Philip Dormitzer, who along with Jansen had helped forge the original alliance with BioNTech, hadn't seen his wife or young children since March, a long eight months. Years earlier, she had almost died of pneumonia. Fearful of contracting the disease or seeing her children become ill, she had encouraged her husband to focus on his vaccine research and to continue interacting with his Pfizer colleagues. The Dormitzer family would reunite only when an effective vaccine was available.[2]

The independent committee meeting got under way and Jansen stood by in her home on New York's Hudson River, waiting to hear the results. In the Connecticut conference room, tension was thick in the air. Bourla and Dolsten tried to make idle chatter, doing their best to avoid the topic at hand, but they failed miserably. They couldn't get their minds off the vaccine.

"What do you think the results will be?" Bourla asked.

Dolsten wasn't sure how to respond. This was his boss, after all. If he gave a high prediction of efficacy and the true number was lower, Bourla might be disappointed. Then again, if Dolsten proposed a low number, it might suggest that he wasn't confident in their vaccine. That was pretty much the last thing Bourla or anyone on edge around the table wanted to hear at that moment.

"Seventy-five percent," Dolsten replied.

Bourla didn't look happy.

"Not more?!" he responded.

Bourla was likely displaying mock anger, but Dolsten wasn't entirely sure. No one in the room was thinking very clearly at that moment.

Time dragged on. An hour. Ninety minutes. By one p.m., Bourla and others were truly worried. They began sending Jansen texts.

What is it?

When are you calling?

Jansen told them the committee was still meeting.

"Hang on," she texted.

Her message only confused Bourla, Dolsten, and the others.

Hang on? Is that good news or bad news?

Finally, shortly after one p.m., the committee gave Jansen the results. About forty-five minutes later, after some perfunctory discussions with the committee members, she and Gruber appeared on a large video screen projected on the wall of the room in Connecticut. Everyone nervously waited for either Jansen or Gruber to speak.

Jansen paused, expressionless, looking at the group. Then she spoke.

"Good news," she said. "We made it . . . we won."

The room burst into a loud cheer. Bourla pumped his fist and Dolsten jumped up.

The interim review had shown the Pfizer/BioNTech vaccine had been more than 90 percent effective.

"Oh my God!" Dolsten yelled. "It's unbelievable, it's unbelievable!"

"I love you!" Bourla screamed out to his colleagues.

The Connecticut group shared hugs and poured glasses of champagne.

Nearly every person who had come down with Covid-19 had been in the placebo group, it turned out. The trial results also demonstrated additional evidence of the vaccine's safety. Nearly two weeks later, more extensive data would show the vaccine to be 95 percent effective. Pfizer would set plans to obtain an emergency-use authorization from regulators allowing it to distribute the vaccines before the end of 2020.

Moments later, Bourla told Şahin and Türeci the great news. Privately, the couple had expected an efficacy figure of about 80 percent. The true number stunned them. They became emotional, jumping up and down while hugging each other tightly. Then they enjoyed their own celebratory beverage: a cup of freshly brewed tea.

Soon they set up a call to relay the results to five members of their senior executive team. It was ten p.m. in Germany. One BioNTech executive, Sean Marett, dialed into the video call in his basement, to avoid waking his children, who were sleeping upstairs. He sat on the edge of a couch, near some children's toys and stray gym equipment. All that day, Marett had paced the house, waiting for the results. His palms were sweating as he waited for the news.

"We got the results," Şahin told the group before relaying the details.

There was complete silence. The executives were stunned. Then, Marett began laughing. Within moments, the entire group began giggling uncontrollably. For several minutes, they couldn't stop. No one could manage to say a word. All they could do was laugh.

In an instant, months of fear, pressure, and nervousness had been released.

• • •

On November 15, the data-safety monitoring committee overseeing the Moderna vaccine's trial was ready to share interim results of the company's own phase 3 study. Hoge, representing Moderna, dialed into the video call. He was terrified. Pfizer's numbers had been so good, and he worried that Moderna's might not be able to match them. What if they didn't come close? Every possible worst-case scenario flashed through his mind as he ratcheted down his expectations.

I'll take eighty percent, he thought.

The committee's meeting began at ten a.m. Around noon, it sent word to Hoge and Tony Fauci, representing the government scientists who worked on the vaccine with Moderna, that the committee members were ready to share the results.

The moment he joined the video meeting, Hoge studied the faces of the committee members.

Is that a smile? Wait, that one looks glum. What does that mean?!

Slowly, Hoge began to realize the expression he was seeing on the faces of almost every committee member was sheer boredom. They had spent over two hours discussing the company's trial data and now they looked like they could use a long break. Some of the scientific experts were checking their emails, it appeared. This was a huge potential turning point in a historic pandemic. It was also the biggest moment in Moderna's history and in Hoge's professional life; he had been up three straight nights, unable to sleep. And these guys can't manage a little excitement or enthusiasm? Oh no, the results must truly be awful, Hoge figured. He scrutinized their faces once again, looking for new clues to the trial results.

Gimme a smile! Someone, anyone!

The chairman of the committee began to address the group, recounting all the reasons the Moderna trial had been conducted and what it aimed to find. His comments could not have been more dry or boring.

The goal?! Dude, we're trying to stop a pandemic, that's the goal!

Hoge thought about cracking a joke, but he saw Fauci in his home office, stoic as everyone else, and thought better of it. Hoge noticed that the chairman's arm was visibly bruised and in an enormous black-and-white air cast. Hoge wanted to ask what had happened, but thought better of that, too.

Next, the committee's chief statistician began speaking. It was as if the committee had searched the world for the only person drier than the committee chairman. The statistician explained the math that went into the figures the committee was about to reveal, how many people had been in the study, and other facts that Hoge and the others knew quite well already. Everyone on the call pretended to be paying attention. The statistician spoke for about three minutes; to Hoge, it felt like three hours.

The whole time, Bancel and a few other Moderna executives were sending messages to Hoge on a group chat.

What's going on?!

Hoge had nothing to tell them.

Then the numbers were revealed: Ninety-five people in the thirty-thousand-subject study had developed Covid-19 with symptoms. Ninety of those people had received a placebo; only five had been given Moderna's vaccine.

Hoge couldn't believe what he was hearing. He started calculating the efficacy figure in his head, zoning out for a moment or two. Then, Hoge began to panic that he had missed some important information that Moderna would have to reveal to investors and others. He furiously scribbled the figures, alert again to what he was hearing.

Hoge heard more good news: Among those ninety-five volunteers, eleven experienced severe cases of infection; they all were people who had received the placebo. Not one had been given Moderna's vaccine, an additional sign of its efficacy.

Hoge stole a moment to text his colleagues on the group chat.

It's a home run.
A HOME RUN.
94.5%

Fauci spoke next: "This is just stunning . . . amazing . . . I'm speechless."

Then the committee asked Hoge if he wanted to say anything. He was in a giddy stupor and wasn't prepared to speak, but he roused himself long enough to thank the committee for its time.

In his home in Boston, Bancel met his wife in a hallway. They embraced. His eighteen-year-old daughter raced down from her second-floor room, while his sixteen-year-old daughter ran up the basement stairs.

"The four of us were crying," he says.[3]

The Moderna vaccine had proved 94.5 percent effective at protecting people from Covid-19, a result on par with the Pfizer/BioNTech shots. Moderna even said its shots were stable for thirty days at refrigerator-freezer temperatures, making them easier to deliver and store than the Pfizer vaccines, which needed to be kept at much colder temperatures.

Like the Pfizer/BioNTech results, the Moderna figures were preliminary, but follow-up results would show both shots to have similar efficacy. The world would have two vaccines to provide protection against the vicious virus. The Dow Jones Industrial Average soared, social media lit up, and millions of people around the world breathed deep sighs of relief. For the first time in over eight months, they could imagine a return to normalcy.

• • •

Adrian Hill, Sarah Gilbert, and the rest of the Oxford team counted down to their own phase 3 clinical-trial results. The previous few months had been rough on the group, as their vaccine had lost its front-runner status, and as questions emerged about how the team was running its trials. But their shots were still needed. By then, the coronavirus had killed 1.3 million people around the world, and Oxford, with its partner, AstraZeneca, had promised to deliver up to three billion shots by the end of 2021 in various countries, including many lower-income nations.[4]

Interim data for the vaccine's phase 3 trials in the United Kingdom and Brazil gave Hill, Gilbert, and their colleagues a chance to move past the troubles. They knew that impressive results would bolster the chances of quick regulatory authorization of their shots, enabling their vaccine to be in arms around the world before the end of the year. Over the weekend of November 22, not long after Pfizer/BioNTech and Moderna shared details from their phase 3 clinical trials, Oxford and AstraZeneca executives received the trial results: They were good, but a bit confusing.

Their vaccine had an efficacy of 62 percent for the largest group of trial participants, nearly nine thousand volunteers, who had received two full-strength doses several weeks apart. This kind of figure would have been celebrated at the outset of the pandemic, of course, but Oxford and AstraZeneca scientists knew their results paled in comparison with those of Pfizer/BioNTech and Moderna.

As they analyzed the data, though, the Oxford team found a reason to cheer. There had been a smaller number of volunteers, 2,741 in total, who had been given an initial, half-strength dose of the vaccine before receiving a second, full dose twelve weeks later. For these people, the vaccine had been 90 percent effective, exciting the researchers. Everyone at Oxford knew why these volunteers hadn't received the normal dose: They had used an Italian manufacturer to produce many of their shots, including doses given to this group of 2,741 subjects. The Italian manufacturer used a different technique than the Oxford researchers to measure the strength of each vaccine dose. Oxford's in-house measurement determined that the potency of this batch was higher than expected, though the Italians disagreed and said it was fine. To be cautious, Oxford had lowered the dosage of those shots, in case its measurement method was indeed accurate. This way, they could ensure the shots weren't too potent. It wasn't a big deal—measurement discrepancies between labs are common, and regulators had been apprised of the half-dose decision months earlier.

Now, though, the Oxford and AstraZeneca teams had to explain the striking discrepancy in the efficacy of their shots. They had received opprobrium for not being sufficiently transparent and desperately wanted to avoid more painful, public criticism. Yet, the two teams were thrilled by the 90 percent result—many of the researchers had privately been hoping for an efficacy figure that might match the results from Pfizer/BioNTech and Moderna. They were proud of their shots and wanted to trumpet their effectiveness.

On the morning of November 23, Oxford and AstraZeneca simultaneously announced the results. In a press release, Oxford called the results a "breakthrough," while AstraZeneca in a separate release said that "the vaccine was highly effective in preventing COVID-19." The very first figure AstraZeneca cited was the efficacy figure of 90 percent. After sharing the lower, 62-percent efficacy figure, AstraZeneca said that combining the two dosages had "resulted in an average efficacy of 70 percent."

Right away, many in the media seized on the higher figure.

The Wall Street Journal blasted a headline: "AstraZeneca-Oxford Covid-19 Vaccine up to 90% Effective in Late-Stage Trials."[5]

Quickly, though, the Oxford/AstraZeneca team faced a wave of criticism. The higher-efficacy figure had resulted from a small subset of their overall study. Some thought the researchers had cherry-picked their data, a no-no in science, and it wasn't clear how they had arrived at the 70 percent figure. Oxford and AstraZeneca couldn't even fully explain why a half dose had provided such strong protection, nor even how it had resulted.

"We stumbled upon doing half dose–full dose," Mene Pangalos, head of AstraZeneca's non-oncology research and development, told Reuters. "Yes, it was a mistake."[6]

But his boss, Pascal Soriot, said "It was not a mistake," something both Gilbert and Hill were adamant about.

"It wasn't a mix-up in dosing," Gilbert told the *Financial Times*.[7]

Slaoui had additional reasons to be disappointed. On the day the results were revealed, he said those in the half-dose group were all under the age of fifty-five, raising new questions about the vaccine's effectiveness in older adults most vulnerable to Covid-19.[8] Later, it became clear that the effectiveness of the half dose likely was due to the especially long intervals between the first and second dosage, a delay that had proved beneficial. By then, though, critics had piled on.

"The world bet on this vaccine," said Eric Topol, a well-known clinical trial expert at the Scripps Research Institute in San Diego. "What a disappointment. . . . If they just were upfront on safety, on efficacy, on dosing, on everything, from the get-go, they'd be in such a better position. But what they've done now is diminish credibility, and I don't know how they're going to regain that."[9]

Hill had spent his career dishing criticism at his fellow researchers. Now, scientists and others around the world were ripping into him and his colleagues.

"The company tried to embellish their results by highlighting a reported ninety percent efficacy in a relatively small subset of subjects in the study," said Geoffrey Porges, a research analyst at investment firm SVB Leerink. "The suggestion by the inventors that the small sample given the lower priming dose was evidence of superior efficacy only brings discredit to the program."

Hill was livid. He thought the criticism was unfair. Yes, his group could have improved their communication and analysis, he told people, but they had acted swiftly to help stop a pandemic. Their vaccine might not be perfect, or even the best of the lot, but it worked and it was saving lives. Why couldn't people see that?

When a fellow scientist called him late in 2020, Hill aired his frustrations.

"Nobody knows what the hell they're talking about," he said, referring to scientists, the media, and pretty much everyone else criticizing the Oxford/AstraZeneca effort.

Hill's voice rose as his defense continued.

"We got a vaccine out the door," he said. "This virus is *killing* people!"

19

Winter 2020–Summer 2021

Never was so much owed by so many to so few.

—WINSTON CHURCHILL[1]

Just after nine a.m. on Monday, December 13, 2020, Sandra Lindsay became the first American to receive a Covid-19 vaccination outside of a clinical trial. A critical-care nurse at Long Island Jewish Medical Center in Queens, New York, who had lost family members to Covid-19, Lindsay reported that her Pfizer/BioNTech shot felt no different from previous vaccinations. She encouraged others to follow her lead, including members of her West Indian community, some of whom were indicating early wariness about Covid-19 vaccines.[2]

A week later, Moderna's vaccine was cleared by U.S. authorities for use in those aged eighteen and older, just like Pfizer/BioNTech's shots. Soon both vaccines were going into the arms of doctors, nurses, and other frontline health workers, as well as residents of nursing homes and those most vulnerable to severe Covid-19 disease. Later, others would be offered both companies' vaccines.

The shots weren't nearly sufficient to quell the pandemic, however. The United States and the rest of the world were suffering through a terrible winter wave of SARS-CoV-2 infections that was worse than the outbreaks experienced in the spring and summer. In December 2020, the U.S. death toll topped 350,000 people, and hospitals were dangerously full as daily infections hit a record of nearly 300,000.[3] Europe, dealing with its own infection surge, enacted tight restrictions ahead of the Christmas holiday period, as did various nations around the globe.

The world needed more effective vaccines, and Gregory Glenn, the pediatrician who ran research and development at Novavax while tending to his chicken coop in rural Maryland, was desperate to help. Glenn was sixty-five years old, Novavax's chief executive officer, Stan Erck, was seventy-one, and Gale Smith was seventy-one. The trio had spent over a decade trying to produce effective vaccines. Finally, they had one that seemed close to the finish line. The U.S. government had ordered 110 million doses of Novavax's Covid-19 shots, which would be distributed upon receiving regulatory authorization. By some measures, the company's vaccine did a better job stirring the immune system than all the others, at least in early trials. The shots generated plentiful amounts of neutralizing antibodies, the immune-system agents assumed to be the most effective at fighting the virus, while also inducing a strong response from T cells.[4]

The Novavax team still needed definite evidence their shots worked, though. Throughout January 2021, the executives awaited results from the company's late-stage clinical trials. Erck maintained a nervous optimism, but some close to him were on edge. His wife, Dr. Sarah Frech, lit candles in front of a West African voodoo doll and rubbed it, an act she hoped might bring her husband's company some long-awaited good fortune.

In late January, Glenn and Erck headed to Erck's second home in South Carolina, to await results from the company's U.K. clinical study. They didn't want to be in the office—another failure would be too devastating and difficult to process there. The old friends preferred to be together in a more relaxed setting.

They were standing around an outdoor picnic table when Glenn's phone rang. It was a Novavax statistician named Iksung Cho.

"Let's get on Zoom," he told the men.

Glenn and Erck opened their computers, joining a few others on the call. Cho said he had data to relay. After all the years of dashed hopes and shattered expectations, the friends weren't sure what to expect.

Cho shared some figures with the group. Complete silence. The men, both graying grandfathers, reached for their reading glasses, but the figures were still too small for them to read. Glenn moved his face closer to the screen and squinted.

Is this eighty-nine-point-three?

It was. Novavax's Covid-19 vaccine's phase 3 trial in the United Kingdom had been revealed. It was 89.3 percent effective at protecting people from the Covid-19 disease. Glenn couldn't believe his eyes. He choked up, unable to speak. Novavax's vaccine truly worked. After all these years, Glenn and his colleagues finally knew success.

At the time, a worrisome variant strain of the coronavirus was circulating in the U.K., making the 89.3 percent figure even more impressive. The vaccine was much less effective in a separate, middle-stage study in South Africa, where another vicious variant was spreading, but the results were on par with those of Moderna and Pfizer/BioNTech elsewhere, most analysts determined.

In June 2021, Novavax's phase 3 study from subjects in the United States and Mexico showed its shots to be 90.4 percent effective at preventing symptomatic disease in adults, more proof that Smith and his colleagues had developed one of the most effective vaccines against the coronavirus. Regulatory clearances were still months away because the company had yet to ensure that its manufacturing processes met regulatory standards. The delays meant it was likely too late for Novavax to grab much of the initial Covid-19 market from Pfizer/BioNTech and Moderna in the West. But Novavax had pledged to deliver 1.1 billion doses globally and the vaccine seemed destined to play an important role in inoculating much of the world, including parts of Africa and other areas in desperate need of vaccine supplies. Some also anticipated that Novavax would help supply eventual booster shots in the West and elsewhere. Writing in *The Atlantic* in June, scientist Hilda Bastian noted that Novavax's shots had a lower rate of side effects than the mRNA vaccines, and they were milder as well, while having roughly the same efficacy.[5]

"The success of the Novavax vaccine should be A1 news. . . . For the moment, it's the best COVID-19 vaccine we have," Bastian wrote.

The little company finally could.

The results left Smith elated. He could barely stop smiling. Smith had spent years developing ways to use insect viruses and cells for vaccines. He had met abject failure working with Frank Volvovitz on AIDS shots at MicroGeneSys, and then devoted sixteen years to a half dozen different vaccines at Novavax, stumbling each time.

Now, he was on the verge of helping to stem a historic pandemic. He also was excited about an all-in-one coronavirus and flu vaccine that he and his colleagues were working to perfect. Thanks to an influx of cash in the wake of the company's Covid-19 achievements and a stock price that was over two hundred dollars, he now ran a research and development team that had doubled in size to nearly forty people. Most of all, Smith, who had recently turned seventy-two years old, appreciated that he still had a spot on the bench at Novavax and an opportunity to perfect his insect-virus approach.

The evening the U.S. results became public, Smith and his wife drove thirty minutes to dine at The Inn at Little Washington, an acclaimed restaurant at the foot of the Blue Ridge Mountains. They enjoyed eight full courses, savoring every bite.

"You go through life hoping to have a chance to make a difference," says Smith. "I'm just grateful to have the strength left to have an impact."

• • •

Adrian Hill's team at the University of Oxford also received long-awaited good news. On December 30, 2020, their jabs were authorized for use by the United Kingdom. Doses were immediately distributed, helping the country fend off a new surge of Covid-19 cases. In late January, the Oxford/AstraZeneca shots were authorized in Europe as well, more reason for Hill and his colleagues to celebrate. After decades of work, they finally had a vaccine going into biceps.

In February 2021, though, a new and serious concern arose: Previously healthy women were developing blood clots after inoculation, and some were experiencing a severe condition known as cerebral venous sinus thrombosis, or CVST. The European Medicines Agency determined that the condition occurred in just one out of every hundred thousand people vaccinated with the Oxford/AstraZeneca shots, but it was yet another painful setback for Hill's program. There would be other slipups during the year, including production shortfalls, questions about the vaccine's effectiveness for the elderly, and worries about its ability to handle new strains of the coronavirus.

Even long-awaited results of a large, late-stage clinical trial of 32,000 people in the United States, Chile, and Peru weren't without controversy. In late March 2021, just after AstraZeneca shared preliminary data indicating that its vaccine was 79 percent effective, an independent study-monitoring board called the information out of date, an extraordinary, public reproach that prompted the NIAID to express its own concerns.

It was all too much for Hill—he couldn't believe the official bodies were undermining his group's vaccine, even as the virus killed thousands a day and too many people were finding reasons to resist inoculation.

"Talk about efforts to maintain confidence in vaccines," Hill emailed a *Washington Post* reporter after the monitoring board leveled its public criticism. "What is going on?!"[6]

A bit later, Oxford/AstraZeneca shared updated data showing its jabs were 76 percent effective at preventing symptomatic disease and 100 percent effective at preventing serious illness and hospitalization across ages and ethnicities. By then, though, the flubs and frustrations had left deep marks on the program. Most were unnecessary and unexpected blunders from a group that should have known better—to many, Hill and his colleagues seemed like a talented Premier League team undone by inexplicable and ugly own goals.

Some members of the media were rather tart in their critiques.

"Like a baby boomer dancing on TikTok it's impossible to look at AstraZeneca's Covid vaccine efforts without a feeling of disbelief bordering on disgust," Adam Feuerstein of STAT said. "One missed step after another, almost all self-inflicted."

By the summer of 2021, Oxford and AstraZeneca hadn't even asked U.S. authorities to allow their Covid-19 shots in America. Still, the vaccine had been authorized for use in more than seventy other countries and were the most widely used shots in many parts of the world. The vaccine was proving a true lifesaver.[7] Of all the various shots, the Oxford/AstraZeneca jabs were among the cheapest and easiest to transport and store, lasting more than six months at normal refrigeration, a key part of why they were so popular. Over 200 million people had received the vaccine worldwide by the summer of 2021, and AstraZeneca announced plans to deliver up to three billion doses by the end of the year, including hundreds of millions for people in poor and middle-income countries.[8]

Hill and Gilbert seemed well past past the mockery and mistakes.

In conversations with peers, the scientists spoke of their frustration regarding the criticisms, but they also expressed pride about how they had helped develop a safe and effective vaccine that was protecting so many people around the world. In April, Vaccitech, a start-up co-founded by Hill and Gilbert that owned intellectual property crucial to their Covid-19 vaccine, sold shares in a public offering giving the two scientists ownership of about 10 percent of the company, which was worth about $500 million.[9]

By then, Hill had shifted back to his original passion: fighting malaria. A malaria vaccine he had developed, known as R21, had begun a phase 3 trial. Earlier in the year, it had showed efficacy of 77 percent, much better than an existing vaccine. Hill and his colleagues hoped their low-priced jabs would be in arms by 2023, combating a disease that takes four hundred thousand lives each year, most of them children in sub-Saharan Africa.[10]

"A lot more people will die in Africa this year from malaria than will die from Covid," Hill noted to a reporter. "I don't mean twice as many, probably ten times."[11]

Later in June, Hill received an honorary knighthood from Queen Elizabeth, while Sarah Gilbert was made a Dame, career-capping honors for both scientists. That evening, Hill attended a barbeque in Oxford with some colleagues and others. He received a round of applause and a champagne toast. Hill, who had just returned from a trip to Gibraltar, where he had remarried, was jovial, optimistic, and proud.

• • •

Dan Barouch was also celebrating.

On February 27, 2021, the U.S. Food and Drug Administration authorized Johnson & Johnson's Covid-19 vaccine for adults aged eighteen and older in the United States, the third shot to receive a green light in the country. The decision was made based on a study of about 44,000 volunteers eighteen and older that found the vaccine to be 66.1 percent effective at protecting people from developing Covid-19, including in parts of the world dealing with dangerous variants of the virus, and 72 percent effective in the United States alone.[12]

It wasn't quite the same level of protection as the Pfizer/BioNTech and Moderna vaccines, of course, but J&J's shots were 85.4 percent protective against severe Covid-19, leading *The Wall Street Journal* to call it "a desperately needed new source of doses as [health authorities] scramble to ramp up inoculations ahead of elusive emerging strains" of the virus that were rapidly spreading.[13]

The J&J shots were "fridge-stable," meaning they could be shipped and stored at the temperature of a regular refrigerator. That made them easier to deploy in poorer nations and others lacking the expensive freezers necessary to keep doses supercold for extended periods, as was required for the Pfizer/BioNTech shots. J&J's single-dose vaccine also held special appeal for those unwilling or unable to return three or four weeks after an initial, prime shot to get booster inoculations required in the regimens of the mRNA vaccines. The J&J vaccine's side effects seemed pretty mild as well.

Newly reported cases, hospitalizations, and deaths related to Covid-19 remained at high levels, so political officials and other leaders were thrilled that J&J pledged to deliver 100 million doses to the United States by the end of June and to send additional supplies to the European Commission and other countries, all on a not-for-profit basis during the pandemic.

Working with J&J's Janssen Pharmaceuticals division, Barouch had helped develop and test the shots, and they were based on Barouch's Adenovirus-26 technology. As such, he emerged as a public face of the program, making television appearances and conducting interviews with the press. Walking the streets of Boston near his laboratory, he was sometimes stopped by strangers thanking him for his efforts. Others emailed or wrote letters, sharing their own words of appreciation.

His thirteen-year-old daughter, Susanna, attended a middle school that conducted a hybrid learning program during the pandemic, allowing in-person attendance for those testing negative from the virus while permitting others to stay home and learn via live video. Fearing the disease, a homeroom teacher elected to work remotely during the 2020–2021 academic year. After the middle-aged woman was inoculated with the J&J vaccine, she emailed Barouch saying she had cried with joy and relief. Two weeks later, she met Barouch's daughter for the first time, another emotional encounter for the family.

The J&J shots proved popular, with 6.8 million doses administered in the first six weeks or so. Public authorities distributed supplies to vulnerable and isolated people, some of whom had limited access to health care. College students appreciated J&J's one-and-done inoculation process, as did sports teams, like the New York Yankees.

Everything changed on Tuesday, April 13, however.

The day began early and uneventfully for Barouch. He woke at five a.m., as usual, and by seven was downstairs in the family's living room in their Newton, Massachusetts, home, practicing violin with his daughters. He finished a session with his ten-year-old daughter, Natalie, and had begun playing with Susanna when he received an urgent text from his wife, Fina, an ophthalmologist who had already left for work and was listening to the news in her car.

She sent a link to a news article. Barouch immediately saw the bombshell: American health authorities were recommending a pause in the use of J&J's Covid-19 vaccine. Six women had suffered blood clots after receiving the shots. All were between the ages of eighteen and forty-eight years old. One had died, while others were or had been in intensive care. It wasn't clear whether the clots were related to the vaccine, but the U.S. Food and Drug Administration and the U.S. Centers for Disease Control and Prevention were worried enough to halt J&J's vaccine rollout, as they investigated the cause of the health emergencies.

Barouch was blindsided—he had no idea there had been so many blood-clot cases. Even J&J hadn't known authorities were considering a pause in the rollout until twenty minutes before the announcement. Desperate for information, Barouch headed to the websites of *The New York Times*, *The Wall Street Journal*, and NPR. He couldn't believe what was happening.

For over a decade, Barouch had argued that using an adenovirus to carry genetic messages into the body was safe and effective, even when skeptics pointed to Merck's disastrous experience relying on these viruses to shepherd its HIV vaccine. Barouch was also relying on adenoviruses for shots he was developing for AIDS and other diseases. Now, there was a possibility his vaccine approach was doing harm, much like Merck's HIV vaccine.

A debate soon erupted about the wisdom of the U.S. authorities' move. A pandemic was ongoing and too many people were hesitant to get vaccinated—now they would be even more reluctant, said critics of the government's decision. Clots associated with birth control pills were much more common, others noted.

"Where was everyone's concern for blood clots when we started putting 14-year-old girls on the pill," one woman wrote on Twitter.[14]

But Barouch's peers in the worlds of science and health were generally supportive of the decision. Alternative Covid-19 vaccines were available. There might be additional cases that authorities weren't yet aware of. And the usual treatment of these blood clots—administering a drug called heparin—was potentially harming the women, so authorities needed to step in.

Barouch was deeply troubled. He kept coming back to Hippocrates's pledge—"First, do no harm." Could the vaccine be hurting people? Were there other cases? He needed to know how bad the news was and if his approach was going to be discredited.

He started calling and texting government scientists, friends, and others to ask how vaccination halts worked, what a government investigation might entail, and how it might end.

"What's the process?" he asked Nelson Michael, the senior scientist at the Walter Reed Army Institute of Research. "What's going to happen?"

Barouch sounded concerned, even agitated. Michael tried to reassure his old friend, but said he was also in the dark about how the investigation would unfold.

"You have been involved in great science, Dan," Michael told him. "Let's hope for the best."

Barouch couldn't let it go. Later the same day, he called Michael again, asking if he had any new information.

On April 23, ten days after the pause began, U.S. health regulators resumed inoculations with J&J's shots, saying the benefits outweighed the risks. They had determined that there had been about 1.9 cases per million people overall, and 7 per million women aged eighteen to forty-nine.

The vaccine's popularity never recovered in the United States, however. By the summer of 2021, J&J had administered about 12.8 million shots, about 8 percent of the U.S. total. It didn't help that tens of millions of doses produced by Emergent BioSolutions—in the same Baltimore factory Novavax was forced to vacate—had to be tossed out because of possible contamination, or that J&J's shots were linked to another rare side effect called Guillain-Barré syndrome. A spate of infections during the 2021 baseball season among Yankees players inoculated with J&J's shots was yet another public relations disaster.

It seemed premature to judge the vaccine's fate, though. J&J was working on modifications to reduce or even eliminate the risk of blood clots.[15] The vaccine was popular in parts of the world, including South Africa, and J&J was still committed to delivering 500 million doses to Covax, the world's main effort to supply Covid-19 vaccines to poorer nations. One study suggested J&J's shots were the most effective at stopping the Delta variant.

By the summer of 2021, Barouch was back in his lab, waiting for results from his team's latest study of their AIDS vaccine, his life's focus.

"We still need a vaccine for HIV," Barouch says. "It remains one of the greatest challenges of our generation."

• • •

Like much of the world in the summer of 2021, Lawrence Garbuz was still dealing with the coronavirus.

It had been over a year since Garbuz, one of the first people diagnosed with Covid-19, was in a New York hospital, fighting for his life. During that time, he had participated in a half-dozen studies about the effects of Covid-19, aimed at gaining a better understanding of the disease. On many occasions, he gave blood, hoping to aid health providers as they had helped him.

Eager to move on from the disease, he tried not to dwell on how he had become sick.

"I gave up a long time ago trying to figure out who gave it to me," he says.

Over the course of the year, Garbuz met many people from his area who said that they, too, had been in the hospital with Covid-19 around the time he was battling the disease, suggesting that Garbuz likely wasn't among the earliest in the New York region to become infected, though he became the reluctant public face of those suffering during the first wave.

"I understand my role," he says. "I view myself as being the canary in the coal mine, but next time people can find another canary."

By then, Garbuz had received two doses of the Pfizer/BioNTech vaccine, experiencing side effects of extremely high fevers for about a day each time, unpleasant reminders for himself and his family of his difficult earlier experience. Like a number of people who suffered during the first wave of Covid-19 infections, Garbuz was still feeling its impact. He tired easily, had some lung problems and nerve pain, and didn't feel himself, sharing many of the symptoms of those with "long Covid."

"I hope one day this will be resolved," he says.

• • •

Jessamyn Smyth was in better spirits.

Smyth, the professor from western Massachusetts who contracted Covid-19 in March 2020, spent nearly a year dealing with symptoms of the disease, while wondering if she'd ever feel herself again.

In late February 2021, she was inoculated with the Pfizer/BioN-Tech shots. Within a week, she noticed her symptoms improving. After her second dose, she felt almost fully healthy, for the first time in nearly a year.

"I was basically fixed," she says.

Soon she was back in the pool. Within eight weeks, she had returned to her original swimming pace. Still, Smyth was up nights, worried that her symptoms would return.

"That's what long Covid does to you," she says. "It gives you a few good days and you think maybe you're getting better, and then it just burns your world down again."

Nearly all her symptoms disappeared, with the exception of some minor flare-ups. Like some others with long-term problems caused by the disease, the vaccine seemed to jigger Smyth's immune system, possibly allowing it to finally do a proper job fighting the virus.

"I'm doing so well," she says. "Pool and open water swimming (oh, to be in the lakes again), biking, finishing books, being myself for the first time in ages in terms of energy and focus and general strength.

"It's an immense relief!"

• • •

On the morning of January 3, 2021, Stéphane Bancel and his wife, Brenda, drove to Moderna's vaccine-manufacturing plant in Norwood,

Massachusetts. There, the couple met a group of nurses who were busy inoculating Moderna's staff. Bancel and his wife waited their turn, sat down in two comfortable chairs, rolled up their sleeves, and held hands. The nurses injected them with Moderna's Covid-19 vaccine.

As the syringe entered his shoulder, Bancel thought of the long journey he had been on, the lives that were being saved by his company's shots, and the months ahead. He was hoping he and his team could relax a bit after their difficult year and eventual vaccine success.

They never had a chance. As new and dangerous variant strains of the coronavirus emerged during 2021, Bancel and his colleagues scrambled to rework their vaccine, develop potential booster shots to handle new variants, and test vaccines for adolescents and children. They also worked to ramp up production and get their vaccines into nations around the world. As their sprint became a never-ending marathon, many at the company were caught unprepared.

By the summer of 2021, Bancel was a billionaire, as soaring Moderna shares gave the company a value of over $160 billion. Stephen Hoge, Juan Andres, and many other top executives also became phenomenally wealthy.

But they were also a mess. Many staffers were physically and emotionally scarred from the previous year. Moderna began 2020 as a relatively small company, at least compared to Pfizer and other drug giants, and the help it had received from the U.S. government was in developing and conducting early tests of its vaccine, not in producing and distributing the shots. As a result, Moderna staffers worked nonstop for over a year. The pressures of developing, testing, and producing their vaccine were intense. During 2021, the toll caught up to many of them.

Juan Andres, the manufacturing chief, was among those on an emotional roller coaster. During the second half of 2020, he had forged a close partnership with Gus Perna, the four-star Army general who coordinated the United States' vaccine response as part of

Operation Warp Speed. Together, the men had solved a series of imposing logistical problems to enable Moderna's shots to be produced and delivered. In December, when Andres learned the first vaccines were being distributed around the country, he began crying uncontrollably in his living room, picturing older members of his family who finally could be protected.

"Now we have a chance," he told his wife, as he held her close.

By March 2021, Moderna had managed to produce 100 million vaccines. The company was on pace to produce up to one billion shots during the year. But Andres couldn't help thinking about what more he could have done. Had the company been able to produce more vaccines, even more lives would have been spared, he believed.

At one point, Bancel spoke with Andres, urging him to be kinder to himself, reminding him that he had already done so much to help fight the pandemic.

"I don't tend to punish myself," Andres says. "But whatever you accomplish, it's never enough. . . . We can do better. . . . People are dying out there."

By the summer of 2021, many Moderna executives found it difficult to sleep, or they developed back pain or other ailments. They all battled exhaustion. Some took aggressive steps to try to maintain their health. Bancel, Hoge, and Andres embraced intermittent fasting, for example, and Andres built a standing treadmill at his desk, setting a goal of 25,000 steps each day.

Hoge's own goal had nothing to do with a vaccine or a new exercise. He just wanted to help his staffers recover their emotional health.

"There are a lot of broken people here," he says. "I feel like we made it to the top of Mount Everest, but if we're not careful we'll die on the way down."

Most of all, Bancel, Hoge, and others were gearing up for what they expected would be an extended and difficult battle against SARS-CoV-2.

"This will be a long haul; we need to sustain the same amount of effort," Hoge says. "There hasn't been a moment of elation. If we miss a day someone dies."

• • •

Uğur Şahin spent much of 2021 working to get the Pfizer/BioNTech's Covid-19 vaccine to people around the world. In the spring, he traveled to China to negotiate with regulators toward a fifty-fifty joint venture with Shanghai Fosun Pharmaceutical Group to deliver 100 million shots to the country. Şahin's vaccine would supplement China's homemade shots, which were effective but were proving less protective than many of those produced in the West.

One afternoon, as Şahin walked through a Chinese airport on his way to a meeting with the authorities, he was stopped by a local lugging a heavy carry-on bag.

"Excuse me," the traveler said. "But when is your vaccine available here?"

In many ways, Şahin's international celebrity, and the successful development of his company's Covid-19 shots, were unlikely, even astonishing, developments. For almost his entire career, lasting over three decades, Şahin hadn't envisioned saving lives with a vaccine, at least not one combating an infectious virus. He fought cancer—that was how he expected to impact the world.

Now that he and BioNTech had helped return humanity to a semblance of normality, however, Şahin was determined to use his unexpected achievement—and the resulting windfall from his company's success—to further his original goals. By the summer of 2021, BioNtech's shares had soared to nearly four hundred dollars a share from just over thirty dollars before the pandemic began. The company was worth about $90 billion and it was sitting on piles of cash from sales of its Covid-19 shots. In 2021, BioNTech was expected to earn nearly

$19 billion from sales of its vaccine, adding half a percentage point to Germany's entire annual gross-domestic product.[16]

To colleagues, Şahin appeared newly energized—he now had the funds to employ an expanded, six-hundred-person research and development operation, to accelerate existing research, and to begin new, ambitious work.

"Now there's a clear path to realize our dreams," he told a BioNTech researcher.

Şahin pushed his team to make progress in cancer immunotherapy vaccines as well as to discover advances in treatments against infectious and autoimmune diseases, including multiple sclerosis. He and the BioNTech scientists were even eyeing challenging diseases like tuberculosis and AIDS. His ambitions raised the tantalizing prospect that the horrors wrought by the deadly coronavirus could, in an indirect way, help vanquish some of the cruelest diseases known to humankind.

Still biking to work, Şahin continued to leave colleagues slack-jawed with his commitment to his research. He even developed novel ways to squeeze more work time from the day. Now, he divided his days into thirty-minute blocks, without a break, as a means of making himself even more efficient, he said. Associates and others knew they had a better chance of reaching him over the weekends, though, which he filled with somewhat less-intense, sixty-minute work blocks that included a few moments of down time.

One day in the summer of 2021, after BioNTech released a new piece of data demonstrating the effectiveness of its Covid-19 vaccine, Şahin surprised an associate by saying that he and Türeci were allowing themselves a reward: a thirty-minute walk.

When they returned to the office, Şahin seemed refreshed.

"This is just the beginning," he told a colleague with a smile.

AFTERWORD

During the summer of 2021, Covid-19 staged a vicious comeback.

Just when vaccines were reducing infections in the West and many people were beginning to imagine a return to a semblance of prepandemic normalcy, a new and especially contagious variant of SARS-CoV-2 known as B.1.617.2, or the Delta variant, emerged. The variant, which swept through India before sparking waves of infection elsewhere, served as a reminder that the coronavirus wasn't nearly finished terrorizing the world.

For most people, Covid-19 vaccines provided sufficient protection from the most dangerous effects of the variant. But large segments of the global population had yet to be inoculated, including about 99 percent of those on the continent of Africa. Even in the United States, only 50 percent or so of the population had been vaccinated, according to the Centers for Disease Control and Prevention. The more a virus circulates in a population, the greater chance it has to mutate into a more dangerous pathogen, potentially one that's resistant to shots, suggesting more danger could be ahead.

"The virus is not going away," says Stephen Hoge, Moderna's president.

Indeed, it will be almost impossible to eradicate SARS-CoV-2 as mankind did with smallpox and a number of other infectious diseases. This coronavirus likely will continue to spread in bats or other animals. Eventually, it could become an endemic virus that leads to seasonal disease, like influenza, as well as more painful, periodic outbreaks. Humankind will likely need to learn to live with the coronavirus, while finding creative ways to encourage unvaccinated populations to roll up their sleeves and receive shots.

But if the virus is discovering creative ways to continue spreading havoc, scientists are demonstrating at least as much ingenuity designing counterattacks to SARS-CoV-2. Researchers are also going all out to prepare for, and protect against, the next inevitable pathogen, raising hopes of a safer future.

During the summer of 2021, for example, Pfizer, Moderna, and other vaccine companies were busy chasing second-generation Covid-19 shots capable of disarming its dangerous variants. At the same time, government scientists were studying ways to combine existing vaccines, to improve the duration of protection while also safeguarding against the dangerous variants. Nelson Michael, director of the Center for Infectious Diseases Research at the Walter Reed Army Institute of Research, calls it the government's "Cocoa Puffs/Trix" experiment, a play on how some children like to mix cereals in the morning.

"It's looking at what's on the shelf, taking a little of this first and then a little of that next, an approach like a kid would do with cereals," he says.

Drew Weissman, the mRNA pioneer, is among those going a step further, testing an all-in-one vaccine to protect against all coronaviruses, including those that cause SARS and MERS, diseases that still haven't been entirely stamped out. And researchers at Walter Reed are testing a supershot that might confer immunity against a wide variety of pathogens, including new strains of the coronavirus. The researchers believe their shots will trigger such a strong immune response that they will potentially fend off many types of viruses and diseases.

"The next pandemic could come from an entirely different family of pathogens," says the vaccine's cocreator, Kayvon Modjarrad, a protégé of Barney Graham. "We need to be prepared."

• • •

One of the few topics of debate related to the Covid crisis that unites the right, left, and many in between relates to its origins. Reasonable people of all political persuasions suspect the coronavirus spilled out of a laboratory, rather than an animal.

There are reasons to be skeptical that the virus emerged naturally. The crisis began in Wuhan, not far from the Wuhan Institute of Virology. In 2019, scientists in that lab were doing advanced coronavirus work, and the institute has experienced safety issues in its past. The possibility exists that the virus evolved in the wild and was brought into the Wuhan lab for study, before escaping through a careless researcher.

From the start, the Chinese government has dragged its feet about cooperating with world bodies working to understand the pathogen's beginnings, sparking concerns. As of the summer of 2021, scientists still couldn't point to a virus circulating in nature that was the precursor of SARS-CoV-2.

"Debate over the viruses's origins will be a drumbeat for years to come," says Simon Wain-Hobson, a microbiologist at the Pasteur Institute in Paris. "We have a Chinese connection and an authoritarian Chinese Communist party. And as a wonderful backdrop, the Wuhan Institute of Virology was performing gain-of-function research on bat coronaviruses. Ian Fleming couldn't have done better."

That said, there's a much higher likelihood that SARS-CoV-2 originated in an animal and spilled over into humans, directly or through an intermediate animal host, a phenomenon called zoonosis. These kinds of infections are quite common. About sixty-thousand people die each year from rabies, for example, and animal viruses were responsible for a series of infectious diseases in humans in recent decades, including SARS-CoV-1.

Animals that are known to be particularly susceptible to coronaviruses, including raccoon dogs and civets, were sold in markets in Wuhan. In late 2019, an epidemic in China was killing millions of pigs, forcing the country to rely on more of these animals as food sources.

After HIV emerged, speculation was rampant that it, too, had been engineered, either intentionally or not, perhaps by the CIA, KGB, or another body. There was no clear viral parent to HIV, either.

In 1990, though, more than a decade after it emerged, a virus that was a close cousin of HIV was found in chimpanzees. A plethora of similar viruses were also discovered in central African monkeys and apes, thus ending the debate.

It may take even longer to discover the origins of the coronavirus in nature.

"Virologists need time," Wain-Hobson says.

• • •

Crises and catastrophes often result in medical breakthroughs. Ambulances and anesthesia emerged from World War I, as did advances in triage, reconstructive surgery, and a vaccine for typhoid. Antibiotics, antimalarial drugs, and penicillin were introduced during World War II. In the Vietnam War, physicians developed ways of resuscitating soldiers using intravenous fluids, methods later applied to civilian patients.

"Society usually makes progress out of necessity," argues Jeremy Farrar, director of the Wellcome Trust.

Good has already resulted from the coronavirus crisis. Many people adopted healthier balances between their professional and personal lives and a new appreciation for family. Hopefully, these shifts will be long-lasting. In the world of medicine, we've learned what can be accomplished when scientific development is done simultaneously, rather than in stages. And progress has also been made on more efficient drug manufacturing and distribution, techniques that can be applied to therapeutics and vaccines, reducing the costs of various treatments.

The pandemic forced scientists to perfect and prove their methods of working with mRNA, accelerating a process already under way. Billions of dollars in profits that have resulted for some of those pursuing mRNA research will likely bring more talent, financing, and improvements in the field.

It's not yet clear whether or not mRNA can work for a wide range of drugs, however. A new generation of technology will likely be required, argues Kenneth Chien, the Moderna cofounder who now is a professor at Karolinska Institutet in Sweden, as companies develop the ability for repeated mRNA dosings that can target specific tissues. Still, the possibilities that will emerge once we're able to instruct our bodies to produce specific antibodies are tantalizing. Jeremy Farrar predicts advances in cancer vaccines, dementia treatments, and more, potentially by immunizing the body against early cancerous cells and other incipient antigens.

"Whole new areas of medicine have opened up," he says. "Out of the horror of Covid will come remarkable advances."

For years, pandemic warnings of health policy authorities were ignored or even mocked. During the worst of the 2020 crisis, Anthony Fauci received death threats and some politicians suggested that doctors were inflating the death toll from the coronavirus as a means of generating higher hospital fees.

The counsel and guidance of public health authorities likely will be needed again, perhaps soon. There's reason to expect new pandemics in the years ahead involving pathogens potentially even more dangerous than SARS-CoV-2. As global warming continues, travel expands, and humans further encroach on nature, animal diseases are likely to continue crossing over to affect mankind, underscoring the paramount importance of investing in preparedness and public health.

• • •

Months before his passing in the fall of 2020, Rabbi Lord Jonathan Sacks noted that the United States and the United Kingdom, two of the countries that had suffered the most from the coronavirus crisis, are also the nations best known for defending liberty and freedom, while prizing, even venerating, individualism. Working at *The Wall Street Journal* during the crisis, I fielded angry emails from readers pledging to resist rather than comply with mask requirements or other perceived infringements of their personal rights.

By contrast, countries that placed a larger emphasis on the collective good, such as South Korea, Taiwan, and New Zealand, avoided some of the worst impacts of the pandemic. A potential reason is that their citizens proved more willing to comply with government mask mandates while sacrificing some privacy and other rights, enabling tracing systems and other measures.

Free will is rightly cherished in the West and individualism plays an enormously important and necessary role in any healthy society. So does self-interest. Some of the investigators at the forefront of the Covid-19 vaccine effort were likely motivated, at least in part, by fame and fortune, suggesting that promoting individual goals can bring broader benefits. Better, though, that the coronavirus crisis results in a renewed emphasis on collective relationships and an appreciation for those who make sacrifices on behalf ofothers.

"I think future anthropologists will take a look at the books we read on self-help, self-realization, self-esteem," Rabbi Sacks argued. "They'll look at the way we talk about morality as being true to one-self, the way we talk about politics as a matter of individual rights. And I think they'll conclude that what we worship in our time is the self, the 'Me,' the 'I.' The antidote to this? A reassertion of the 'We.'"

ACKNOWLEDGMENTS

Teams of dedicated individuals were needed to produce effective Covid-19 vaccines. I relied on an equally devoted group to help produce this book.

Lauren Sherman Doberman was my scientific tutor, adviser, and sometimes savior. Getting mRNA into cells was nothing compared with helping a guy like me understand it all. (Most of our sessions felt like an episode of *The Office*: "Why don't you explain this to me like I'm five.")

I was truly blessed that Peter Krell and Jason McLellan were kind enough to read my manuscript, spot errors, and provide insights. Four of the sharpest eyes I've ever encountered.

From day one, my publisher, Adrian Zackheim, and editor, Merry Sun, were enthusiastic, encouraging, and insightful; I'm grateful for your continued support. Thanks also to the rest of the team at Penguin: Jessica Regione, Megan McCormack, Megan Gerrity, Linda Friedner, Nicole Celli, Jane Cavolina, Meighan Cavanaugh, and Mike Brown. Margot Stamas and Suzanne Williams are my marketing maestros. Anastassia Gliadkovskaya and Ethan McAndrews contributed invaluable research assistance. Thanks to Connor Guy, for truly expert editing.

When I finished high school, I thought I was done with biology. I guess I wasn't. I was blessed to be able to turn to the following researchers and members of the scientific community, who answered endless questions with uncommon patience: Ken Chien, Eli Gilboa, Smita Nair, David Boczkowski, John Shiver, Katalin Wolff, Patrick Remington, Jim Hagstrom, Cliff Lane, Danny Douek, Henry Masur, Jaap Goudsmit, Nelson Michael, Hans Hengartner, Susan Weiss, and Kathryn Holmes. Michael Kinch and Larry Pitkowsky were kind enough to read my manuscript and provide valuable thoughts.

I'd like to thank Matt Murray, *The Wall Street Journal*'s managing editor, Charles Forelle, the paper's financial editor, and Ken Brown, the *Journal*'s financial enterprise editor.

Ari and Robin Moses provided great liquor and even better company. I truly benefited from Ari's sage advice. Mike and Yonit Sinreich contributed additional amusement and helpful distraction.

Thanks to Jerry, Alisha, Hannah, and Aiden Blugrind, who opened their hearts and home . . . and Aiden's desk when he went to camp. Tova and Aviva provided love and support. Monica Aranda was always there for me, Israel Blugrind rooted me on, and Sara Fuchs shared helpful thoughts. Special thanks go to Moshe and Renee Glick for steadfast encouragement and support. I treasure our friendship.

I'm grateful for the support of friends, colleagues, and family members, including Ezra Zuckerman Sivan, Jack Sivan, Shara Shetrit, Adam Browler, Howard Simansky, Marc Tobin, Stu Schrader, James Reichman, Hal Lux, Joshua Marcus, David and Shari Cherna, Suzanne and Stephen Loughrey, Judah and Avigaiyil Goldscheider, Carol Buchman-Krutiansky, Kirsten Grind, and Alex Engel.

Spending time with the Lakeview and Swayze minyanim, and AABJ&D's Sunday sluggers, were highlights of a difficult year. Much appreciation to Andrea and Ronny Sultan, Ed Zughaft, and Elizer Zwickler. Steve Forbert, Bob Marley, Johannes Brahms, Miles Davis, and Luther Vandross provided comfort deep into the night.

Writing this book gave me time to spend with my mother, Roberta Zuckerman, and Gary Steinman, the IGF protein's biggest promoter. For that I'm truly thankful. I continue to rely on lessons taught by my late father, Alan Zuckerman, whose approach to writing and research continues to echo in my own.

One of the few benefits of the pandemic was being locked down with my sons, Gabriel Benjamin and Elijah Shane, who continue to give me so much pleasure.

Lastly but definitely not leastly, Michelle Zuckerman was my rock, providing encouragement when I wavered, humor when I was down, and suggestions when I was stuck. Thank you for your love.

NOTES

INTRODUCTION

1. World Health Organization, "WHO Coronavirus (COVID-19) Dashboard," July 29, 2021, https://covid19.who.int/.
2. Julie Bosman, "A Ripple Effect of Loss: U.S. Covid Deaths Approach 500,000," *New York Times*, February 21, 2021, https://www.nytimes.com/2021/02/21/us/coronavirus-deaths-us-half-a-million.html.
3. Thalia Beaty, Eugene Garcia, and Lisa Marie Pane, "U.S. Tops 4,000 Daily Deaths from Coronavirus for 1st Time," Associated Press, January 8, 2021, https://apnews.com/article/us-coronavirus-death-4000-daily-16c1f136921c7e98ec83289942322ee4.
4. Carl Zimmer, "The Secret Life of a Coronavirus," *New York Times*, February 26, 2021, https://www.nytimes.com/2021/02/26/opinion/sunday/coronavirus-alive-dead.html.
5. Alison Galvani, Seyed M. Moghadas, and Eric C. Schneider, "Deaths and Hospitalizations Averted by Rapid U.S. Vaccination Rollout," Commonwealth Fund, July 7, 2021, https://www.commonwealthfund.org/publications/issue-briefs/2021/jul/deaths-and-hospitalizations-averted-rapid-us-vaccination-rollout.

CHAPTER ONE

1. Randy Shilts, *And the Band Played On: Politics, People, and the AIDS Epidemic* (New York: St. Martin's Press, 1987).
2. Jon Cohen, *Shots in the Dark: The Wayward Search for an AIDS Vaccine* (New York: W. W. Norton, 2001).

3. Michael Kinch, *Between Hope and Fear: A History of Vaccines and Human Immunity* (New York: Pegasus Books, 2018).
4. Cohen, *Shots in the Dark.*
5. Faye Flam, "Flossie Wong-Staal, Who Unlocked Mystery of H.I.V., Dies at 73," *New York Times*, July 17, 2020, https://www.nytimes.com/2020/07/17/science/flossie-wong-staal-who-unlocked-mystery-of-hiv-dies-at-73.html.

CHAPTER TWO

1. Peter Coy, "Microgenesys Triumph Good for Sufferers, Unsettling for Investors with AM-AIDS-Microgenesys," Associated Press, August 20, 1987, https://apnews.com/article/785a7c18905797e3fa4f878cbb007c83.
2. Coy, "Microgenesys Triumph."
3. Lyn Bixby and Frank Spencer-Molloy, "The Struggle for Money to Fuel a Research Mission," *Hartford Courant*, February 8, 1993, https://www.courant.com/news/connecticut/hc-xpm-1993-02-08-0000106194-story.html.
4. William Hathaway, "Parasite Links Men in Daring Venture," *Hartford Courant*, October 6, 1996, https://www.courant.com/news/connecticut/hc-xpm-1996-10-06-9610060087-story,amp.html.
5. Bixby and Spencer-Molloy, "The Struggle for Money."
6. Lyn Bixby and Frank Spencer-Molloy, "State Entrepreneur's Quest Stirs National Controversy," *Hartford Courant*, February 7, 1993, https://www.courant.com/news/connecticut/hc-xpm-1993-02-07-0000106224-story.html.
7. Hathaway, "Parasite Links Men."

CHAPTER THREE

1. "Hilleman Isolates Mumps Virus," The History of Vaccines, https://www.historyofvaccines.org/content/hilleman-isolates-mumps-virus; Laura Newman, "Maurice Hilleman," *British Medical Journal* 330, no. 7498 (April 2005): 1028.
2. Jon Cohen, *Shots in the Dark: The Wayward Search for an AIDS Vaccine* (New York: W. W. Norton, 2001).
3. Donald G. McNeil Jr., "Trial Vaccine Made Some More Vulnerable to H.I.V., Study Confirms," *New York Times*, May 18, 2012, https://www.nytimes.com/2012/05/18/health/research/trial-vaccine-made-some-more-vulnerable-to-hiv-study-confirms.html.
4. McNeil Jr., "Trial Vaccine."
5. Rebecca Ng, "Sarah C. Gilbert Interview," Immunopaedia, https://www.immunopaedia.org.za/interviews/immunologist-of-the-month-2018/sarah-c-gilbert-interview.
6. David D. Kirkpatrick, "In Race for a Coronavirus Vaccine, an Oxford Group Leaps Ahead," *New York Times,* April 27, 2020, https://www.nytimes.com/2020/04/27/world/europe/coronavirus-vaccine-update-oxford.html; Meera Senthilingam, "Does This

Doctor Hold the Secret to Ending Malaria?," CNN, June 2, 2016, https://www.cnn.com/2016/06/01/health/cnn-frontiers-adrian-hill-malaria-vaccine/index.html.

CHAPTER FOUR

1. Andrew Kilpatrick, *Of Permanent Value: The Story of Warren Buffett* (self-pub., Andy Kilpatrick Publishing Empire, 2007).
2. Matthew Cobb, "Who Discovered Messenger RNA?," *Current Biology* 25, no. 13 (June 2015): R526–R532, https://doi.org/10.1016/j.cub.2015.05.032.

CHAPTER FIVE

1. Daniel Victor and Katherine J. Wu, "Nobel Prize in Medicine Awarded to Scientists Who Discovered Hepatitis C Virus," *New York Times,* October 5, 2020, https://www.nytimes.com/2020/10/05/health/nobel-prize-medicine-hepatitis-c.html.
2. Gina Kolata, "Kati Kariko Helped Shield the World from the Coronavirus," *New York Times*, April 8, 2021, https://www.nytimes.com/2021/04/08/health/coronavirus-mrna-kariko.html#click=https://t.co/zsCgQ1uADw.
3. Kolata, "Kati Kariko."

CHAPTER SIX

1. Bill DeMain, "The Story Behind the Song: Space Oddity by David Bowie," *Classic Rock*, February 13, 2019, https://www.loudersound.com/features/story-behind-the-song-space-oddity-david-bowie.
2. Wallace Ravven, "The Stem-Cell Revolution Is Coming—Slowly," *New York Times*, January 16, 2017, https://www.nytimes.com/2017/01/16/science/shinya-yamanaka-stem-cells.html.
3. William Broad and Nicholas Wade, *Betrayers of the Truth* (New York: Simon & Schuster, 1982).
4. Catherine Elton, "Does Moderna Therapeutics Have the NEXT Next Big Thing?," *Boston Magazine*, February 26, 2013, https://www.bostonmagazine.com/health/2013/02/26/moderna-therapeutics-new-medical-technology/3/.

CHAPTER SEVEN

1. Stéphane Bancel, "The Other Side Speaker Series w/ Stéphane Bancel," interview by Jodi Goldstein, Harvard Innovation Labs, April 19, 2016, YouTube video, https://www.youtube.com/watch?v=-P53wVGfvjw.
2. Damian Garde, "Ego, Ambition, and Turmoil: Inside One of Biotech's Most Secretive Startups," STAT News, September 13, 2016, https://www.statnews.com/2016/09/13/moderna-therapeutics-biotech-mrna.

3. James D. Watson, *The Double Helix: A Personal Account of the Discovery of the Structure of DNA* (New York: Simon & Schuster, 2001).
4. Catherine Elton, "Does Moderna Therapeutics Have the NEXT Next Big Thing?," *Boston Magazine*, February 26, 2013, https://www.bostonmagazine.com/health/2013/02/26/moderna-therapeutics-new-medical-technology/3/.
5. Tim Loh, "The Vaccine Revolution Is Coming Inside Tiny Bubbles of Fat," *Bloomberg*, March 3, 2021, https://www.bloomberg.com/news/articles/2021-03-04/the-vaccine-revolution-is-coming-inside-tiny-bubbles-of-fat.

CHAPTER EIGHT

1. "Structural Biology," NIH Intramural Research Program, https://irp.nih.gov/our-research/scientific-focus-areas/structural-biology.
2. Rafael Lozano et al., "Global and Regional Mortality from 235 Causes of Death for 20 Age Groups in 1990 and 2010: A Systematic Analysis for the Global Burden of Disease Study 2010," *Lancet* 380, no. 9859 (December 2012): 2095–2128, https://doi.org/10.1016/S0140-6736(12)61728-0.
3. Michael Blanding, "Shot in the Arm: Groundbreaking COVID-19 Vaccine Research by Alumnus Dr. Barney Graham Began at Vanderbilt Decades Ago," Vanderbilt University, March 17, 2021, https://news.vanderbilt.edu/2021/03/17/shot-in-the-arm-groundbreaking-covid-19-vaccine-research-by-alumnus-dr-barney-graham-began-at-vanderbilt-decades-ago.
4. Lawrence Wright, "The Plague Year," *New Yorker*, December 28, 2020, https://www.newyorker.com/magazine/2021/01/04/the-plague-year.
5. Ryan Cross, "The Tiny Tweak Behind COVID-19 Vaccines," *Chemical & Engineering News*, September 29, 2020, https://cen.acs.org/pharmaceuticals/vaccines/tiny-tweak-behind-COVID-19/98/i38.
6. Elisabeth Mahase, "Covid-19: First Coronavirus Was Described in the BMJ in 1965," *British Medical Journal* 369, no. 8242 (April 2020): m1547, https://doi.org/10.1136/bmj.m1547.
7. Ivan Oransky, "David Tyrrell," *Lancet* 365, no. 9477 (June 2005): 2084, https://doi.org/10.1016/S0140-6736(05)66722-0; Mahase, "Covid-19: First Coronavirus."
8. Oransky, "David Tyrrell."
9. Yanzhong Huang, "The SARS Epidemic and Its Aftermath in China: A Political Perspective," in *Learning from SARS: Preparing for the Next Disease Outbreak* (Washington, D.C.: National Academies Press, 2004), 116–36.
10. Jon Cohen, *Shots in the Dark: The Wayward Search for an AIDS Vaccine* (New York: W. W. Norton, 2001).

CHAPTER NINE

1. "Research Not Fit to Print," *Nature Biotechnology* 34 (February 2016): 115, https://doi.org/10.1038/nbt.3488.

2. Damian Garde, "Ego, Ambition, and Turmoil: Inside One of Biotech's Most Secretive Startups," STAT News, September 13, 2016, https://www.statnews.com/2016/09/13/moderna-therapeutics-biotech-mrna.

CHAPTER TEN

1. "Uğur Şahin ve Özlem Türeci'nin baba ocağında gurur var!" [There is pride in Uğur Şahin and Özlem Türeci's paternal hearth!], A Haber, November 13, 2020, https://www.ahaber.com.tr/gundem/2020/11/13/ugur-sahin-ve-ozlem-turecinin-baba-ocaginda-gurur-var.
2. Uğur Şahin and Özlem Türeci, "BioNTech Founders Türeci and Şahin on the Battle Against COVID-19," interview by Steffen Klusmann and Thomas Schulz, *Der Spiegel*, January 4, 2021, https://www.spiegel.de/international/world/biontech-founders-tuereci-and-sahin-on-the-battle-against-covid-19-to-see-people-finally-benefitting-from-our-work-is-really-moving-a-41ce9633-5b27-4b9c-b1d7-1bf94c29aa43.
3. Joe Miller, "Inside the Hunt for a Covid-19 Vaccine: How BioNTech Made the Breakthrough," *Financial Times*, November 13, 2020, https://www.ft.com/content/c4ca8496-a215-44b1-a7eb-f88568fc9de9.
4. "Uğur Şahin ve Özlem Türeci'nin baba ocağında gurur var!"

CHAPTER ELEVEN

1. Sheila Weller, "'I Have HIV': This Researcher Is Fighting the Disease—and the Stigma Attached to It," Johnson & Johnson, November 29, 2018, https://www.jnj.com/personal-stories/im-a-researcher-living-with-hiv-and-fighting-the-disease-and-stigma.
2. Alan Cowell, "Ebola Death Toll in West Africa Tops 1,200," *New York Times*, August 19, 2014, https://www.nytimes.com/2014/08/20/world/africa/ebola-outbreak.html.
3. Brian Blackstone, Reed Johnson, and Betsy McKay, "Zika Virus Is Spreading 'Explosively,' WHO Chief Says," *Wall Street Journal*, January 28, 2016, https://www.wsj.com/articles/who-to-decide-if-zika-virus-is-a-global-health-emergency-1453989411.
4. Siddhartha Mukherjee, "The Race for a Zika Vaccine," *New Yorker*, August 15, 2016, https://www.newyorker.com/magazine/2016/08/22/the-race-for-a-zika-vaccine.
5. Dara Mohammadi, "Adrian Hill: Accelerating the Pace of Ebola Vaccine Research," *Lancet* 384, no. 9955 (November 2014): 1660, https://doi.org/10.1016/S0140-6736(14)61738-4.

CHAPTER TWELVE

1. Jeff Clabaugh, "Novavax Replaces CEO," *Washington Business Journal*, April 19, 2011, https://www.bizjournals.com/washington/news/2011/04/19/novavax-replaces-ceo.html.

2. Rahul Singhvi, "Trial by Fire," University of Maryland Ventures, December 5, 2017, https://www.umventures.org/news/trial-fire.
3. Natalie Grover, "Novavax Hopes to Crack Elusive Vaccine for Common Respiratory Virus," Reuters, August 10, 2015, https://www.reuters.com/article/us-novavax-vaccine/novavax-hopes-to-crack-elusive-vaccine-for-common-respiratory-virus-idUSKCN0QF0CA20150810.

CHAPTER THIRTEEN

1. Damian Garde, "Here's the Slide Deck Moderna Uses to Defend Its $7.5 Billion Valuation," STAT News, March 27, 2018, https://www.statnews.com/2018/03/27/moderna-slide-deck/.
2. Ryan Knutson and Kate Linebaugh, "Novavax's Long Road to a Covid-19 Vaccine," March 1, 2021, *The Journal* (podcast), produced by *Wall Street Journal*, podcast audio, https://www.wsj.com/podcasts/the-journal/novavax-long-road-to-a-covid-19-vaccine/6c0098ff-8479-4bc1-8f52-50f47ff8db59.
3. Knutson and Linebaugh, "Novavax's Long Road."

CHAPTER FOURTEEN

1. Dina Fine Maron, "'Wet Markets' Likely Launched the Coronavirus. Here's What You Need to Know," *National Geographic*, April 15, 2020, https://www.nationalgeographic.com/animals/article/coronavirus-linked-to-chinese-wet-markets.
2. Drew Hinshaw, Betsy McKay, and Jeremy Page, "Over 47,000 Wild Animals Sold in Wuhan Markets Before Covid Outbreak, Study Shows," *Wall Street Journal*, June 8, 2021, https://www.wsj.com/articles/live-wildlife-sold-in-wuhan-markets-before-covid-19-outbreak-study-shows-11623175415.
3. Rui-Heng Xu et al., "Epidemiologic Clues to SARS Origin in China," *Emerging Infectious Diseases* 10, no. 6 (June 2004): 1030–37, 10.3201/eid1006.030852.
4. Natasha Khan, Fanfan Wang, and Rachel Yeo, "Health Officials Work to Solve China's Mystery Virus Outbreak," *Wall Street Journal*, January 6, 2020, https://www.wsj.com/articles/health-officials-work-to-solve-chinas-mystery-virus-outbreak-11578308757.
5. Jeremy Page and Lingling Wei, "China's CDC, Built to Stop Pandemics Like Covid, Stumbled When It Mattered Most," *Wall Street Journal*, August 17, 2020, https://www.wsj.com/articles/chinas-cdc-built-to-stop-pandemics-stumbled-when-it-mattered-most-11597675108.
6. Fanfan Wang and Stephanie Yang, "SARS Experience Guides China's Effort to Contain New Virus," *Wall Street Journal*, January 10, 2020, https://www.wsj.com/articles/sars-experience-guides-chinas-effort-to-contain-new-virus-11578681205.
7. Jasper Fuk-Woo Chan et al., "A Familial Cluster of Pneumonia Associated with the 2019 Novel Coronavirus Indicating Person-to-Person Transmission: A Study of a

Family Cluster," *Lancet* 395, no. 10223 (February 2020), 514–23, https://doi.org/10.1016/S0140-6736(20)30154-9.

8. Page and Wei, "China's CDC, Built to Stop Pandemics."
9. Charlie Campbell, "Exclusive: The Chinese Scientist Who Sequenced the First COVID-19 Genome Speaks Out About the Controversies Surrounding His Work," *Time*, August 24, 2020, https://time.com/5882918/zhang-yongzhen-interview-china-coronavirus-genome.
10. Natasha Khan, "New Virus Discovered by Chinese Scientists Investigating Pneumonia Outbreak," *Wall Street Journal*, January 8, 2020, https://www.wsj.com/articles/new-virus-discovered-by-chinese-scientists-investigating-pneumonia-outbreak-11578485668?mod=article_inline.
11. Ryan Knutson and Kate Linebaugh, "mRNA Vaccines Are Taking On Covid," *The Journal* (podcast), produced by *Wall Street Journal*, podcast audio, April 19, 2021, https://www.wsj.com/podcasts/the-journal/mrna-vaccines-are-taking-on-covid-what-else-can-they-do/a8ca75b4-0b53-45b1-828e-8afee95310f1.
12. Dr. Sabine L. van Elsland and Kate Wighton, "Two Thirds of COVID-19 Cases Exported from Mainland China May Be Undetected," Imperial College London, February 22, 2020, https://www.imperial.ac.uk/news/195564/two-thirds-covid-19-cases-exported-from-mainland.
13. Brianna Abbott and Stephanie Armour, "CDC Warns It Expects Coronovirus to Spread in U.S.," *Wall Street Journal*, February 25, 2020, https://www.wsj.com/articles/cdc-warns-it-expects-coronavirus-to-spread-in-u-s-11582653829.
14. Brianna Abbott, "Test Kits for Novel Coronavirus Hit a Snag in the U.S.," *Wall Street Journal*, February 13, 2020, https://www.wsj.com/articles/test-kits-for-novel-coronavirus-hit-a-snag-in-the-u-s-11581565817.
15. Mike Esterl, "Flu Pandemic Is Declared—First Time in 41 Years," *Wall Street Journal*, June 12, 2009, https://www.wsj.com/articles/SB124471165680705709; Jeremy Brown, "What Past Crises Tell Us About the Coronavirus," *Wall Street Journal*, January 31, 2020, https://www.wsj.com/articles/what-past-crises-tell-us-about-the-coronavirus-11580403056.

CHAPTER FIFTEEN

1. Leslie Brody, "Covid-19's 'Patient Zero' in New York: What Life Is Like for the New Rochelle Lawyer," *Wall Street Journal*, March 5, 2021, https://www.wsj.com/articles/covid-19s-patient-zero-what-life-is-like-for-the-new-york-lawyer-11614686401.
2. Gina Kolata, "How the Coronavirus Short-Circuits the Immune System," *New York Times*, June 26, 2020, https://www.nytimes.com/2020/06/26/health/coronavirus-immune-system.html.
3. Pam Belluck, "What Does the Coronavirus Do to the Body?" *New York Times*, March 26, 2020, https://www.nytimes.com/article/coronavirus-body-symptoms.html.

4. Jennifer Levitz, "'She Is Going to Make It, Damn It': One Doctor's Quest to Save Her Patient from Covid-19," *Wall Street Journal*, June 26, 2020, https://www.wsj.com/articles/young-coronavirus-spike-boston-hospital-icu-doctors-patient-covid-19-11593171722.
5. Antonio Regalado, "A Coronavirus Vaccine Will Take at Least 18 Months—If It Works at All," *MIT Technology Review*, March 10, 2020, https://www.technologyreview.com/2020/03/10/916678/a-coronavirus-vaccine-will-take-at-least-18-monthsif-it-works-at-all/.
6. Robert Kuznia, "The Timetable for a Coronavirus Vaccine Is 18 Months. Experts Say That's Risky," CNN, last modified April 1, 2020, https://www.cnn.com/2020/03/31/us/coronavirus-vaccine-timetable-concerns-experts-invs/index.html.

CHAPTER SIXTEEN

1. Stephanie Baker, "Covid Vaccine Front-Runner Is Months Ahead of Her Competition," *Bloomberg Businessweek,* July 15, 2020, https://www.bloomberg.com/news/features/2020-07-15/oxford-s-covid-19-vaccine-is-the-coronavirus-front-runner.
2. Pedro M. Folegatti et al., "Safety and Immunogenicity of a Candidate Middle East Respiratory Syndrome Coronavirus Viral-Vectored Vaccine: A Dose-Escalation, Open-Label, Non-Randomised, Uncontrolled, Phase 1 Trial," *Lancet* 20, no. 7 (July 2020): 816–26, https://doi.org/10.1016/S1473-3099(20)30160-2; Baker, "Covid Vaccine Front-Runner."
3. Nathan Vardi, "Ugur Sahin Becomes a Billionaire on Hopes for Technology Behind COVID-19 Vaccine," *Forbes*, June 1, 2020, https://www.forbes.com/sites/nathanvardi/2020/06/01/ugur-sahin-becomes-a-billionaire-on-hopes-for-technology-behind-covid-19-vaccine/?sh=7b901fb433fb.
4. "Mission Possible: The Race for a Vaccine," *National Geographic*/Pfizer, April 6, 2021, YouTube video, https://www.youtube.com/watch?v=jbZUZ9JYNBE.
5. "Mission Possible: The Race for a Vaccine."

CHAPTER SEVENTEEN

1. Chris Smyth et al., "Coronavirus Vaccine Could Be Ready by September," *Times* (London), April 11, 2020, https://www.thetimes.co.uk/article/coronavirus-vaccine-could-be-ready-by-september-flmwl257x.
2. Stephanie Baker, "Covid Vaccine Front-Runner Is Months Ahead of Her Competition," *Bloomberg Businessweek,* July 15, 2020, https://www.bloomberg.com/news/features/2020-07-15/oxford-s-covid-19-vaccine-is-the-coronavirus-front-runner.
3. David D. Kirkpatrick, "In Race for a Coronavirus Vaccine, an Oxford Group Leaps Ahead," *New York Times*, April 27, 2020, https://www.nytimes.com/2020/04/27/world/europe/coronavirus-vaccine-update-oxford.html; "Oxford University Is Leading in the Vaccine Race," *Economist*, July 2, 2020, https://www.economist.com/britain/2020/07/02/oxford-university-is-leading-in-the-vaccine-race.

4. Ludwig Burger et al., "Special Report—How a British COVID-19 Vaccine Went from Pole Position to Troubled Start," Reuters, December 24, 2020, https://www.reuters.com/article/us-health-coronavirus-britain-vaccine-sp-idUKKBN28Y0XU.
5. Baker, "Covid Vaccine Front-Runner."
6. Sarah Gilbert, "If This Doesn't Work, I'm Not Sure Anything Will," interview with Tom Ireland, *Biologist*, July 2020, https://thebiologist.rsb.org.uk/biologist-covid-19/if-this-doesn-t-work-i-m-not-sure-anything-will.
7. David E. Sanger, "Trump Seeks Push to Speed Vaccine, Despite Safety Concerns," *New York Times*, April 29, 2020, https://www.nytimes.com/2020/04/29/us/politics/trump-coronavirus-vaccine-operation-warp-speed.html.
8. Helen Branswell, "Vaccine Experts Say Moderna Didn't Produce Data Critical to Assessing Covid-19 Vaccine," STAT News, May 19, 2020, https://www.statnews.com/2020/05/19/vaccine-experts-say-moderna-didnt-produce-data-critical-to-assessing-covid-19-vaccine/.
9. Matt Levine, "Money Stuff: It's a Good Time to Raise Vaccine Money," *Bloomberg*, May 19, 2020, https://www.bloomberg.com/news/newsletters/2020-05-19/money-stuff-it-s-a-good-time-to-raise-vaccine-money.
10. Jared S. Hopkins, "How Pfizer Delivered a Covid Vaccine in Record Time: Crazy Deadlines, a Pushy CEO," *Wall Street Journal*, December 11, 2020, https://www.wsj.com/articles/how-pfizer-delivered-a-covid-vaccine-in-record-time-crazy-deadlines-a-pushy-ceo-11607740483.
11. Peter Fimrite, "Studies Show Coronavirus Antibodies May Fade Fast, Raising Questions About Vaccines," *San Francisco Chronicle*, July 17, 2020, https://www.sfchronicle.com/health/article/With-coronavirus-antibodies-fading-fast-focus-15414533.php.
12. Peter Loftus and Gregory Zuckerman, "Novavax Nears Covid-19 Vaccine Game Changer—After Years of Failure," *Wall Street Journal*, February 23, 2021, https://www.wsj.com/articles/novavax-nears-covid-19-vaccine-game-changerafter-years-of-failure-11614096579.

CHAPTER EIGHTEEN

1. Sharon LaFraniere et al., "Blunders Eroded U.S. Confidence in Early Vaccine Front-Runner," *New York Times,* December 8, 2020, https://www.nytimes.com/2020/12/08/business/covid-vaccine-oxford-astrazeneca.html.
2. "Mission Possible: The Race for a Vaccine," *National Geographic*/Pfizer, April 6, 2021, https://www.youtube.com/watch?v=jbZUZ9JYNBE.
3. Sharon LaFraniere et al., "Politics, Science and the Remarkable Race for a Coronavirus Vaccine," *New York Times*, November 21, 2020, https://www.nytimes.com/2020/11/21/us/politics/coronavirus-vaccine.html.
4. "Pushing Boundaries to Deliver COVID-19 Vaccine Across the Globe," AstraZeneca, February 2021, https://www.astrazeneca.com/what-science-can-do/topics/technologies/pushing-boundaries-to-deliver-covid-19-vaccine-accross-the-globe.html.

5. Jenny Strasburg and Joseph Walker, "Astra-Zeneca-Oxford Covid-19 Vaccine Up to 90% Effective in Late-Stage Trials," *Wall Street Journal,* November 23, 2020, https://www.wsj.com/articles/astrazeneca-oxford-covid-19-vaccine-up-to-90-effective-in-late-stage-trials-11606116047.
6. Ludwig Burger, Kate Kelland, and Alistair Smout, "Decades of Work, and Half a Dose of Fortune, Drove Oxford Vaccine Success," Reuters, November 23, 2020, https://www.reuters.com/article/us-health-coronavirus-astrazeneca-oxford/decades-of-work-and-half-a-dose-of-fortune-drove-oxford-vaccine-success-idUKKBN2832NC?edition-redirect=uk.
7. Clive Cookson et al., "How AstraZeneca and Oxford Found Their Vaccine Under Fire," *Financial Times,* November 27, 2020, https://www.ft.com/content/cc78aa2f-1b10-446a-88d9-86a78c5ce461.
8. LaFraniere et al., "Blunders Eroded U.S. Confidence."
9. LaFraniere et al., "Blunders Eroded U.S. Confidence."

CHAPTER NINETEEN

1. Peter Curry, "The Few: Winston Churchill's Speech About the Battle of Britain," History Hit, October 31, 2018, https://www.historyhit.com/the-few-winston-churchills-speech-about-the-battle-of-the-britain/.
2. Melanie Grayce West, "New York City Kicks Off Covid-19 Vaccine Drive," *Wall Street Journal,* December 14, 2020, https://www.wsj.com/articles/queens-nurse-gets-first-vaccine-shot-in-new-york-city-11607958012?mod=article_inline.
3. Paulina Villegas et al., "U.S. Surpasses 300,000 Daily Coronavirus Cases, the Second Alarming Record This Week," *Washington Post,* January 8, 2021, https://www.washingtonpost.com/nation/2021/01/08/coronavirus-covid-live-updates-us/.
4. Peter Loftus, "Novavax Covid-19 Vaccine Produces Positive Results in First-Stage Study," *Wall Street Journal,* August 4, 2020, https://www.wsj.com/articles/novavax-covid-19-vaccine-produces-positive-results-in-first-stage-study-11596571200.
5. Hilda Bastian, "The mRNA Vaccines Are Extraordinary, but Novavax Is Even Better," *Atlantic,* June 24, 2021, https://www.theatlantic.com/health/archive/2021/06/novavax-now-best-covid-19-vaccine/619276/.
6. William Booth, Carolyn Y. Johnson, and Laurie McGinley, "AstraZeneca Used 'Outdated and Potentially Misleading Data' That Overstated the Effectiveness of Its Vaccine, Independent Panel Says," *Washington Post,* March 23, 2021, https://www.washingtonpost.com/world/astrazeneca-oxford-vaccine-concerns/2021/03/23/2f931d34-8bc3-11eb-a33e-da28941cb9ac_story.html.
7. Jenny Strasburg, "AstraZeneca's Covid-19 Vaccine Is Safe, 79% Effective in Late-Stage U.S. Trials," *Wall Street Journal,* March 22, 2021, https://www.wsj.com/articles/astrazeneca-covid-19-vaccine-is-79-effective-in-late-stage-u-s-trials-11616397735.
8. Nick Triggle, "Covid: Under-30s Offered Alternative to Oxford-AstraZeneca Jab," BBC, April 7, 2021, https://www.bbc.com/news/health-56665517; "Pushing Boundaries to Deliver COVID-19 Vaccine Across the Globe," AstraZeneca, February 2021,

https://www.astrazeneca.com/what-science-can-do/topics/technologies/pushing-boundaries-to-deliver-covid-19-vaccine-accross-the-globe.html.

9. Jenny Strasburg, "If Oxford's Covid-19 Vaccine Succeeds, Layers of Private Investors Could Profit," *Wall Street Journal,* August 2, 2020, https://www.wsj.com/articles/if-oxfords-covid-19-vaccine-succeeds-layers-of-private-investors-could-profit-11596373722.
10. "Promising Malaria Vaccine Enters Final Stage of Clinical Testing in West Africa," University of Oxford, May 7, 2021, https://www.ox.ac.uk/news/2021-05-07-promising-malaria-vaccine-enters-final-stage-clinical-testing-west-africa.
11. Francis Elliot and Tom Whipple, "Malaria Vaccine Another Success Story for Jenner Institute Team Behind Covid Jab," *Times* (London), December 5, 2020, https://www.thetimes.co.uk/article/malaria-vaccine-another-success-story-for-jenner-institute-team-behind-covid-jab-9r55m7jj3.
12. Thomas M. Burton and Peter Loftus, "J&J Covid-19 Vaccine Authorized for Use in U.S.," *Wall Street Journal,* February 27, 2021, https://www.wsj.com/articles/j-j-covid-19-vaccine-authorized-for-use-in-u-s-11614467922.
13. Burton and Loftus, "J&J Covid-19 Vaccine Authorized for Use in U.S."
14. @sigh__oh, Twitter post, April 13, 2021, 8:35 a.m., https://twitter.com/sigh__oh/status/1381949214574448640?lang=en.
15. Parmy Olson and Jenny Strasburg, "J&J, AstraZeneca Explore Covid-19 Vaccine Modification in Response to Rare Blood Clots," *Wall Street Journal,* July 13, 2021, https://www.wsj.com/articles/j-j-astrazeneca-explore-covid-19-vaccine-modification-in-response-to-rare-blood-clots-11626173015.
16. Carolynn Look, "BioNTech Vaccine to Give German Economy Extraordinary Boost," Bloomberg, August 10, 2021, https://www.bloomberg.com/news/articles/2021-08-10/biontech-vaccine-to-give-german-economy-extraordinary-boost?cmpid=BBD081621_CORONAVIRUS&utm_medium=email&utm_source=newsletter&utm_term=210816&utm_campaign=coronavirus.